MILADY
SalonOvations™

IN THE BAG

Selling in the Salon

MILADY
SalonOvations

IN THE BAG

Selling in the Salon

Carol Phillips

Milady Publishing Company
(A Division of Delmar Publishers Inc.)
I(T)P™ An International Thomson Publishing Company

New York • London • Bonn • Boston • Detroit • Madrid • Melbourne • Mexico City • Paris
Singapore • Tokyo • Toronto • Washington • Albany NY • Belmont CA • Cincinnati OH

NOTICE TO THE READER

Milady Staff
Publisher: Catherine Frangie
Developmental Editor: Joseph Miranda
Senior Project Editor: Laura V. Miller
Project Editor: Annette Danaher
Sr. Art/ Design Supervisor: Susan C. Mathews
Production Manager: John Mickelbank

For more information contact:
Milady Publishing Company
(A Divison of Delmar Publishers Inc.)
3 Columbia Circle, Box 15015
Albany, NY 12212-5015

International Thomson Publishing
Berkshire House
168-173 High Holborn
London, WC1V7AA
England

Thomas Nelson Australia
102 Dodds Street
South Melbourne 3205
Victoria, Australia

Nelson Canada
1120 Birchmont Road
Scarborough, Ontario
M1K 5G4, Canada

International Thomson Publishing GmbH
Konigswinterer Str. 418
53227 Bonn
Germany

International Thomson Publishing Asia
221 Henderson Bldg. #05-10
Singapore 0315

International Thomson Publishing Japan
Kyowa Building, 3F
2-2-1 Hirakawa-cho
Chiyoda-ku, Tokyo 102
Japan

1 2 3 4 5 6 7 8 9 10 XXX 01 00 99 98 97 96 95 94

Library of Congress Cataloging-in-Publication Data
Phillips, Carol
    In the bag : selling in the salon / Carol Phillips.
    p.   cm.
    Includes index.
    ISBN 1-56253-236-7
    1. Beauty shop supplies industry—Management. 2. Beauty shops—
  Management. 3. Retail trade—Management. 4. Selling—Cosmetics.
    I. Title.
HD9999.B252P48 1995
680—dc20
                                         94-6811
                                           CIP

DEDICATION

To Mom and Dad

Thanks for showing me that

beauty and brains can mix

CONTENTS

CHAPTER 4
DYNAMITE DISPLAYS 49

CHAPTER 5
SELECTING A PRODUCT LINE 59

CHAPTER 6
INVENTORY CONTROL SYSTEMS 67

CHAPTER 11
RETAIL KILLERS AND SALES BUILDERS 139

CHAPTER 12
THE STEP-BY-STEP SELLING SEQUENCE . . . 145

CHAPTER 13
CLOSING THE SALE 163

CHAPTER 14
SELLING TO MEN 173

CHAPTER 15
SELLING SERVICES 181

CHAPTER 16
SELLING PRODUCTS 191

CHAPTER 17
EIGHTY-FIVE COMMON CONSUMER QUESTIONS . 219

CHAPTER 18
TELEPHONE SAVVY 231

PART THREE
BUILDING YOUR BUSINESS AND THE
FOUNDATION FOR SUCCESS   241

CHAPTER 19
BUSINESS BUILDERS 243

ACKNOWLEDGMENTS

Jody Byrne. Thank you for recognizing the salon and our radically different approach to retailing. I appreciate the opportunities, support and advice you have freely shared with me.

Cathy Frangie. Finally we made it! Thank you for the opportunity to share my message. You made this massive project come together beautifully.

Joe Miranda. Thank you for being my lifeline on the other end of the phone. You were the calm in the storm.

Frank Jackson. Thank you for the picture perfect fotographz.

Rebecca James. Thank you for all your inspiration, constant guidance and for being an incredible writing influence. Gee Toto we're not in Kansas any more.

Betty Link. Thank you for your encouragement, listening with your heart and for showing me how to be more adept.

Martha Slater. My angel on earth. Thank you for sharing your gentle spirit with me.

Linda Fox. Thank you my soul sister. Thanks for being there through everything over the years and across the miles. (Wish I had paid more attention in Mrs. H's class.)

Ricky Levin. Thank you for having the black cat cross my path. You are one of the few who understand.

Chris Boyle. Thank you my love. You were there to ignite the creative muse. The balloons, boxes and bubbles were perfect. I look forward to sharing a lifetime of rewards.

Special Thank You to the Manufacturers and Distributors. Thank you for giving me a platform to share in The Bug's message with your accounts at shows, conventions, and workshops over the years. I am looking forward to helping thousands of additional salons get the product off the shelf and in the bag.

Also, thank you to the following professionals for their expertise and very helpful input while reviewing this manuscript:

Ken Young, Oklahoma City, Oklahoma
Jo An Paganetti, New York, New York
Henry Gambino, Philadelphia, Pennsylvania
Tom Rough, Chicago, Illinois

INTRODUCTION

SALON TALES

Behind me I could hear the action of the precision cutting shears coming together. The shears and their operator were creating a transformation on the six o'clock client, a young woman with drab brown hair who appeared to be in her mid-thirties. The wide-eyed reflection in the mirror revealed the customer's inner apprehension as she watched lock after lock of split and neglected ends hastily being removed from her hair.

I love people watching, especially clients and the salon industry personnel servicing them. The nature of the beauty industry is an intimate and very personal one. This intimacy between technicians and customers always proves to be an enlightening and educational experience.

Trying not to make the stylist nervous, I attempted to blend into the salon's surroundings. I wanted to inconspicuously watch, curious to see what would transpire during this young woman's visit. A nudge of foreboding told me that what I was about to observe was happening in salons throughout the country. While my conditioner was processing I watched this whole episode, looking into the station's mirror and peering over the top of the book I was pretending to read.

Things seemed to be going "normally"—no conversation, no questioning, and no consultation, except for the obligatory "How do you want your hair styled?" at the onset of the service. Part and divide. Comb. Snip. Comb. Snip. Comb. Snip. For about twenty-five minutes, the stylist worked that hair. After surveying the finished cut, which met with his approval, he picked up the black turbo blow-dryer. He started to remove the moisture from the hair but clicked off the blower when he realized he forgot to put on a styling aid. The stylist rummaged through the products on the station and finally came across the one he was seeking. He turned the can upside down and squirted out a giant glob of mousse, which he proceeded to peck and finger-comb through his customer's hair.

Once the heat had evaporated the moisture, the stylist turned off his blow-dryer. He picked up his shiny silver brush and expertly swept it through the client's hair—brushing, fluffing, twisting, smoothing, and finally curling. I could hear the buzz of the clippers trimming the now exposed neckline so I knew the service was about to come to an end. A few squirts of finishing spray and he was done. To top it all off, he lightly hand-molded the hair, putting every strand in its place.

He handed the woman the basic salon rectangular hand mirror. She was spun around in the hydraulic chair to inspect his handiwork. A slow swivel to the right and stop. It was apparent to me the client was struggling with the hand mirror. She couldn't quite get the hang of looking into two mirrors to see her reflection. Indifferent to her dilemma, he proceeded to twirl her to the left. She finally nodded in approval, and he repositioned her toward the front of the station. He unhooked the well-worn shampoo cape and, in a sweeping toreador gesture, tossed it aside.

Ending his service he said, "Thanks for coming in. Have a good one." (Have a good what?) And in the blink of an eye he positioned himself behind the front reception desk. After lighting up a cigarette, he started flipping through a magazine.

Meanwhile, the customer was wiping off the remnants of

1

her haircut at the station. She stood there flicking off the hair that stubbornly refused to let loose of her sweater and fall to its final resting place amid the multicolored pile of hair trimmings that represented the day's work for the stylist. She put on her dark gray overcoat and gathered up her belongings. After bundling up, she made her way to the front desk and paid her $18. She headed for the door, when she stopped in her tracks. Momentarily frozen with one hand on the door handle she looked back over her shoulder and quietly asked, "Excuse me, do you have a ladies' room?" "Yeah," her stylist replied, not wanting to be interrupted from reading the two-month-old *People* magazine. "It's straight back, through two doors and it's on the left. Don't mind the mess."

Well, I now thought I had a few minutes to read while waiting for the time to go off. She was his last customer, so there was no one else to observe and learn from.

As she was exiting the back room, she passed some inset shelves on the left wall where an array of bottles and jars caught her eye. The collection of professional products was minimal, to say the least, and coated with a film of salon residue. "Do you have any of the stuff you used on my hair today?" she shyly inquired from the back of the salon. I put my book down thinking this might get interesting. The stylist finally got up from his stool and casually strolled back to where she was standing. The client by now was examining a bottle of sculpting gel she had removed from the display. "Yeah, I think we do." After shifting a few bottles, he managed to locate the appropriate shampoo for her hair type.

"Do you have conditioner?" she eagerly asked.

"Yeah, let me find it," he responded in an obvious I've-had-a-long-day attitude.

The lack of communication during the cut and style was bad enough, but not to be excited by a warm-blooded ready-to-buy client was more than I could stand. I was ready to jump up and assist her even if my hair was wrapped in a plastic bag.

"What else did you use on my hair? I really like the finished look. I want the same thing at home so I can duplicate it tomorrow." By now I was white knuckled, clutching the armrest because the stylist seemed totally oblivious to this golden opportunity.

Within ten short minutes the client walked out of the salon with shampoo, conditioner, gel, mousse, finishing spray, curling brush, and a blow-dryer—a grand total of over $140

in ten minutes. (It took him forty-five minutes to do the haircut and style for which he was paid $18.) What would have happened if the client didn't request the ladies' room? Yes, that's right, she would have left the salon, jumped in her car, and headed straight for the nearest store that sold beauty products and given them her money.

My hunch was right. This stylist had the technical skills—his cut was great—but he almost blew an additional $140 sale simply due to lack of communication. Don't let opportunities pass you by. *Selling is communication and communication is selling,* and that is what this book is all about.

The cost of running a business has never been higher. Staff turnover, rent, product expenses, utilities, taxes, owner burnout, and general industry apathy make staying in business a real challenge. In the state of California approximately five thousand new salons open each year; the same amount also go out of business. What's wrong with this picture?

I'm not trying to be negative, but you need to utilize every option available for making a success of your business. (Success in your terms, not just monetarily.) Selling should be at the top of your strategy list to help you achieve your goals. You could literally double your sales with a retail/selling game plan. You can't afford not to retail.

Selling is simply getting the customer to say yes to you, your products, and your services. Most cosmetologists feel it is easier to sell a service than a product. You may give the best service, but if you can't sell you are certainly missing the boat.

You see, being a success is a matter of choice, not chance. You are born either male or female. Never in the history of evolution was there a born salesperson, hairdresser, esthetician, manicurist, massage therapist, or image consultant. But somewhere along your life's path you chose to become involved in the beauty business. You chose your career, now you can choose to grow in your selling skills.

IN THE BAG PHILOSOPHY

I have never felt that selling is some high-pressure, slap-on-the-back philosophy. The real trick to getting the product in the bag is:

• Knowing what products and services you offer.

• Knowing how to present the information.

- Finding solutions to the client's beauty problems.
- Tuning into people and understanding what makes them tick.
- Designing your physical work space to support your selling efforts.
- Giving the client the opportunity to buy.

It is not:

- Being pushy or shoving products down the customer's throat.
- Selling something the client doesn't want or need.
- Being overbearing or obnoxious.
- Telling clients anything just to make the sale.
- Being dishonest.
- High pressure/high pitch.

Retailing can literally send shocks of panic through cosmetologists. I've seen palms get clammy and beads of perspiration pop out on the forehead and upper lip. I've heard voices crack and squeak when cosmetologists go into the sale. But the truth of the matter is that you sell every day, even if you think you are not. Have you ever had a client ask, "Where did you get your training?" "Where did you go to school to learn to do that?" Of course you have. The client was asking you to sell yourself and your skills.

There is no hidden mystery to successful selling. Many people feel there is a veil around retailing, a mystery that some people are gifted at selling. Not true. If you can talk you can sell. The mystery comes from lacking the nuts and bolts, the knowledge and skills necessary to make the sale. Just as you once had to learn the step-by-step technique for cutting, perming, coloring, facials, manicures, and massage, there are guidelines for selling.

How do I know that the ideas in this book work? My positions behind the counter as a makeup salesperson, behind the chair as a cosmetologist and esthetician, and behind the desk as a salon owner have been the best teachers imaginable. I learned selling skills the hard way through years of observing people, daily application, trial and error, research, studying techniques, and of course the university of hard knocks.

I opened the doors to my salon two months after my twenty-first birthday, unfortunately, with next to no money and no business plan. I did have, however, a handful of loyal customers and tons of determination. At twenty-one, you don't think about failing, you just lunge forward. If I could only get the doors open I knew I could make it work. If I had known the obstacles that were ahead I would have done things differently. Major roads leading to the salon were closed for the first two years; a shopping center was being constructed nearby so there was background noise of jackhammers and bulldozers; the small Midwestern town had no labor pool and three major industries—oil, aircraft, and agriculture—had taken a nosedive; my competition was copying my product line and underselling the price. These are just a few of the obstacles I faced.

I started my first business in an extremely poor period in economic history. In 1982, interest rates were hovering around 20 percent. Financing was next to impossible to obtain. I remember sitting in a meeting for securing financing to open the salon and a very mature man looking over my loan application. He patted me on the hand and asked, "Tell me, honey, why don't you want to get married and have babies?" His granddaughter was about my age and he couldn't fathom why I wanted to go into business.

The salon did open with almost fifteen hundred square feet and one employee besides myself. Most of the fixtures, equipment, supplies, and inventory had not yet arrived. When my handful of loyal clients wanted their appointments I worked out of the front office for the first six weeks.

The phone company was on strike so the business telephone had to be temporarily installed in my apartment to guarantee a phone number. (A secure number was needed so I could print business cards and literature and start promoting the salon.) For the first three weeks my employee had to sit by the phone at the apartment scheduling appointments. Between customers at the salon I would run over to a pay phone and call Annie to get the appointment updates.

When I went into business I knew how to do the actual treatments—give a facial, makeup lessons, waxing, and massage. I was lacking, as are most students coming out of beauty school today, the skills necessary for seriously running and managing a business.

Due to a lot of hard work and determination the business grew and so did the number of employees. At the time I was behind the chair six days a week and the average service was seventy-five minutes and $30. Being limited with two hands and a finite number of hours in the day, I had to find a way to make the entire space and the entire staff generate additional income.

During this period I became aware of "inspirational dissatisfaction." I was so dissatisfied with the salon's financial situation I became inspired to improve. There had to be a way to generate additional sales without booking more appointments before or after normal hours. Then it hit me! I had better teach the staff to sell. Retailing had to have our attention. I had to find a way to get the bottles and jars to work for me. You don't have to be a brain surgeon to figure out that a $100–125 retail sale in ten to fifty minutes is more profitable than $30 for a seventy-five minute facial. In my book, there is no comparison for profitability. You need both service and retail sales.

My first job in high school was as a counter salesperson in a local Merle Norman makeup studio. Thank goodness for my two years of training and learning to sell beauty products. My high school job prepared me to lay the necessary foundation for my salon's revenue-producing game plan. I knew the products we offered were as good as those in any other store. I just needed to develop a system for setting the salon up to help generate product and service sales.

After investing hours and hours, I put together a way to train the staff to sell, to be effective communicators, to actively listen and fill a need or solve a problem. The first batch of product I purchased was under $100. We kept selling and turning the inventory by reinvesting the product's profits into more product to sell. At one point, I had more product than the distributor.

Success followed and within three short years the salon was supported by our retailing efforts. Eventually the clients were conditioned to shop at the salon. I laugh when I think of some of the clients. I swear many of them became so ingrained with the salon's education and service they would even consult with us on the choice of a husband.

By this time, word got around in the industry that my company's retail sales were dramatically higher (over 50 percent of gross revenue) than the national average (10 percent of gross). I knew I had hit a nerve when calls started coming in from other owners who wanted to know the secret. They wanted to know how they could get their staff to do the same thing. That's when I started lecturing and consulting.

The hard work paid off. I was rewarded in January 1988 when *American Salon* magazine named me retailer of the year. Milady Publishing caught that article and as a result you are now holding in your hands this book. The foundation lessons of *In the Bag* are the building blocks that I used to build the salon's sales.

Hardest Part of Retailing

Whenever I teach a retailing class, the first question I ask the audience is "What's the hardest part about retailing?" The following is a list of the standard responses I receive in every seminar. The great news is that for every objection listed below, you will find the answer or solution in this book.

- "Knowing what to say." (chapter 12)
- "Need more time to sell." (chapter 10)
- "Completing the sale." (chapter 13)
- "Keep on selling after the customer says no." (chapter 12)
- "Need to be more assertive." (chapter 9)
- "Don't know what to do with a wishy-washy client." (chapter 10)
- "Need more product knowledge." (chapter 17)
- "Don't want to be pushy." (chapter 18)
- "Need to know how to back up the service with product sales." (chapter 8)
- "Need to make myself get started." (chapter 22)
- "Afraid of the word no." (chapter 12)
- "Don't know all of the product selling points." (chapter 16)
- "What do I do when the client has product at home?" (chapter 12)
- "Never had any selling training." (the whole book)
- "There is not enough product to sell." (chapter 6)
- "It's hard to compete with the department stores." (chapter 3)
- "It's not my job to sell products." (chapter 1)
- "Lack of self-esteem." (chapter 9)
- "Lack of goals and ambitions." (chapter 2)
- "Just not motivated." (Appendix I)

- "Just too sensitive to retail; the rejection is too much." (chapter 11)

- "Customer had too many other things on her mind." (chapter 1)

- "No money to be made." (chapter 2)

- "Client doesn't have enough money." (chapter 12)

- "Client can get the product cheaper somewhere else." (chapter 5)

- "I don't sell because I've got some tough customers." (chapter 10)

- "Booked solid all day." (chapter 13)

- "The salon's so small I don't have room to stock massive amounts of product." (chapter 6)

- "Maintaining enthusiasm." (chapter 22)

- "Need more customers." (chapter 2)

- "Selling to men." (chapter 14)

- "Marketing the products." (chapter 4)

- "Managing my time." (chapter 22)

HIGHLIGHTS OF THE BOOK

In the Bag is divided into three major parts. The first part shows you how to set the stage for selling. It details the business side of the business. The second part reveals everything you need to know for developing your selling skills. The third part is devoted to building your business through promotions and advertising and building the foundations for personal success.

You can read a book, attend a seminar, watch a video, but you have to be willing, ready, and open for growth. When you're ready results can happen. I have a sign in my office that says "WHEN YOU ARE THROUGH IMPROVING YOURSELF, YOU ARE THROUGH." We are not even close to finishing; we're just getting started.

PART ONE
Setting the Stage for Selling

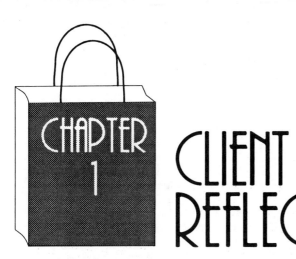

CHAPTER 1

CLIENT REFLECTIONS

In this business you have many hats to wear for each client. You will be called upon to be part psychiatrist, part healer, part teacher, part artisan, part preacher, and part chemist. You spend your days touching more than just the outside physical appearance of the men and women who come into your salon. You touch the innermost being of the individual. You work on, advise, stroke, and nurture the very center of the client's identity.

The goal of this chapter is to teach you to look at your business with clients uppermost in your mind, heart, and eyes. What makes them tick? What emotions are coursing through their veins?

perception of defined beauty. Are people now any different than in days gone by?

Self-adornment has its roots deep in the daily activity of humans. Primping was a form of communication. Self-decoration was evident before humans used words to express themselves. Cave men and women wore jewelry, hair accessories, and paint before they wore clothing. Visual signals denoted rank, hierarchy, and personal possessions among ancient tribes. The art of adornment displayed the visual resumé, the status, the level of wealth of the wearer. All the painting and powdering, subtly or not so subtly, was and still is the basis for attraction, either to please others or oneself.

BEAUTIFUL EVOLUTION

For thousands of years men and women have been plucked, painted, powdered, scrunched, shaved, dyed, cut, curled, rolled, waved, teased, sprayed, tressed, tinted, bleached, brushed, tousled, rinsed, braided, twisted, knotted. They have been perfumed, massaged, primped, pampered, blushed, curled, lined, smudged, adorned, tweezed, waxed, packed, scrubbed, soaped, steamed, pinched, sloughed, softened, smoothed, slathered, pierced, pushed, nipped, filed, buffed, and polished. (Fig. 1.1)

The beauty business is probably the second oldest profession in the world. Archaeologists have found evidence of Egyptian perfumes and beauty parlors dating back to 4000 B.C. and makeup paraphernalia back to 6000 B.C. Every culture and period in the history of the civilized world has had their own

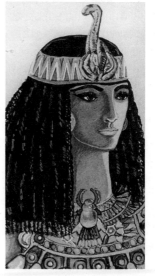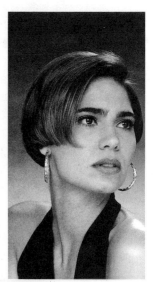

Fig. 1.1 Beauty through the ages.

If human beings have had thousands of years to perfect the art of looking good, why do so many men and women walk around looking as they do? (Putting aside economics and those that truly can't afford the price tag for beauty.) I'm curious about the millions of Americans—especially those that can afford the time and money for self-beautification.

When I first moved to southern California I wanted to see what the Beautiful People looked like, so I took a weekend and went to five different movie theaters, each in a different area of Los Angeles and Orange County. Boy was I shocked! My expectation was that I would see hordes of beautiful blondes, shapely bodies, and fashion-conscious men and women. Of the hundreds of men and women I observed, very few had developed a personal "look" or defined self-expression. I was shocked to see bad perms, awful haircuts, poorly conditioned hair, no makeup, and shorts and T-shirts for miles. Quite honestly, looking around the theaters I could have been Anywhere, USA. Which leads me to wonder why people do look the way they do.

Why Oh Why the Same Old Style?

Many people hang onto the same old look because it is easier to stay the same. It is less stressful than hassling with themselves and the people around them postchange. "Why did you have to mess with your hair? It looked okay the way it was."

Fear of past mistakes also keeps people from making a change. It's easier to do nothing than make more mistakes. Think of all the bottles and jars you have got sitting around, the ones you have purchased that were the wrong color or consistency or simply didn't work as promised. If you have made mistakes as a trained professional, think of how many your clients may have made. Avoidance is easier than admitting you might make another shopping error.

Because of the lack of qualified professional help, many people have not had the opportunity to learn. They have not been taught that a few minutes of the right effort could produce outstanding results.

Many are fearful of the unknown. They cannot see the end result of the service or product. The effort is not worth the risk involved with change. Change is conflict.

Many suffer from an abused, neglected, or battered self-image.

The Big C Word——Change!

Beauty is an emotional and psychological battleground. The big *C* word here isn't commitment; it's change. Change produces a myriad of feelings in everyone.

Client: "My stylist wants to change me, to make me over." *Stylist:* "Why do they still want to hold onto the same old look?"

Client: "Gee I must not be pretty the way I am." *Stylist:* "Can't they see if they would only change they could look so much better?"

Client: "I am holding on to my hair length because that's who I am and I'm not going to let him cut it all off." *Stylist:* "A few inches off and she would look fantastic."

You have chosen a career that thrives on change. Every day you are emotionally charged up over new looks, trends, products, techniques, colors, even packaging. Without new excitement and stimulation the beauty industry would shrivel up and blow away. Where change is essential for you, it takes on a whole new meaning for your client.

As fashion shifts every six months, so do the new collections for beauty looks. Every six months you should be ready for some new looks and products. Don't assume that if you are ecstatic for a change your client will receive your suggestions with open arms and wallet. Certain clients leap to be the first in line for the hottest new look. Others hang back until a look, technique, or product has a proven track record. For many it takes great strength to let go of a favorite style.

Change is letting go of the comfortable. Change can be as difficult as throwing away your favorite pair of slippers, the ones that have taken you years to break in, the snuggly ones. Change requires time for assimilating the new and improved look. Have you ever had a client say, "After you cut my hair all off, I didn't recognized myself when I passed a mirror. It just didn't look like me."? It takes a period of time for clients to become comfortable and familiar with a new look.

Inside Out or Outside In

Clients' outer reflections are a direct link to their innermost beings. How clients view their inside is often expressed through their physical appearance.

Clients will seek appearance changes in their life from the outside in or the inside out. People who have been working on their souls, minds, and hearts will get to a point when they are ready and willing to face changes on the outside. They are harmonious with their inner selves. They are then ready to tackle change on the outside.

Clients experiencing a significant amount of unattended internal turmoil will opt for making radical changes on the outside before confronting the internal conflict. This is the client who wants an overhaul because her husband just left her for someone younger, or someone who believes a new nose will solve all of life's problems. These clients believe that if they make themselves better looking on the outside, all will be well internally. Listen closely in your consultations to determine the client's core beliefs. The client must have realistic expectations for a satisfactory end result. You can make an impact on someone's outlook, but be aware of their true motives.

You will know when the time is right to suggest a new style for many of your clients. You will see subtle changes, tiny clues indicating that change is in the air. A hair part may switch from left to right. You may see them sporting a bold new lip color they would never have tried before.

Major life cycle changes also spur clients into "new and improved me." Listen for life cycle clues such as job changes, moving, marriages, divorce, babies, promotion on the job, class reunions, major milestone birthdays (especially thirty and forty). This is why you see swarms of your clients prior to most of life's big events.

Fatal Reflection

The most handsome man in the country had never seen his own good looks. One day while walking through the forest he came across a refreshing pool of water. When he bent down for a drink of cool water, he caught his reflection in the pool. Up until that moment he had never seen his reflection. Narcissus finally realized why he created commotion when he went into villages. He fell in love with his own reflection. Over and over he tried to embrace himself, but his arms disappeared into the reflection. Realizing he couldn't hold onto his image, Narcissus knelt to kiss it and fell into the water. He was swallowed up by his own reflection.

This ancient Greek myth of Narcissus led to the superstition that seeing your own reflection is bad luck. What do we say when a mirror is broken? Seven years of bad luck. Freud described narcissism as a morbid preoccupation with oneself.

Mirror Mirror

Remember the queen in *Sleeping Beauty?* She consulted the spirits by asking "Mirror mirror on the wall who's the fairest of them all?" She was none too happy with the truthful response.

There is a fine line between self-improvement and narcissism, yet every salon is jammed with mirrors, constantly reflecting what clients do and do not like about themselves. (Fig. 1.2) The only place filled with more mirrors than a salon is a fun house at an amusement park. For many of your clients, especially women, what they see is no laughing matter. For many, in varying degrees, it is upsetting and painful to look in the mirror. Really look into the mirror, and truthfully study the reflection.

Mirrors can be friends or foes to your clients. Mirrors do make people self-conscious. When facing a mirror you are forced to look into it. You can't help it. A mirror in your presence demands attention.

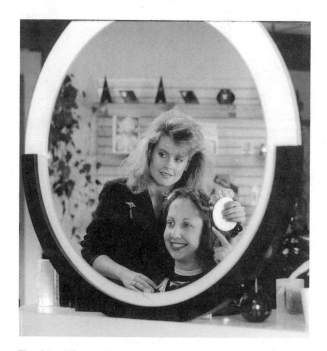

Fig. 1.2 Mirror, mirror on the wall. (Photo by Michael A. Gallitelli on location at Rielms Hair Salon, Latham, NY.)

Mirrors make clients self-critical. The constant evaluating and measuring up causes anxiety. Mirrors are our measuring sticks. Do we conform to the rigid standards of society and ourselves?

Mirrors reflect and accentuate our positive or negative self-talk. When you catch a quick glance in the mirror do you flood yourself with negative comments? God, I hate my... Can't stand those... Boy are they ugly.... Are you sabotaging yourself with these negative thoughts and feelings? Your customers are doing the very same thing.

SELF-IMAGE

Maxwell Maltz, noted psychologist and plastic surgeon, was one of the first to reveal that "self-image is the key to understanding human personality and human behavior. Change the self-image and you change the personality and the behavior." You mean if you change the way someone looks and sees herself, you can change her life? What a responsibility! More than any other area a person's self-image can affect her destiny. You expand the boundaries of self-image and you broaden the area of the client's possibilities for individual achievement.

Six Levels of Self-Development

You are dealing with delicate feelings people have about themselves. They use their outsides, consciously or subconsciously, to express their inner self. Most personal conflicts in life stem from the bruising of self-image. Clients will seek your services and be more receptive to suggestions and sales as they work through the different levels of self-image. These levels are self-esteem, self-deception, self-acceptance, self-improvement, self-worth, and self-confidence. (Fig. 1.3)

Self-esteem
Self-esteem is developed through the years. The view or mental picture clients hold of themselves is a compilation of experiences and expressions collected over the years.

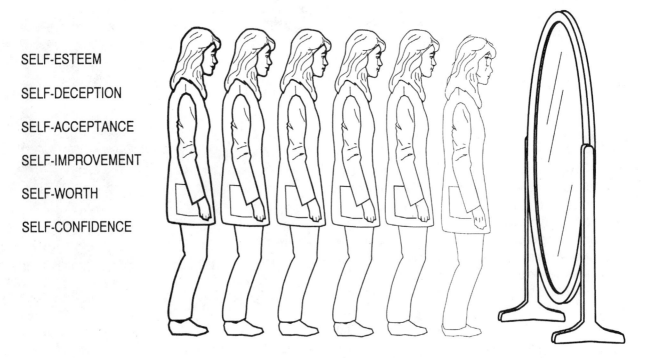

SELF-ESTEEM

SELF-DECEPTION

SELF-ACCEPTANCE

SELF-IMPROVEMENT

SELF-WORTH

SELF-CONFIDENCE

Fig. 1.3 Six levels of self-development.

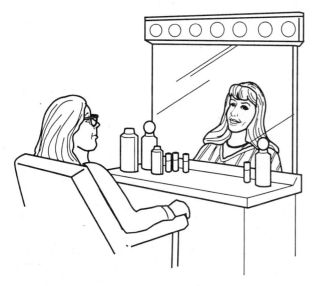

Fig. 1.4   What do we really see when we look into the mirror?

Self-deception

Do your clients really look into the mirror? Do they see themselves as others see them? (Fig. 1.4) Your clients are their own worst critics. Most women do not look in the mirror and assess the whole package. They pick apart the pieces and dissect the body and appearance. The dissecting distorts the individual uniqueness and positive qualities, until the reflection is a mere jigsaw puzzle of self-deception. Hair too unruly. Nose too fat. Thunder thighs. Blotchy skin. Dark bags under eyes. Their self-evaluation is misconstrued. Picture looking through a shiny brass kaleidoscope. See the unique colorful fractions? Now slightly shift the rainbow-filled picture and see how it becomes distorted. The magnificent picture is blurry.

Most of your clients will look in a mirror several times a day, yet they can't identify their face shape. A group of fashion professionals was asked to trace their bodies on a pattern sheet. When the drawings were hung on the wall the women couldn't identify their own body silhouette. Not one woman in the class could recognize herself in the drawing. We look, but we don't see.

Self-acceptance

Self-acceptance is the launching pad for self-development and growth. Self-acceptance doesn't discount the need for growth and change. In fact, it is just the opposite.

Carl Rogers, a psychologist, says, "The curious paradox is that when I accept myself just as I am, then I can change."

Self-improvement

The client has taken a realistic look in the mirror. She has accepted that she has positive attributes and some areas that need improvement. The customer is then ready, emotionally and physically, to take action toward a new look.

When clients are ready for self-improvement you will notice them softening and hopefully removing the emotional barriers and mental stumbling blocks that stand in the way of the transformation. Self-improvement is accepting the responsibility to do something about the way you look and feel. Self-improvement means the client is willing to risk change and try something new. A recent Carnegie Foundation study showed that the major predictor of sound mental health is people's willingness to risk. Picasso said, "Every act of creation is first of all an act of destruction."

Self-worth

The client has decided she is worth it—the physical effort, the emotional risk. She has come to a point where she is going to invest time and money in herself, be it beauty education, new products, new clothes, new looks, whatever. She has made the conscious leap of faith and is willing to risk change. This is the client that is willing and ready to loosen her hold on the past and improve the present.

Self-confidence

Self-confidence is radiated when the connection between the client's true inner person and outer expression is shown to the world. This is the point when your client looks in the mirror and the reflection she sees is the harmonious marriage of the inner person and the outer expression.

Selling to the Six Levels of Self-Development

Clients at the stages of *self-acceptance* and *self-improvement* can be your most exciting and rewarding customers. It may take time and patience, but once they have taken your advice, they may then evolve into clients with *self-worth*. They will continue to come back to you, be open to your advice, and invest in products and services to improve their looks. And ultimately, they have the opportunity of developing into that head-turner, the *self-confident* woman. This doesn't mean that the client has stopped learning. The self-confident customer is now a quick read. It will take only minutes for her to understand the idea or product that is right for her.

Self-esteem and *self-deception* are flip sides of the same coin. The customer with self-esteem can be complacent and unwilling to accept a radical change. You will have to introduce new ideas slowly and patiently. The self-deceptive client is the most difficult. However, if you select her best feature and work on it for the most dramatic effect, she is likely to go out into the world and receive compliments that will reinforce your work. Even if she can't see the improvement for herself, she will enjoy the newfound attention and may accept further change. The self-deceptive client will need plenty of tender loving follow-through from week to week.

Client Relationships

Men and women will always be searching for quality products and services, treatments and techniques that will help them look and feel their best.

The relationship between stylist and client is a unique one. The stylist is rarely face-to-face with the customer. This is an interpersonal relationship enacted through mirror images. The emotions are revealed to the mirror, not in body-to-body, face-to-face contact. (Fig. 1.5) The mirror becomes a buffer. It filters the risk involved with sharing private feelings and thoughts. Clients find it easy to talk, share, and even unload their private thoughts and desires. The client/stylist relationship takes on a precarious tone, one similar to an encounter with someone on the plane or train. You feel safe revealing personal secrets to the casual acquaintance. The safety factor is that you have limited contact and momentarily you will be out the door.

Think about it. Most of your hair services are performed on a six-to-eight-week cycle. You are with the client for a brief period of time, yet mountains of personal trivia are revealed. You establish a closeness with your clients They share with you how they really want to look, and they trust you to make them look better. If they can trust you with their hair, skin, and nails, then they can trust you with their feelings, desires, and dreams. Our business is one of the very few designed to cater to

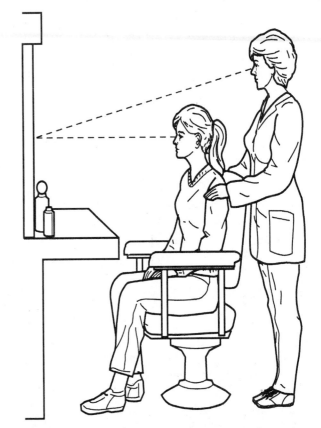

Fig. 1.5 Through the looking glass. All communication is directed to mirror and through mirror—no face-to-face contact.

people's desires, a business constructed to transform people into the image they wish they could be.

With the exception of your true friends, do you socialize with your clients? Probably not. How do clients react to you when they see you at a restaurant, movie, or mall? One of my special clients actually waved me away as I approached her table in a restaurant to say hello and compliment her on the way she looked. I was hurt that she didn't want to acknowledge me. The very next morning she called the salon to apologize. She told me that she didn't want her friend to know she was seeing my staff for corrective treatments.

The relationship you establish is a delicate and precious one. You are serving and selling the public, yet you know many personal secrets. There is a fine line between social and business relationships.

A TRIP TO THE SALON

Over the years television, movies, and the media have depicted hairdressers and cosmetologists as flamboyant, often outrageous and opinionated dictators of feminine fashions. People who work their wizardry only to have clients bolting from the salon screaming after they've caught their reflection in the mirror.

Do you realize how frightening it can be for a client to walk into the salon? Have you ever wondered how traumatic it can be for a client to even walk in the front door of your establishment? When was the last time you put yourself in the client's position? The next time the salon is empty, I want you to go the front door, walk into the salon, and stroll around. Sit in every chair a client may sit in and imagine what it would be like to be a potential client. What feeling do you pick up? Does it feel slightly uncomfortable for you? Imagine your client's reaction. In your mind are you seeing flashes of actual events that have happened in the salon?

Many emotions are working their way through clients' minds and bodies as they take the walk to sit "in the chair,"

especially if they are in for a haircut, perm, or color. You simply cannot wash the end result down the drain if by chance the client isn't pleased. The results are going to be visible for quite some time. You are altering the way clients view themselves.

If the client is in for a body massage, you are asking her to take off all her clothes. If the client is having a facial, the technician is going to examine the skin under a magnification mirror intensified ten times the normal skin. You bet it's intimidating especially if it's a first appointment at the salon.

Every day you are in your natural habitat, a place where you spend eight-plus hours a day. You are comfortable with every nook and cranny and every activity that occurs there. Customers may feel as anxious and stressed going into a salon as they would visiting their doctor or dentist. Such anxiety is not great if you want to sell them more products and services. It is critical to keep a soft spot for the fears your clients may be experiencing visiting your place.

Being sensitive to the client's needs is one link in setting the stage for effective and profitable retailing. Designing the salon environment is critical to support your sales goals.

EVALUATING YOUR BUSINESS

CHAPTER 2

BUSINESS FOCUS

Before we can plot your future growth in sales, we need to take a long, focused look at your business today. This chapter will help you define your current business operations and evaluate the direction for expanding your sales by uniquely positioning your company. We'll take a look at golden opportunities, clients' perceptions, and competitive edges. After those evaluations, we'll shop for the perfect client and define your strengths.

Marketing is defined as the act of buying or selling in a marketplace; it is all business activity. Marketing is more than simply advertising your product/service. In my opinion it is everything that happens from the time the customer picks up the phone to call you to your follow-up after the sale. Customers are constantly receiving impressions about your business, which reflects marketing, which affects sales. Every impulse or impression is a potential golden opportunity.

Golden Opportunities in Your Salon

Jan Carlzon, president of Scandinavian Airline Systems (SAS), faced a seemingly impossible task—to turn an $8 million loss around for the airline. In his plan to turn around the company, Carlzon realized that the ten million passengers the airline carried were in contact with five SAS employees per trip. He soon calculated that ten million passengers times five employees equals fifty million moments of truth, or staff/customer contacts. These golden opportunities were when each employee

had the potential of leaving a positive or negative impression regarding SAS. The pivotal success turning point for SAS was when the company's top priority became managing these moments of truth.

How many of your employees have contact with a single client? You might be shocked to discover the quantity of contacts. I've divided the salon experience into eight golden opportunity areas. Each area has examples of what can happen, the make or break points, the moments of truth that can take place in beauty businesses every day. Remember each one is an opportunity for leaving a positive or negative impression with the client. Every contact can have an impact if the client will 1) leave with a positive impression of the experience, 2) return to your business, and 3) recommend you to her friends. The following eight golden opportunity areas are too important to overlook when building your sales.

The Eight Golden Opportunities

1. *The client decides to take action*
   - Can the client pronounce your salon's name?
   - Is your salon name easy to spell?
   - Can your number be found in the telephone book?
   - What has the client heard about your business?
   - Is your salon clearly identifiable?
   - Does the client have clear directions on how to find you?
   - Does the client know what to expect when she arrives?

- How many telephone rings before the call is answered?
- Does the person answering the phone know how to schedule appointments?
- Does the person speak clearly and distinctly into the phone?
- Is the person trained to answer consumer questions?
- Is the call handled efficiently?
- What is the tone of the conversation?

2. *The client physically arrives*

- Is your business sign posted in an easy-to-view location?
- Is your building numbered?
- Can you see into the salon or is the window covered with drapes or blinds?
- Are you listed on the building directory or marquee?
- Is there sufficient parking available?
- Is the client greeted upon arrival?
- What is the first impression the client receives upon entering?
- Is the client made to feel welcome?
- Does the staff introduce themselves to the client?
- Does the client know where to go once she enters the salon?
- What is the overall mood of the salon?
- How long does the client have to wait before service begins?
- Is the client offered any refreshments?
- Does someone offer to take the client's coat?
- Is the client instructed what to do?
- Is the client escorted where she needs to go?
- Is there room for the client to sit down?
- What does the salon smell like when the client enters?

3. *The physical layout of the salon*

- What's the first thing a client will see upon entering the salon?

- Is the salon clean? (baseboards, chairs, dryers, light fixtures, displays, counters, mirrors, coffee area, reception desk, stations, testers, walls, sinks, floors, windows, ashtrays)
- Are professional-only magazines in view of the client?
- Are there old dog-eared magazines in the reception area?
- What feeling does your color and decor emit?
- Are there piles of hair on the floor?
- Do you see dirty cups and glasses?
- Are there empty containers and treatment bottles in view?
- Are the bathrooms clean?
- Are there sufficient supplies in the bathrooms?
- Are the shampoo bowls comfortable?
- Is the salon crowded and hard to walk through?
- Is lighting even and consistent throughout the salon?
- Are the departments clearly defined and easy to locate?
- Does it look like a salon?

4. *Treatment and service execution*

- Is the treatment area organized?
- Is the work area set up and ready to go?
- Do you have to search for supplies?
- Are the products too hot, cold, messy, or runny?
- Does the technician discuss proper home care?
- Does the client's makeup get smudged during the service?
- Does the client's clothing get soiled during the service?
- Are the counters and work area clean?
- Is there an initial consultation before beginning the service?
- Is the client instructed on what will happen during her visit?
- Does the client know what to expect during the procedure and after?

- Does the client clearly express her desired results?
- Is the client left unattended? If so, is she told so?
- Is the technician working on multiple clients?
- Does the technician seem experienced, efficient, and knowledgeable?
- Is the client satisfied with the finished product?
- Is there an initial consultation before beginning the service?
- Is the salon temperature comfortable for the client?
- Is the noise level acceptable to the client's ear?
- Is the music selection reflective for the clients or staff?

5. *Product sales*
   - Are you out of stock on items?
   - Is the product dusty and dirty?
   - Does it look like it has been on the shelf too long?
   - Are the products organized?
   - Do you know the product prices?
   - Are there point of purchase displays to pique the client's interest?
   - How frequently is stock rotated?
   - Can you find the product you are looking for?
   - Is there sufficient inventory?
   - Are the products clearly categorized?
   - Is the product display inviting?
   - Does it look like you are in the business of selling products?
   - Are price stickers covering up important information?

6. *Staff exposure*
   - Does staff gossip in front of clients?
   - Are workers' hairstyles up-to-date and fashionable?
   - How are they dressed? Fashionable? Funky? Chic? Casual? Polished? In need of pressing? Shoes?
   - How are their accessories? Makeup? Skin care? Nails?
   - Do they acknowledge all clients?
   - Are they friendly and approachable?

- Does the staff appear cliquey?
- Are they helpful to and supportive of each other?
- Did they introduce themselves to the client?
- Do they appear knowledgeable in their craft?
- Do they appear to be team players?
- Do you get a genuine feeling of caring from the technician?
- Does the conversation get sidetracked with unprofessional dialogue?
- Does the staff reveal their personal problems in front of the clients?
- Do they treat all clients equally?
- Is it apparent that they like their job?

7. *Checkout time*
   - Do you have enough cash in the drawer to make change?
   - Are prices posted or accessible?
   - Was the client asked to schedule another appointment?
   - Does the staff know how to ring up a credit card sale?
   - Does the staff know how to run the cash register or computer?
   - Can they make change?
   - Can the client get to the desk or is it too crowded?
   - Does the staff suggest home care products?
   - Do they ask the client if she has any questions regarding home care and maintenance?
   - Does the staff know how to prepare a receipt?
   - Can the client find her coat and belongings?
   - Is there room to pay?
   - Is the counter too tall, short, narrow?
   - Was the client thanked for her business?
   - Are there shopping bags in which to place purchased products?

8. *Management activities*

- Have you provided the staff with sufficient supplies to do their duties?
- Do you take business calls while servicing a client?
- Does the staff have the proper training for excellent customer service?
- Do they have good technical skills? Communication skills?
- Is there follow-up after the sale?
- Are you a good listener?
- Do you praise and acknowledge a job well done?
- Are you supportive of the entire staff?
- Are you happy to see every client that patronizes your business?
- Do you get too wrapped up in the business of business and overlook a customer?
- Can you maintain a positive outlook even in up and down cycles?
- Do you allow time for sufficient planning and organizing to properly execute a new idea or concept?

What's Happening in Your Business?

Your first challenge is to go back over the previous list and add to it any activities you observe in your business. (I presented this exercise as part of a speech at a National Cosmetology Association (NCA) convention and in fifteen minutes the group came up with over two hundred golden opportunities.)

Your second challenge is to take the eight detailed areas and walk through your salon with the eyes of a customer. Really scope out what's happening in your business. Sit in every chair your clients may use. Look around from each position to get a view of areas exposed to clients. Rate each topic on a scale of one to five. Highlight your strong golden opportunities and make notes on changes that need to be made.

1,000 Club

For you to distance yourself from the competition you do not have to perform one task 1,000 times better. You perform 1,000 tasks 1 percent better. Will your effort pay off? Carlzon, the president of SAS, was able to turn an $8 million loss into a $71 million moneymaker in less than one year concentrating on the details! I'd say it pays to pay attention to details. Join the 1,000 club today! Commit to paying attention to the little things.

HOW CLIENTS PERCEIVE YOU

The perfect place to gather information about your business is from your existing and former clients. Circulate a client survey soliciting their opinions, preferences, and perceptions. Quite often business owners wear blindfolds regarding their "baby" and as a result may not be aware of customer preferences. Don't miss out on a chance to improve your sales. Ask the people who support your company for their opinions.

The best reason for customer surveys is that they reveal what the client thinks and feels about your company versus what you perceive. Over the years I have found this undertaking the best investment before planning any major projects.

Everyone in the salon business was talking full-serve and day-spa business as the wave of the future. So naturally I checked into expanding my salon to accommodate many new services. I was ecstatic when I found the perfect building to relocate the salon. It was the ideal situation: parking, architectural style, pool, private kitchen, outside patio, water fountains, exercise area—you name it, this place had it. I could not believe my good fortune when the building came up for sale. I was ready to take the plunge and thought it would be worth the extra capital to relocate. Then I distributed a client survey, and as a result I saved over $350,000. I thought the clients would jump at the chance for a salon like I was planning with all the amenities, but their responses revealed that the business required to make the salon profitable would not warrant the additional expenses. It turned out there was a big difference between my perceptions and what the clients thought. If and when you are contemplating major and even minor changes, get opinions from the people that support your business. Check with the people who give you their hard-earned cash for your products and services. The investment for circulation of a questionnaire is minimal compared to the alternative.

Customer survey:

1. Makes clients feel important because you have asked for their opinions.
2. Demonstrates your desire to offer the best products and services for them. Client input gives you the direction for fulfilling their needs.
3. Tips you off to your strong and weak areas.
4. Directs you toward potential sales triggers.

You will find a sample survey in Figure 2.1 (pages 22–24). Use any or all of the questions in your quest for building your business. You will note that the first area is for the name and address. I suggest you fill them out by hand. Many of the clients will return the survey with the cover not still attached. The clients that leave the cover letter attached are perfect sales candidates based on their responses especially to the "I'd like to have" questions.

Make it easy to fill out and offer them a token gift for taking the time to assist your efforts. A complimentary lipstick or minitreatment works wonders for increasing your response rate.

Make your customer survey as simple or as complex as you desire. It can serve as a salon evaluation, can tell you your clients' product, service, and educational requirements, and can enlighten you to potential sales. Allow your customers the opportunity to share their insights about your business.

HOW DO YOU STACK UP AGAINST THE COMPETITION?

A great way to generate new ideas for your company is to do a little comparison shopping. You will not only get new ideas for your operation but also a firsthand account of how you stack up against the competition. Feel free to shop other salons, department stores, specialty boutiques, and drug and grocery stores. Comparison shop locally and take time when you travel to investigate other stores. Scout out places where your clients currently purchase services and products and stores where they have previously shopped.

Salon owners should even hire someone to shop their own business. I recommend sending in a client to go through all the regular services and procedures a new client would experience. You can reimburse the shopper for any product or service expenses, or simply give her a gift certificate up front.

If you're not personally comfortable shopping the competition ask a friend or family member to be your eyes and ears. Select someone who will give you an honest assessment. When you have selected the detective and target store, clue the person into what you want to know: general feel of store, facility layout, strengths and weaknesses, display sets, product selection, customer service, well-educated and informative personnel. See Figure 2.2 (pages 26–27) for recording the detective's findings.

When I was designing my salon, I combined the information gathered from customer surveys and comparative shopping analyses. I discovered another key salon in my area was designed in a red and black Oriental theme and concentrated on a holistic skin and body approach. That was fine, but I knew I had to create something completely different. I was determined to make my salon stand apart from the crowd. So the original color scheme for the salon was gray, white, chrome, and clinical. The goal was to showcase the contrast in image and salon philosophy. Taking the time to research the market helped me carve out a niche for my new venture.

Defining Your Strengths

Why would I, as a potential client, come in to see you? Service? Relaxation? Trust? Products? Results? Why should I come in to see you versus your competition down the street? How would you respond to that question? What would you say? Personality? Dedication? Better quality? Knowledge? Service? More professional? Friendship? Now, out of all the things listed above, how many would apply to your business? To your competition? Are they similar? *Almost* every beauty business would fit those descriptions. (By the way those responses were given to me from an audience of over five hundred, and they all agreed that their business fit 95 percent of the characteristics.)

What are the differences between Wendy's and McDonald's hamburgers? The difference is that anywhere in the country you can purchase consistently prepared food at a reasonable price in every McDonald's store. Wendy's will make the burger your way. Do you notice that Wendy's and McDonald's go in on the same street corner? These businesses are not afraid to battle bun-to-bun on the same

(text continues on p. 25)

SAMPLE CLIENT SURVEY

Name _____

Address _____

    As a special client, I value your feelings, reactions, and opinions. (Your business name) is ready for a change and I would greatly appreciate your input. Thank you for taking the next few minutes to fill out the needed information. When we receive your survey, as a token of our appreciation, please feel free to select a new lipstick on your next visit to the salon.

    Thanks for your input.

Signed,

(Salon Owner)

CLIENT QUESTIONNAIRE

Why do you go to (business name)? Please rate (1-20) in order of importance to you the following:

_____Good service	_____Atmosphere	_____Convenient to home
_____Location	_____Socially	_____Convenient to office
_____Products	_____Feel "cared for"	_____Pricing
_____Relaxation, antistress	_____Staff—people and personalities	_____Facility
_____Professional advice	_____Improve self-esteem	_____Pampering
_____Treatments	_____To look better	_____Results
_____Convenient hours	_____Other _____	

Please circle the services you have had:

Haircut	Haircolor	Perm	Conditioning Treatment
Skin Treatment	Makeup Application	Makeup Lesson	Manicure
Pedicure	Artificial Nail	Body Massage	Body Treatment

If you have discontinued any services please tell us why.

What day(s) are convenient for you to visit the salon? Please circle your response.

| Monday | Tuesday | Wednesday | Thursday | Friday | Saturday | Sunday |

What time(s) are convenient for you to visit the salon? Please circle your response.

| Before 8:00 A.M. | 9:00 A.M.–noon | noon–4:00 P.M. | 4:00 P.M.–7:00 P.M | after 7:00 P.M.. |

Fig. 2.1 Client questionnaire.

If you are currently using our home care products, what are your favorite three?

HAIR	SKIN	MAKEUP
1.	1.	1.
2.	2.	2.
3.	3.	3.

What products if any have you tried and found to be less than satisfactory?

If you could change the current packaging of your products, what would you design?

What products would you like to have available that are not currently carried in the salon?

What services would you like to have available that are not currently offered in the salon?

Circle any of the following services you might consider having and the expected price.

Aromatherapy massage: Unique therapeutic massage that incorporates essential oils for harmonizing the body.

One hour $40 $50 $60

Color analysis: In-depth consultation and workshop to identify colors and clothing textures that work best for you.

One hour $50 $60 $70

Image consultation: Putting it all together with looks, styles, shapes of clothes, colors, body proportions, and appearance.

Three hours $100 $200 $300

Networking lunches: Scheduled lunches to meet other outstanding women in the community.

One hour $5 $10 $15

Videos of your personal styling lesson (makeup/hair) so you will have an at-home reference of your new look.

$30 $40 $50

Body facial: Cleansing, smoothing, and moisturizing of body skin from head to toe.

One hour $30 $40 $50

Back Facial: Cleansing, smoothing, and hydration of the back. Especially good for problem skin.

One hour $25 $30 $35

Fig. 2.1   Client questionnaire.

Mud pack: Mineralization of the skin with deep cleansing revitalizing mineral clays.

One hour	Face	$10	$20	$30
One hour	Body	$35	$40	$45

Body polish: Smoothing and buffing treatment from the neck down to remove dead cell buildup. Makes the skin silky smooth.

One hour	$35	$40	$45

Swedish massage: Soothing and relaxing massage to relieve overall body stress.

One hour	$45	$55	$65

Shiatsu massage: Ancient Oriental pressure point body massage.

30 minutes	$30	$40	
One hour	$60	$70	$75

Foot reflexology: Pressure point massage on the feet and lower legs. Great for relieving stress. Reflexology results can be felt throughout the entire body.

30 minutes	$20	$25	$30

Would you consider scheduling for yourself or giving as a gift certificate any of the following? Please check those you would consider.

_____**Makeover Package:**
Haircut, style, perm or color make up application, manicure

_____**Skin Purification Treatment:**
Sauna, aromatherapy massage, shower, mud body pack

_____**Antistress Treatment:**
Sauna, body polish, Swedish massage, herbal relaxation wrap

_____**Day of Fitness:**
Body polish,body paraffin,sport manicure and pedicure, foot reflexology, Swedish massage, sauna, and shower.

_____**On-the-Go Treatment:**
Facial, leg waxing, lash tinting, and manicure administered at the same time

_____**Indulgence Package:**
Continental breakfast and cappuccino, hair cut and style, color consultation, facial, Swedish message, body polish, makeup application, manicure, pedicure, gourmet lunch, limousine transportation to and from the salon

Fig. 2.1   Client questionnaire.

Would you be interested in attending any of the following seminars or workshops? The classes would be approximately one to two hours each. Please circle the seminar topics that appeal to you:

_____Personal Image and Self-Projection   _____Nutrition

_____Wardrobe Planning   _____Teen Skin Care

_____Teen Makeup   _____Skin Care

_____Beautiful Hands   _____Hair Styling Class

_____After-five Looks   _____Color Analysis

Makeup for   _____Day   _____Evening   ____Sport   _____Office

How would you rate us on the following overall (1–10)?

_____Salon   _____Staff

_____Products   _____Prices

_____Facility   _____Technical skills

_____Listening skills   _____Timeliness

_____New trends   _____Cleanliness

_____Services: _____Hair   _____Skin   ____Body   _____Nails

Please feel free to make any additional suggestions or comments:_____

_____

_____

Fig. 2.1   Client questionnaire.

corner because they have defined what sets their business apart.

USP

A critical step on the road to building your business is to define what makes your company different from similar businesses in your area. A Unique Selling Position clarifies what makes your business different from the competition. Maybe I should ask you if you have any competition. More and more every day? You need to be very clear on your Unique Selling Position, on what sets you apart.

Now if I asked you what makes your salon different from all the other salons how would you respond? Don't get caught up in simply saying you offer a "quality service and product." Chances are if I called another salon they would tell me the same thing. There are over 200,000 salons in the United States today. What sets yours apart? This may be tough to answer, but if you omit defining your strengths, you may end up just another fatal corporate statistic. Make your company stand apart from the crowd. Don't settle for being just like everyone else. You have unique talents and services. Position them.

Before planning your marketing strategy it is critical that you define your Unique Selling Position. Take time now to write

COMPARISON SHOPPING CHECKLIST

Store Name:_____   Location:_____

Shopper: _____   Date:_____

1. How did you feel upon arriving at the location?

    _____Welcomed   _____Intimidated

    _____Intrusive   _____Comfortable

    _____Uneasy   _____Relaxed

2. How would you describe the overall image?

    _____Positive   _____Contemporary   _____Snobbish

    _____Young   _____Glamorous   _____Stylish

    _____Trendy   _____Homey   _____Dated

3. How did the facility make you feel?

    _____Relaxed   _____Inferior   _____Beautiful

    _____Important   _____Self-conscious

4. What was the color scheme?   _____

5. When you arrived were you greeted?   _____

6. Were the facilities clean?   Yes/No

    _____Stations   _____Retail area

    _____Makeup station   _____Chemical area

    _____Reception area

7. Services

    Did the staff appear knowledgeable?   _____

    Did they conduct an initial consultation?_____

    Were you satisfied with the end results?_____

    Rate the service overall (1–10):   _____

    Did the service begin on time?   _____

Fig. 2.2   Comparison shopping list.

8. Products

      Were you instructed on home care procedures?   _____

      Were testers available for you to try?   _____

      Were products displayed?   _____

      Did you have access to product merchandisers?   _____

      Was there an adequate selection of products?   _____

      How were the products priced? Low, medium, high?   _____

9. Personnel

      How would you rate the following (1–10)?

Staff knowledge	_____	Appearance	_____
Friendliness	_____	Helpfulness	_____
Service skill	_____	Timeliness	_____

10. What was your overall reaction?

11. If you ran the business, what would you do differently?

Fig. 2.2 Comparison shopping list.

out some of the things that make your business unique. You do a great service—big deal, so does some of your competition. You have good products—so do most places. Those are necessary qualities to have, but you have to be very specific and clear in what makes you and your enterprise different. Some examples are: We never run more than five minutes behind. No appointment is necessary. Everyone on staff has won a major styling competition.

    The USP for my salon was, "We would educate customers on how to take care of their skin and body and teach them the proper techniques for achieving the look at home." Our goal was to be an informational and educational salon.

CHALLENGE: Write out your Unique Selling Position before you go any further in this chapter. If you do not have a defined USP, your marketing plan will be diluted and tough to implement. Don't take a shotgun approach with your money, time,

and talent because you are not clear about what you have to offer.

    Once you have identified your USP you should write it out and display it everywhere that is appropriate in your business—advertisements, posters, store signs, and especially your business cards. Keep in mind what you would say to a caller who inquired why he or she should come in and see you.

SHOPPING FOR CLIENTS

Now that you have a clear picture of what sets your business apart, it's time to shop for clients. Before you can establish a business-building campaign you need to know who your current customers are, or if you are a new business, what type of clients you want to attract to your business. You can then design a campaign around the information.

Chances are that if I asked you who your customers are, you might respond with "Well, we see everyone from twelve to ninety years old, men and women, rich to poor, working and nonworking, city dwellers and country people." I'm glad you have that diverse a client base, but for targeting your market the gap is too wide.

After you have identified your Unique Selling Position, your next goal is to identify your ten best customers. Whether I am working with clothing boutiques, plastic surgery groups, or manufacturing companies, I still take them through the following exercise.

Finding Your Ten Best Customers: A Basis for Sales and Marketing

If you could carbon copy ten of your best clients, who would you choose? If you had your choice of the type of client you would like to work with who would that be?

Answer the following shopping list of questions, then fill in the chart in Figure 2.3.

1. List the names of your ten best clients.
2. Are they male or female?
3. What are the client's approximate ages?
4. Are they married or single?
5. Are they working or nonworking?
6. If they work outside of the home, list their occupations.
7. Do they have children? If so, what are the ages?
8. Do they belong to clubs and organizations? If so, list them.
9. What magazines, newspapers, and books do they read?
10. What television shows and radio stations do they enjoy?
11. Estimate their incomes.
12. How did they originally find out about your business?
13. What are your customers' zip codes?
14. What types of cars do they drive?
15. Where is their favorite place to shop?

Once you have completed your shopping list, look for patterns, similarities, and contrasts. This client profile will help you key into where you should be targeting your marketing efforts. Keep this chart handy. You will need to refer back to the ten best list during your planning stages and you will find it so helpful, you will want to update it yearly.

Each challenge is a brick in the foundation of your sales success. Don't shortchange yourself by skipping the exercises. Each one will provide you with answers you will need throughout the rest of this book. You should have filled in the golden opportunities chart, made a commitment to conducting a client survey, scheduled a shopping tour, defined your USP, and profiled your ten best customers.

Did it seem that you had a lot of homework, or should I say salon work, in this chapter? It is impossible for me to give you the formula for selling success without taking into consideration your unique business personality. You should now have a personality profile of your company that will launch you in the perfect direction!

Name	M/F	Ages	M/S	Work/No	Occ	Kids Ages	Club	Read	TV/ Radio	$$	1st Visit	ZIP	Car	Shop
1.														
2.														
3.														
4.														
5.														
6.														
7.														
8.														
9.														
10.														

Fig. 2.3 Ten best list.

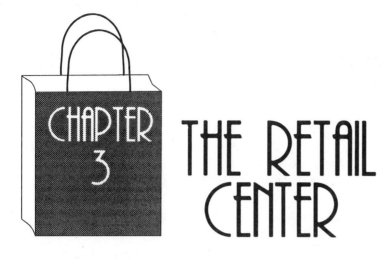

THE RETAIL CENTER

The key to getting clients to spend their hard-earned money in your salon is not only to meet their needs and desires but to create an environment in which it is fun to shop. In this chapter we will go over the fine details of creating the mood and setting for maximizing your sales.

CLIENTS ARE KEY

The salon had been open a year. During the initial time of testing and trials I enrolled in some business classes. One day, our class was to have a guest speaker from the Center for Entrepreneurial Management in New York City. The class was packed with budding students ready to take over the capitalistic free world with their bigger and better mousetraps.

Professor Fran Jabara introduced Mr. Joe Mancuso, our guest speaker. He rose from his chair, walked to the podium, braced himself, and in a very commanding voice asked the group, "What is the very first thing you must have before going into business?" Collectively the group shouted, "Money" knowing we were right on target. Our previous classes had been dedicated solely to the importance of proper capitalization for a start-up business. He responded, "No, not the first thing." During the next ten minutes the students, yours truly included, kept shouting responses: ideas, product, venture capital, location, attorney, business cards, order forms, employees, business plan, energy, positive attitude.

Mr. Mancuso was over six feet tall and cut a very imposing figure. He walked from the podium to the folding table to his immediate right and sat down on one hip. With his foot swinging in the breeze he waited patiently for us to wake up and smell the coffee. He just sat there, his eyes twinkling with an inner knowledge. Finally he walked up to the audience. He put his hands on his hips and loudly proclaimed, "the first thing you need before going into business is a customer."

I'll never forget that day. My perception of my business did a 180 degree turn. I realized that I had designed my salon, product and service menu, and pricing structure based solely on the competition. The flavor of the salon, services offered, the inventory mix, and even the prices were based on what other salons were doing or not doing. Maybe that's why all salons are basically the same, doing the same thing the same way.

My focus switched that day. I went back to the salon after class and walked through the place vowing to concentrate my attention and actions with the client in mind from that point forward. Running with the pack had to stop. I had to view my business as a client would. I had to redesign the salon from a client's perspective.

Comparing Service Experiences

Think back to a time when you went out to eat and the entire evening had a special feel or memory. Did your favorite restaurant cater to your senses? How were you greeted? Was it warm and friendly? How about the temperature of the restaurant? Was it comfortable or chilly? When you were served food, was the presentation appealing to the eye as well as to the palate? As you were sipping your cocktail, how was the music in the background? Was it soft and lifting, barely discernible? Overall was your impression of the evening warm and positive?

This memorable dining experience lingers in your mind because all of the senses were caressed and stimulated. People purchase experiences. And that is true of the beauty business.

SELLING THE SENSES

To maximize sales, you need to evaluate the environment you offer clients. You need to literally set the stage for their shopping experience; to do that you must sell the senses.

Stimulating Sight

Seventy-eight percent of what people buy is what they see. Setting the selling stage to stimulate sight encompasses many areas. Everything the client can see will leave an impression. The more positive strokes you score the better your chance at retaining clients and attracting new ones. Remember you sell through sight.

Mr. Clean
Cleanliness is at the top of the list. Unfortunately the services you perform and the constant foot traffic in the salon make endless cleaning a must. What is the image you are sending to the client? Are the floors clean or are clients walking through hair to get to the station? Keep the chair free of clutter and debris. Pick up any used coffee cups lingering around. The station should be spotless and sparkling clean. The mirror should be free from smears and hair spray residue. The salon needs to be cleaner than the client's home.

Employees' Appearance
What message is the staff sending to the public? Is it one of style and professionalism? Is the appearance too casual for the clients? Go back to your ten best list and evaluate the style of clothes your clients are wearing.

Salon Decor
Every piece of equipment, fixture, chair, desk, table creates an image. What is the flavor of your salon? The look you select for your business is critical. The decor creates the feel and ambiance of the business. Does yours say something different to the client? The theme of your salon needs to be carried out through all areas.

Lighting
Salon lighting must be flattering to you and your clients. Are you hit with a blast of light when you enter the salon? When you look in the mirror is the reflection your actual coloring or are you cast in a green glow? Clients should see subtle differences in lighting as they walk through the salon. Proper lighting allows clients to read brochures, inspect product packaging, and read home care instructions.

Display
The products you put on the shelf will help to stimulate buying. Think of the last dinner you had where the dessert menu was carried out on a tray. The waiter presented a visual menu. It sure is a lot harder to turn down dessert when it is looking so tasty on a tray in front of you. Displays work the same way. All of chapter 4 covers ways to stimulate sales through displays.

Videos
One way to stimulate sight is to have a video recorder playing in the salon. Start a current video library. Position your monitor so the client can view the videos from key locations within the salon.

Magazines
Check the dates on magazines. Make sure the periodicals are for the current month. Get rid of any magazine older than the current month. You represent the fashion and beauty industry. Old magazines won't do if you want your clients to keep up to date with hair, makeup, nail, and clothing styles.

Keep a selection of style books for the clients to browse through. Put together a portfolio of before and afters you have executed. Pull sheets from magazines to show new looks and options and compile them in a photo album.

How are you selling through sight?

Tantalizing Touch

When clients enter the salon you can touch them physically as well as internally through the emotions. In setting the selling stage you will need to concentrate on both areas of stimulation. Let's work from the outside in. Every salon has a "feel." What does your salon reveal to clients as soon as they enter the front door? Is the salon relaxed, upbeat, happy, tense, crazy, ethereal, or what? The salon itself is sending a message to clients. Pay close attention for negative energy flowing through the salon. Clients can "read" the overall tone of a salon within a few seconds of entering.

The textures of counters, fabrics for chairs, and even hand shakes all work toward stimulating the sale through touch. Even stepping onto a cold floor after a message leaves an impression. Place testers around the salon to get the clients' hands involved.

How are you selling through touch?

The Sound of Music

Music plays a very important role in your selling success. If you are serious about increasing your retail sales, you will need to eliminate the radio from the salon. Now don't panic if you can't cut hair without music; you'll still be able to work. I have a personal rule as an educator and lecturer, and that is if I take something away from you, I must give you something to replace it.

Yes, you will need to eliminate the radio for two reasons. One is that when the news comes over the air waves, your clients' attention is instantly diverted to the news broadcast. You may be into the close of a home care recommendation and you have lost them. The second reason for silencing the radio is commercials. I was doing a salon training program when I overheard a competing salon's commercial blast the air waves. "Yes, you can have a new look, new do, new perm for spring. All for $32.95." A client was at the front desk paying her service bill and was writing a check for $78.00 for a perm. The client's reaction was, "Why am I paying you all this money when I can get it for half price down the street?"

Now, if you cannot have the radio, what can you play? Cassette tapes are fine, compact discs are great—anything but the radio.

Vexing Volume

There seems to be a daily, even hourly, power struggle in some salons as to how loud the music should be played. The rule here is that the music should be background, mood-setting music, not Saturday night at the hop. Establish a base level for volume control. You need to be able to hear the clients' conversation and the phone ringing.

Music Selection

When it comes to sales the rule here is that the music selection should reflect the client base, not the staff. The type of music you play in the salon should be harmonious to the blend of clients. If your salon caters to young, hip clientele, then by all means head-banging music is fine. If, however, you are trying to attract the upscale working woman, this music is far from acceptable. I like to vary the mood and flavor of the music throughout the day. Rotate the selections. In the morning you can play more pop or classical music. After lunch the tempo may need energizing.

Some top-selling tunes can make your clients feel pretty, sexy, and gorgeous. (I should add if your clients are mostly women.) Instrumental music is more effective for sales because you are not competing with lyrics for clients' attention.

Facial and Body-work Music

If you offer facials and body therapy be careful in your music selection process. Have you ever had a client finish a treatment, stagger up front to pay, look a little glassy eyed, and express the desire for someone to drive her home? New technicians program music for these services, and the music is too harpy or New Age. The music literally zones clients out. By the end of the treatment they are so far gone they can't make decisions, like to schedule another appointment or invest in products. You can play relaxing tunes, but at the end of the session, bring the client back to reality. Within the last ten to twenty-five minutes switch the tempo.

Paying close attention to the music selection will be music to your clients' ears. The sound you will hear will be the cash register.

How are you selling through sound?

"Scentational" Smells

The power of smell is the strongest of all your senses. Smell has a direct link to your brain. Smell can be a silent salesperson. It works quite mysteriously and has the power to trigger memories and desires.

Think of what you had for lunch three weeks ago on Thursday. Can't remember? Don't fret, neither can I. Now think of fresh baked bread that's just about to come out of the oven. Do you smell it? Can you remember the smell of your house as a child during the holiday season? The evergreen, the cinnamon, the cookies, hot cider brewing on the stove? Just the mere thought of these wonderful things can produce physical reactions and stimulate mental images. When you are strolling through the mall, what store do you know you are approaching? If you guessed Victoria's Secret you are right. They have mastered the art of selling through smelling. The mixture of aromas creates an anchor, and you are drawn to the smell, especially if you have had a pleasurable shopping experience in their store.

When Georgio of Beverly Hills introduced its signature scent, it literally blasted the fragrance into the street. On a visit to Rodeo Drive I discovered two holes in the lions perched about the entrance to the store. They emitted the fragrance into the street at intervals to entice shoppers into the store. Mrs. Fields had the kitchen exhaust turned so that the smells from the ovens wafted into the street. Who can resist the home-baked smell of their chocolate macadamia nut cookies? What a brilliant selling idea.

Your salon needs to have a smell to it. Not the perm or nail chemical smell, but a pleasant olfactory trigger. You can anchor your clients to the salon by different methods.

You can place diffusers throughout the salon that emit essential oils into the air. Use vanilla, cinnamon, or orange-based extracts. You can switch the scent for the holidays and add bayberry, evergreen, or pine.

If your salon is small and intimate, you can place containers of potpourri around the salon. If your operation is larger than seven hundred square feet try one of the other techniques.

Establish a no-smoking policy for staff and clients. I was on my way home from teaching an in-salon staff meeting when I kept smelling smoke. After a few miles I pulled off the highway. I was afraid the car was on fire. I popped the hood and proceeded to examine under it for the source of the fire smell. There was nothing, so I looked under the car and walked around it several times praying that it wouldn't blow up. I saw no smoke or flames so I jumped back in the car and headed home. Well the smell was still lingering and quite frankly I was getting worried so I pulled off again. This time I started rummaging through the car when I bumped a shopping bag. The salon I had been in had a clothing boutique, and I had purchased a few items. When I hit the sack a cloud of smoke rose from it. The only thing I had been smelling for forty miles was the cigarette smoke clinging to the clothes. It had scared me to death.

Stamp out smoking in your salon. If it can be done in restaurants and on airplanes it can be done in salons everywhere.

If your budget will allow, create your own salon signature fragrance or inventory an unusual retail item that can represent the salon's image.

Appoint a sentinel for food smells. When staff dines in the salon, the food smells linger. No one should eat lunch in view of clients. Not only is it bad for sales, but it will probably make your clients hungry.

I know of a couple of salons that have invested in commercial popcorn makers. This can be a nice touch or unique salon selling position. Try it and see what happens in your salon. If the flavor of your salon is more relaxed and casual popcorn is okay, but I would not recommend it if you are trying to project an upscale, elegant image.

Check with your local heating and air conditioning person. Some companies now offer a charcoal air filtering system to reduce unpleasant aromas in the salon.

How are you selling through smells?

Tasty Temptations Make Customers Welcome

You may not be able to get your teapot and cups and saucers to dance like Disney did in *Beauty and the Beast*, but you can still offer your clients something to tickle their taste buds. My favorite is custom blended coffee. I got tired of offering and drinking plain old coffee, so one day I purchased come coffee beans and blended away. I hit on an absolute winner. I swear to this day some of our clients come in just for the coffee. I'll let you in on the winning coffee combo. Take one-third Irish cream beans, one-third orange beans, and one-third amaretto beans. Mix them together and fill your coffee filter. After we started serving the coffee mix, we could tell the pleasant effect it had on the clients. A few even came in a couple of minutes ahead of their appointments to sit and sip their coffee. That was fine with me as they were sitting and looking at product.

Offer a variety of flavored teas, sodas, and bottled water. Don't put out a coffee piggy bank to subsidize the expense. If necessary build the refreshment bar into the overall cost of the service.

Some hotels have taken to putting out an urn of polished shiny apples. The last hotel I was in even had a decorator cookie jar on the registration desk with homemade chocolate chip cookies inside. Even if half the world seems to be on a diet, a sweet treat now and then is delightful. Add a sweet treat to an even sweeter treatment and you've got a winning combination.

Trash the Styrofoam cups. If you want to present the ultimate environment for selling you'll need at least a few china cups and saucers. Serve your soft drinks and bottled water in real honest to goodness glass glasses. But be sure to always sanitize cups and glasses in hot water.

How are you selling through taste?

Even Pretty Salons Can Lack Punch in Merchandising

Years ago I was flown in to give a retail evaluation on a salon. The salon was gorgeous. When you entered it you were greeted by a flooring of beautiful Italian marble, sofas and hand-braided rugs graced the floor, the twenty-five stations were custom built for the location, three of the walls overlooked a posh park and residential neighborhood. The facial and massage rooms were functional and comforting. The fifteen nail stations were artfully positioned in the nail boutique area. They even had several maids just to pick up after the clients and staff. This salon was raking in the bucks in service. They were bringing in $50,000–60,000 a week. Guess what their retail dollars consisted of? I'll help you out. You might think that with that ritzy and posh place, the percentage of retail sales would be staggering. Their monthly average was $3,000 in retail sales—$3,000 for an income of a quarter of a million in service per month!

The owner wanted my input as to how to help increase the retail business. My first target area was the imported armoires in the reception area. They were glassed in and locked; the shelves were dirty and had next to no product on them. I knew it was a no-win situation when I suggested the first thing was to take off the doors or at least open them up so clients could get their hands on what little product was there. The owner flatly refused to alter the decor of the salon under any circumstances.

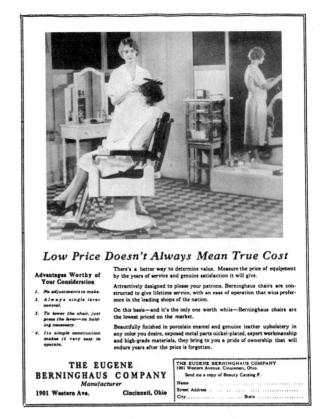

Fig. 3.1 This vintage salon ad emphasizes how good quality and function are needed for results.

After all, she had spent a fortune decorating the palace. Half a million in fixtures and no retail sales. What a shame!

So the moral of the story is to design or evaluate your salon from the image you want to project (Fig 3.1), but don't sacrifice retail sales for pictures and pretty do-dads. You probably have heard the old saying "the surgery was a success, but the patient died." Be careful when you design a new salon or remodel. A decorator may make it look pretty, but if the space isn't generating dollars the business dies.

CREATING A RETAIL SELLING ENVIRONMENT

Every salon has four walls, a ceiling, a floor, and a front door. Why do some salons sell more product than others? It depends on the relationship between the client, the staff, and the feel of the salon. Let's take a look at designing a salon with the ultimate sales possibilities.

Fabulous Floors

Can the floor sell for you? Well, not really, but the wrong flooring cover can detract from sales. If clients' attention is directed down to the floor due to color, dirt, or wild patterns, the client is not looking at you, the products, or the services being performed in your store.

The key thing to evaluate is your traffic flow. In what direction do the clients walk when they are in the salon? What is the first thing you are hit with when you enter a department store? As soon as you walk through the doors, you are facing the cosmetic counters. The strategic positioning of these islands of gold forces you to make a decision. They make you turn left or right to walk around the counter.

Think of the typical bowling alley salon. What happens when the clients breeze through the front door? They whiz through and dash straight back for your chair? Right? The layout of the bowling alley salon gives clients free access to the back or service area without having to stop at the reception desk, and worse not seeing your merchandising areas. (Fig. 3.2)

Set up the reception area so that the client has to make the same department store decision to turn quickly after entering.

Top It All Off

The choice of ceiling height and decoration can add to your retail sales or detract from the products and services. Have you gone into an old department store? You walk through the circular doorway and your eye is attracted to what? Depending on the store you will notice the huge pots and decanters resting on the tops of the counters or you will notice the huge hanging chandelier in the rotunda of the store. Is the store selling either of these things? Usually not.

If the ceiling in your salon is over ten feet tall, the client's eye will be directed up and over the product height. One easy way to correct this is to make the ceiling the same color as the flooring, going no more than two shades lighter. The goal of darkening the ceiling is to bring the eye down to product merchandising level. You can direct the client's attention by use of color and focus.

Fig. 3.2 Typical bowling alley salon (long and narrow).

Goal: create ample shopping opportunities within the salon. No remodeling necessary, wanted client to pass products at least 3 times while visiting salon.

Before: Common salon arrangement. Stations banking walls, reception desk and chairs in front of salon. The disadvantage with this setup is the retail zone. There is none!

After: Same salon now with an eye for retail.

A. Retail zone within 1st 10 feet of entry. Designed using 12" by 12" glass cubes. You can also use slat wall or grids for same linear shelf space. Keep base of shelving knee height. Use 4–5 rows of shelving.

B. 2 Display tables 24" or 36" rounds. Showcase any New and Improved products, feature of the month or seasonal items. Place your promotional testers and display on each table. Use the same theme throughout.

C. Retail Zig Zag Display cubes. Used to break up bowling alley look and to put retail product within steps of each station. This product is to be pulled when taking client through home care consultation. This zig zag pattern creates more privacy reducing the "warehouse" feel. Suspend posters above merchandising cubes. Keep base of shelving knee height. Use 3 rows of shelving.

D. Point of purchase on each station. Every station should have a featured item. Place a tester of the product plus 4–6 retail bottles of the same. Rotate products every 4–6 weeks to coincide with salon's traffic patterns.

E. Retail cubes by station. Use 3 rows across and 3–4 rows high.

F. Retail cubes by dispensary. This area of product puts retail bottles in direct line of sight when a client enters the salon.

G. Lucite shelves (3) for retail product at manicure station. Display retail products that are universal to sell. Nail techs can easily recommend hand and body lotion as well as mascara, body shampoo, eye creams, lipstick colors.

H. Wall mounted promotional displays, posters and signage. Feature product posters and/or manufacturer artwork. Use space to tell clients of specials, events, featured products or services.

Special Note: To create 5 times the retail space, the only thing sacrificed was one reception chair!

****Special Thanks to Red Merrow, Design Director for Belvedere for salon renderings.

Before

After

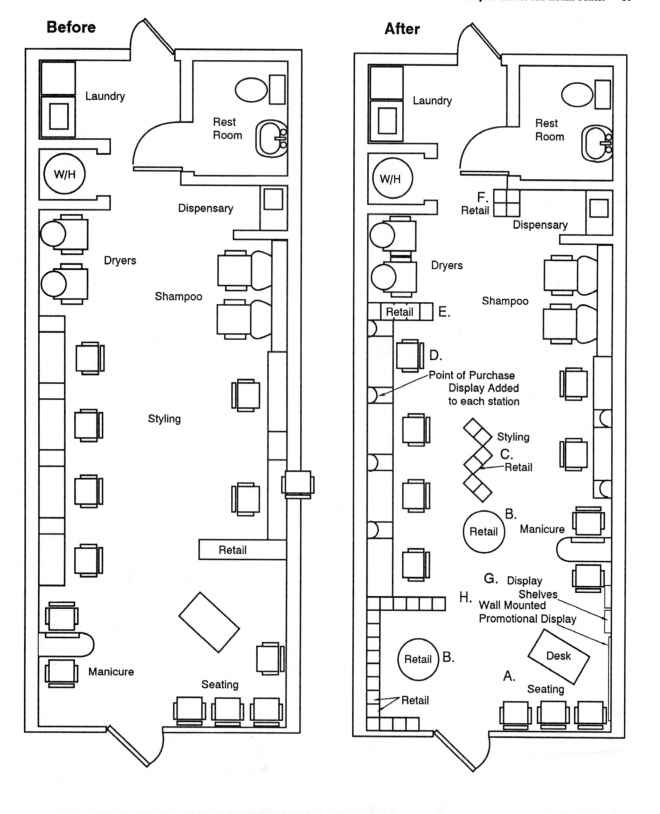

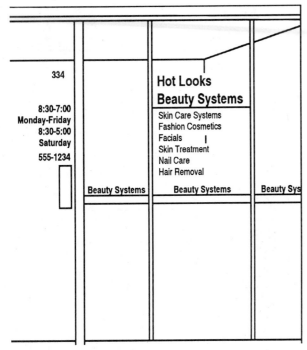

Fig. 3.3   The front window must highlight important facts.

Windows That Broadcast Your Business

Good retailers make it as easy as possible to shop in their store. (Fig. 3.3) The front door of the salon should have the following information:

1. The salon name and logo prominently featured.
2. Your street address and unit number clearly visible from the sidewalk or street.
3. Hours of operation. Let consumers know when the salon is open. List the days of the week and the hours per day.
4. Your phone number in large type.

Special Note

After today, please eliminate the phrase "Walk-Ins Welcome," especially on the front door or window of the salon. "No appointment necessary" is fine. What is a walk-in? It's a live breathing human being who just hasn't called in advance for an appointment.

One of my first retailing jobs was in a flower shop. We had a sign board attached to the outside corner of the building. We used to put up letters that spelled BOKA C & C 4.95. Do you have any idea what that means? I'll help you out. What we tried to say was Bouquet, Cash and Carry (not delivered) for $4.95. The serious problem with this sign was that we were talking in flower store jargon. That was the code we would write on the sales ticket if somebody bought a simple fresh-cut bouquet of flowers. It sure was dumb to assume a customer would have any clue to what we meant. I feel the same way about Walk-Ins Welcome. Please help me eliminate this from the beauty business.

Border Patrol for Identification

One of my favorite window treatments is to create a continuous border over every window. This technique is fantastic if you have two to three or more window panels. I want the client to be able to identify that the entire stretch of glass is part of your business, not the store next door or a separate business. Take your logo or salon name and have it duplicated in vinyl letters, or hand painted across the windows. Think of the client driving by and trying to find your store. Help them out with your window treatment.

Wonderful Walls

Use your walls to create additional excitement in the salon. (Fig. 3.4) These can be covered with textured material or painted. One of my favorite techniques is to paint the walls around the makeup area in flesh tones. I painted one wall in a neutral beige, another ivory, another yellow beige, and another pinky beige. If clients need additional reassurance that the product selected was appropriate for them I would escort them with mirror in tow to the wall that reflected their skin tone. The color changes were subtle, but most effective for increasing sales.

Another way to use your walls as a sales tool is to color code or departmentalize your different zones in the salon. Try a decorative border that wraps around the salon to lead the client through the different departments. The border can even have service descriptive words or symbols through the strip.

Structural walls can be turned into instant indoor billboards. These can house either lighted shadow boxes or transparency frames.

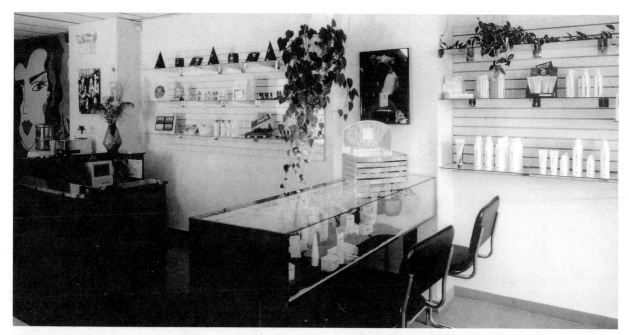

Fig. 3.4 Use the salon walls to create added excitement. (Photo by Michael A. Gallitelli on location at Rielms Hair Salon, Latham, NY.)

If one of your Unique Selling Positions is to support local artists or if you are a patron of the arts it is great to hang true artwork on the salon walls. Other than that I would limit the pretty posters and prints for use in your home, not the salon. Use posters from your product suppliers to decorate the walls. Feature before and afters. Hang letters from satisfied clients. Enlarge and frame articles written about you and the salon. These "works of art" should be gracing the walls.

Keep in mind that the space you are renting needs to generate income and the two areas that will make the cash register ring are your service and retail sales. Constantly ask yourself, "Does this support the income of the salon? Does this action benefit the client? Is this just for pretty's sake, or does it have a purpose?"

Choosing Your Colors

Color is not only a spark in your decor, it has an emotional and mental reaction to the client. Every color gives off vibrations, good or bad, and can affect the way clients feel in your establishment.

Do certain colors sell better than others? The answer to that is most definitely yes, and no. The first thing to evaluate is the overall feel of the salon. Does the coloring reflect the style and image you want to project? Once the color has been selected determine whether it flatters the skin.

Let's take a look at how color can affect your sales and your clients' reaction to the salon.

Black

The national color for hairdressers. Black is the combination of all colors. Black is mysterious, sophisticated, and dramatic. Now, I've yet to see a salon done in all black, but you can combine certain colors with black for different reactions. Some people see black as evil. You can use black, but use it wisely.

Black and White

High contrast colors. Extremes of color spectrum. Great colors for clients with healthy self-image. Maybe too strong and intense for shy or insecure clients.

Black, White, and Silver

High contrast, high tech. Great for modern, deco look. Silver adds to the perceived price of services and products.

Black, White, and Gold

As soon as you add gold to your colors the prices go up. Gold is a royal and expensive accent color. A product with gold on it can easily be $5 to $15 more expensive. This trio of tones is beautiful, but the consumer will perceive your prices to be expensive to extremely expensive. If you are pricey that's great, just don't scare off potential clients by looking high priced if you're not.

White

The opposite of basic black. White through the history of Western culture has been represented as the pure color. White is the epitome of good—the white doctor's coat, the nurse's uniform, white bridal gown, waving the white flag. White opens up a lot of possibilities in the salon. Most people feel safe with white.

A word of caution about using white in the facial, electrolysis, and massage rooms. White does represent clinical and sterile, but what's the first impression a client gets when they walk into a facial room? They see the lounge and the electrical equipment and the first impression is that it looks like a doctor's office. Now I don't know about you, but I hate going to doctors. Soften the medical approach in these rooms with accent colors. Add peach, pink, seafoam green, or terra cotta to warm up the place.

Gray

Gray connotes stable, steel strength. Gray is the combination of black and white. Gray can be nondescript, not taking a stand but in the middle of the road.

When I opened the salon, my color choice of the day was gray, white, and chrome. My favorite colors? No way! But when I needed to establish the difference between myself and others I felt I needed a contrast. My primary competition's salon was done in red, black, and oriental accents. My off-the-hip decision was to design the salon as far from theirs as possible. It worked. But the real moment of truth came when I remodeled the salon five years later and completely altered the color scheme and feel.

I wanted to warm up the place. It had taken on a too-medical look. As soon as we changed from the chrome, gray, and white to peach and terra cotta with gold accents, the clients' reaction was overwhelmingly positive. I even had one client loudly proclaim that for the first time in five years she was not afraid to walk up to the reception desk to pay. "For years when I left the salon and was up front, I looked cold and tired. Now the colors are as flattering to me as my own home. I'll hang around and look at products." Lesson learned the hard way. Client comfort comes first.

Red

Red is the dominant color in the color spectrum. It is outgoing, passionate, and signals attention to the world. Think of the little red sports car screaming for attention. Red in the salon can be used, but judiciously. Red can actually raise body temperature, produce heat in the tissues, and increase hormonal activity.

If you are trying to attract men to the salon, a warm orange red works best, but for the female gender a cooler red is preferred.

Blue

Blue is the overwhelming favorite of many people, especially men. Blue represents the need for peace and tranquility. Think of the blue sky, blue ocean waves lapping against the shore. Blue is credited with a calming effect and can lower blood pressure. Dark blue is a trustworthy color. Think of the navy and police officers in their blue uniforms. A word of caution. Putting too much blue in the salon can be depressing for introverted personalities over extended periods of time.

Purple

Purple is an interesting result of mixing the two extremes of passionate red and serene blue. Purple has been a significant color of royalty and high position. Purple is the color for spirituality and artistic expression.

I can remember my aunties hanging a wreath in the front door of my grandmother's house laced with purple ribbons when my granddaddy died. In the South, this color can represent death, so use it very carefully.

Green

Green generates healing and health. Green is a vital color and those that favor it are nature driven. Think of the internationally famous Body Shop. Could it be any other color?

If your salon is located in the big city or concrete jungle, you might want to add a touch of green. People who exist in that type of environment tend to be green "starved" and could use a sprinkling of the green to warm up their atmosphere.

Yellow

Yellow has the highest visibility. Yellow can be a cheerful addition to the salon. Use it to attract attention to key areas such as the retail zone. Yellow is the color of choice for safety. Think of the insecure clients coming to the salon. Maybe the electrolysis room or waxing room could have yellow accents to counteract the high stress, high tension treatments.

Pink

Use only if you don't expect any male clients to frequent your establishment. It wasn't too long ago that salons were decorated in fluffy pink Cape Cod curtains with white lattice work borders on the walls. Men still have a strong reluctance to going into female terrain for their services.

Pink is the color of intuition and can have a calming effect. Violent inmates were placed in pink holding cells and within minutes they calmed down. Pink lovers are lovers of life and are tender and caring. Your warmed-toned clients however, could be put off by the sappy pink tone.

Brown

The color of the earth. Brown is a folksy color. Brown or light muted brown tones can work well in the salon to create a comfortable hominess to the business. If your salon is set in an area where there are more trees than people, brown may be the perfect palette for you.

A word of caution for the retail zone: darker shades of brown may clash with the merchandise and packaging. Lighten up the color to tan or an eggshell hue as a background for product display areas.

Brown has a regional preference and reaction. If your salon is in the New York area brown doesn't sell well. The same is true for Florida due to the large amount of transplanted New Yorkers.

Orange

Orange is a misunderstood color. Orange is a toned down version of red, yet in some eyes orange is a funny color. Orange can give your salon the energy and psychological qualities of red without the intensity. Orange can be festive, bright, and cheery when it is light. Be careful toning down orange and shy away from murky, flat orange tones. They will produce negative reactions from your clients.

Softened forms of orange will work well in salons—salmon, peach, rust, terra cotta. If your salon is too cold or spends many months in the frozen tundra, add some warmth with these tones.

Color Roundup

Since there are over five thousand different colors it would be impossible to select a handful that sell best. Go back to your ten best list and review your findings to question 15. Where is their favorite place to shop? See if there is a color pattern there as well. Your ten best list will help you design the best environment for producing sales and client comfort.

Light Up Your Sales

Use lighting to strengthen retail sales and service zones in the salon. (Fig. 3.5) There are two basic types of lighting, direct and diffused lighting. Diffused lighting directs its glow over a wide area; direct lighting has a narrow field of light intensity. Create visual excitement by varying the lighting throughout the salon. Unfortunately many salons rely solely on overhead fluorescent lighting. This provides a much-needed light source but doesn't offer any variation in light and dark attention spots in the salon.

Use mounted track lighting to give you flexibility to increase excitement in the retail zones. A series of lights can be maneuvered and directed to different product displays and merchandise areas. For intensifying key promotions and products use a single spot stream of light to capture the client's eye. The ideal location for retail lighting is overhead and slightly in front of the products you wish to single out. This position helps reduce glare and makes the product more noticeable.

One key rule is to make sure the client looks healthy and natural in the lighting. Fluorescent light will give off a cool

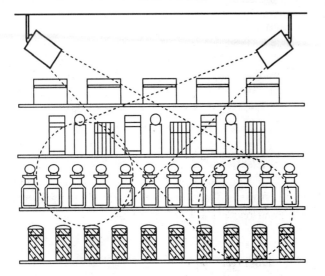

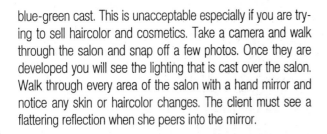

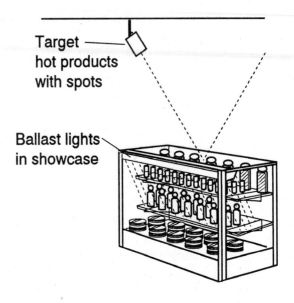

Fig. 3.5   Light up sales.

blue-green cast. This is unacceptable especially if you are trying to sell haircolor and cosmetics. Take a camera and walk through the salon and snap off a few photos. Once they are developed you will see the lighting that is cast over the salon. Walk through every area of the salon with a hand mirror and notice any skin or haircolor changes. The client must see a flattering reflection when she peers into the mirror.

Lighten Up These Areas
Pay close attention to overhead lighting when the client is sitting in the styling chair. The overhead lights can cast dark shadows on the face. No client wants to be forced to look into the mirror only to see extra dark circles under the eye and wrinkles popping out at them.

The most flattering lighting is one that comes out directly from the wall with alternating warm and cool lights. You will need some overhead lighting, but you should have flattering lighting face the client.

For your makeup areas, have lighted makeup mirrors on the station or a showcase that has adjustable lighting options—the kind of mirror that can go from day to office to sunlight. Not only will this help clients see their skin and makeup more clearly, this helps to reinforce the need for different product colors for different occasions and lightings.

Therapy rooms should have dimmer switches to control the volume of light. These inexpensive switches can help you create the right mood for the client.

WHAT'S THE STRONGEST PRODUCT-SELLING AREA?

The answer—first ten feet of your salon. That's right, the very first ten feet in the front door. What is typically within the first ten feet of salons? A few chairs or couches, coffee table, magazine rack, coffee pot, coffee cups, a few plants, hopefully a bit of retail product, the reception desk, a few retail shelves behind it, and the phone.

I had next to no money going in when I first opened my salon. I had a good friend who owned a plant store. After Sandy had been into the salon and saw the spectacular natural sunlight exposure she thought it would be dynamite for plants. Well, since I didn't have much else to fill up the space, she backed up the floral van and unloaded a few dozen blooming goodies. I knew I was in serious trouble when a client inquired as to the price of the dieffenbachia plant. Right then I knew the plants had to go. You couldn't see the products for the forest we had created.

Guard the first ten feet at all costs. Don't decorate, don't load it down—use that key zone to set the tone for your services and product.

Merchandising Fixtures

Once clients enter the salon they should be greeted with a series of fixtures that display merchandise available for sale. For these fixtures to be truly effective they need to be designed with product visibility, storage, and easy access for clients and staff in mind. They need to hold and show the merchandise being sold. There are endless possibilities from premade counters to custom-made cabinets for salons. The main styles of fixtures for retail are open showcases, closed showcases, museum cases, demonstration areas, and wall units.

The Open Showcase

This is a unit that is open and accessible for the clients. The ideal retail zone has a mixture of self-serve areas and staff-assisted counters. The open unit is for frequently purchased items—cleansers, shampoos, body products. These items are physically taller and larger. They will show up on open shelving. (Fig. 3.6)

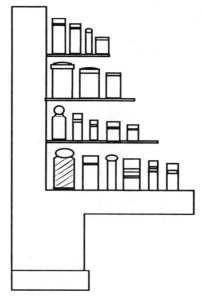

Fig. 3.6   Open showcase.

The Closed Showcase

This is a traditional department store-type counter. The closed unit houses smaller retail items that should be dispensed by a staff member. These products would include eye shadows, blushes, lipstick, concealers, powders, jewelry, scarves, belts, and expensive handbags if you stock accessories. The primary function of the closed showcase is to max out product visibility. You need to get the product out and visible so the client will want to buy it. (Fig. 3.7)

The Demonstration Showcase

This showcase is used as a demonstration or lesson console. They have stools for the client to sit on during the selling sequence. These have more stock and storage space behind the face of the counter as compared to the closed showcase, which has minimal back bar storage. (Fig. 3.8)

I personally prefer the demonstration showcase or lesson console to be next to or attached to the main display counters. You can set up a free station to also serve as an extension of your main lesson zone.

Museum Case

No, these aren't for displaying mummies, but to tease the client with product specials or new introductions. These cases typically don't hold massive volumes of product. They serve to tie-in displays in the retail zone or other service areas within the salon. They have a solid base and a clear Lucite cube or box that fits over the merchandise. (Fig. 3.9)

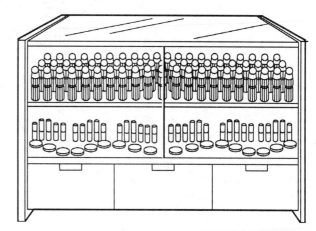

Fig. 3.7   Closed showcase.

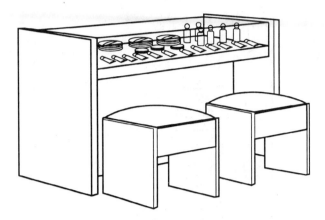

Fig. 3.8 Lesson console.

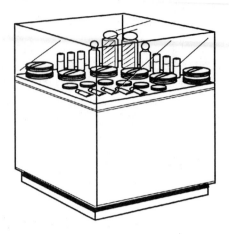

Fig. 3.9 Museum case.

Off the Wall

Wall units can be freestanding display fixtures pressed up to the wall or a fixture attached to the wall directly. Slat wall is commonly used to give a salon extra shelf space for product merchandising. Wall units become another self-serve area for clients. They need to be filled with product and organized for easy shopping. (Fig. 3.10)

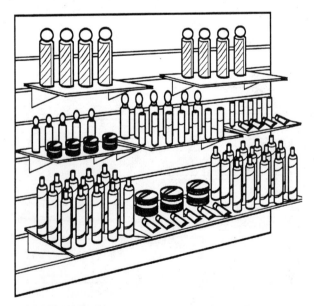

Fig. 3.10 Wall unit.

Doing a Lot With a Little Space and Big Budget

How do you take 150 square feet and turn it into a highly profitable retail zone? You take the fixtures just mentioned and position them for an island kiosk. The best move I made for the salon structurally and for sales was to purchase new fixtures. (Figs. 3.11a, 3.11b) The up-front investment would have choked a horse, but it was worth it. As soon as we changed the color scheme and updated the fixtures for sales, retail sales went through the roof with 40–50 percent increases right away. I had clients telling us that they didn't know we stocked certain items. I was flabbergasted because I had been stocking the items for years. They just didn't see them.

Establish a Boutique within the Salon

The retail zone can be the most profitable area in the salon. This setup could generate thousands of additional retail dollars.

Doing a Lot with a Little Space and Little Budget

Even if you only have one wall in your salon that you can use for retail, it is a start. Take that precious space and merchandise it. Take one wall and stake out a four-by-six-foot area for merchandising. This relatively small area can stock up to twenty-four linear feet of shelving space. The five shelves are four feet long and six inches deep. This will give you visibility and client access to the products you have available for sale.

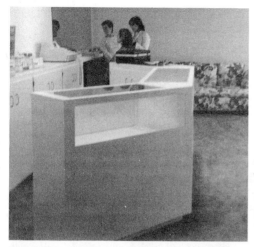

Fig. 3.11a A sad state of affairs. I could get the salon's doors open, but I just didn't have money for good fixtures, let alone enough product to fill the cases.

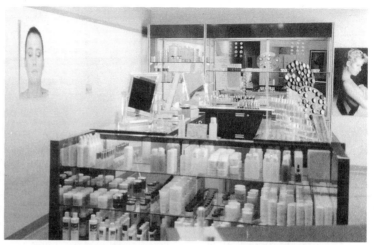

Fig. 3.11b Same space four years later. The showcases fit in 150 square feet. There is one open showcase, one closed showcase, and two lesson consoles with stools, plus one wall unit. Serious retailing possibilities. (Photos from Carol Phillips' private collection.)

Eleven Merchandising Maps

Once you have the fixtures and counters in place, where do you put all of the merchandise on the shelves? Here are eleven key stocking tips for increasing sales. (Fig. 3.12)

Eye to Eye

Keep all retail items at eye level and no lower than the knee. Any product above eye level or, worse, out of reach is out of the selling map. Clients will not look on the floor for beauty products. Keep the products sandwiched between the eyebrows and the bend of the knee.

Keep It in the Family

When you arrange your inventory, display by brand of product. Keep the family together to pack as much visual punch as possible.

Face Out

Make sure the face or the front of every bottle is facing out so the client can read the front label. If the back of the bottle is loaded with information the client might need, to turn one bottle out.

Categorically Correct

Stock the type of product going from left to right on one shelf. Take one shelf and start out at the far left with your basic shampoo for normal hair, next put dry, chemically treated, oily, fine, then any specialty shampoo. The shelf directly underneath will house the corresponding conditioner.

Neat Freaks

This one may sound a little wacky to you but don't keep the shelves filled to capacity and in perfect order. If it is the middle of the day and your merchandising wall has every product slot filled, the impression the client has is that "no one else has purchased anything, so why should I?" Don't confuse this with throwing dust rags in the wind. Just don't replace a product as soon as one is off the shelf in the bag.

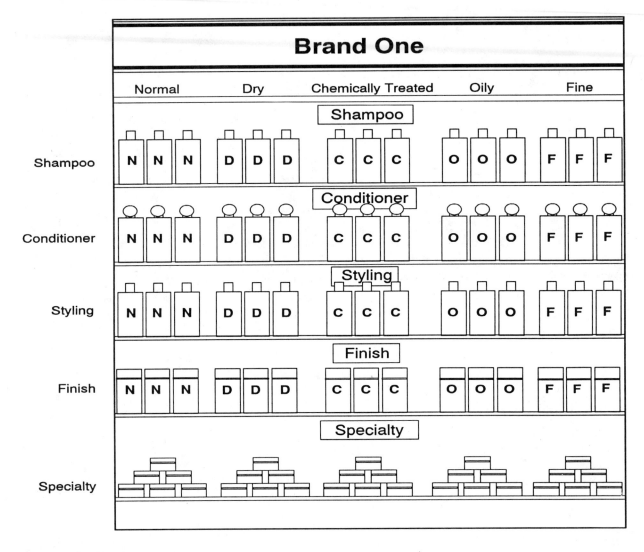

Fig. 3.12 Stocking tips.

Color Bands
Keep the same color or product stocked together. All blue bottles from Company X are placed together, not all the blue products you stock for every company.

Multiple Sizes
If you stock large items, stair step the sizes—the tallest one in the back, then the next size directly in front of the largest and so on.

Makeup Color Collections
Line your color items up cool to warm, left to right with lightest tones first, then medium, then darkest tones in same color—baby pink, light pink, rose, burgundy.

Stock Rotation
Always restock the shelves pushing the oldest product to the front. Replace the units from the back, scooting the previously stocked items forward.

Keep It Simple

Look at the shelves. The products should be inviting, and it should be easy to understand the different categories. Put signs, color bars, header banners, anything to help the client understand the wall of bottles and jars.

Mr. Clean Strikes Again

Keep the inventory super clean. The residue of hair spray can play havoc with tons of items on the shelf. Make dusting and cleaning a staff duty if necessary. But in order to sell more merchandise the goods have to be spotless. Organize your fixtures and counters.

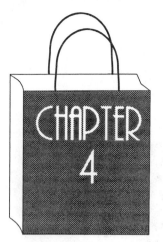

CHAPTER 4

DYNAMITE DISPLAYS

In this chapter, you will learn to create unique and effective displays. Let every spot in the salon support your goals and sales. Displays should tantalize and tease your clients like a masterful burlesque dancer, one who piques your interest and curiosity but leaves you wanting more.

Department stores have mastered visual appeal. When you visit a department store you are silently being sold as soon as you enter. You see promotional tables, banners, jumbo shopping bags, flags, a store theme. The merchandising area is color coordinated to increase the visual impact. Salons need to constantly generate the same excitement within their own retail zones. Displays make your clients look at products. If they see the same products arranged the same way, after one or two visits they stop looking. They stop buying.

SILENT SALESPEOPLE

Displays can help you sell without you having to utter a single word. (Fig. 4.1) Effective displays will entice the client to look at a product or stimulate a question that needs to be answered by a technician, which will lead to a sale. These silent salespeople are on duty every day; they don't need coffee breaks, and they don't show up late for work. Evaluate your salon. Use the information in this chapter to increase your service and retail sales. Use your flare and creativity when designing a display campaign.

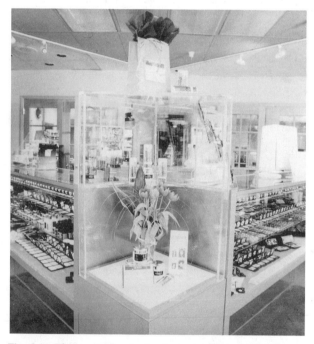

Fig. 4.1 Display shelf—silent salesperson. This tower teases the clients by showing them the feature products of the month (first exposure to the special). (Special thanks to Barbara Gauthier, Sherman Oaks, CA, for letting me remerchandise her retail area. Barbara has made a serious financial commitment to retailing with her inventory and fixtures. The retail area just needed a little adjusting to help increase the retail profit potential.) (Photo by Frank Jackson.)

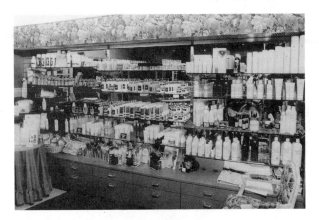

Fig. 4.2a Merchandise wall—before. This wall of product makes a serious statement to shopper: "This salon is serious about your home care needs. We have everything you will need." (Photo by Frank Jackson.)

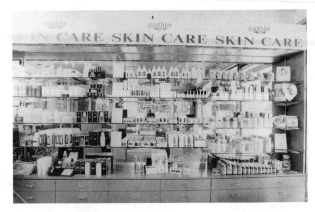

Fig. 4.2b Merchandise wall—after. The product was merchandised by brand and percentage of sales. Shelf talkers were added to assist shoppers by describing products. No additional inventory was shipped in. All the product was in the salon either on the shelf or in drawers. Notice the credit card product of the month special (second exposure to the special). (Special thanks to Barbara Gauthier, Sherman Oaks, CA.) (Photo by Frank Jackson.)

Merchandise Versus Teaser Displays

The difference between merchandise and teaser displays is as great as the differences between the North and the South during the Civil War.

Merchandise display is stocking products in volume. These displays visually tell your client that you are in the product business. You have goods to sell, have committed dollars in inventory, and are open for business. (Figs. 4.2a, 4.2b)

Teasers are ministages for promotions or product features. They are enticing and are used to pique the client's interest and curiosity.

You will have both areas in the salon. You have your stationary merchandise display fixtures, cabinets that stay in the same place in the salon. The merchandise has a designated pattern of placement. The product map is rarely altered. Your teasers will have the flexibility and mobility to maneuver around the salon. These will be switched every few weeks to maintain excitement.

Display Hot Spots

Displays can be used effectively in many areas of the salon. Here is a list of places to promote your services and product.

Hair Stations

Take all personal paraphernalia off the station. You will need room to work and room for small displays. You can place a sign in the mirror stressing the promotion. Keep all station products organized. Have one or two featured products on your station. These are items that have never been used. If your station setup has room for a few shelves for retail product that is great. It is best to have your specialty products close at hand. Keep styling aid displays close to the station. When you instruct the client on proper home care you can simply reach over and pluck one from the shelf to place on your station in front of the client. Keep your used styling products out of direct view of the client. The used station products are yours. We want the client to visually possess the brand new bottle. (Fig. 4.3)

Chemical Area

If you have a designated chemical area, display essential home care products for maintaining chemically treated hair. Use shelving and posters to stress the importance of treating hair that has undergone a chemical process. Display daily

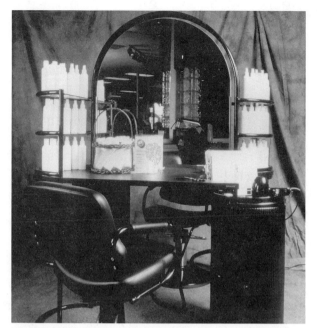

Fig. 4.3 Hair station—perfect combo, service and retail. This business-balanced workstation is ready for both hair services and retailing home care products. Place popular hair care products on each shelf on the left; separate each shelf by hair type: chemically treated, normal, and fine. Don't forget to add the product of the month. Here you will find a see-through small basket with ready-to-sell products. Next to the basket is a Lucite tester stand with a product information card and tester bottle. (Special thanks to the Belvedere Company for use of hair station equipment.) (Photo by Frank Jackson.)

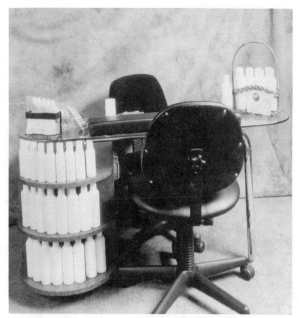

Fig. 4.4 Manicure station. This glass-topped manicure stand has plenty of work space plus merchandising areas. To the client's left are three shelves for stocking retail products. Use the space for the very popular hand and body lotions, body shampoos, body scrubs. To the client's right is the product of the month basket and tester bottle. I like to include a nail home care kit on the station. Grab this to show the client the best way to maintain gorgeous hands and nails. Easy way to retail home care kits. (Special thanks to the Belvedere Company for use of manicure station.) (Photo by Frank Jackson.)

conditioners, intensive conditioner, thermal styling products, color balancing shampoo—any product the client might need to keep the hair in ultimate condition.

Shampoo Area

Don't hide the back bar products. Make sure the client can see the brand of items you are using. This is the time to reinforce brand awareness. They will have seen the products up front; make sure the customer can see the same products in the shampoo area. I guess it goes without saying that you need to be using the same back bar items as you are trying to retail.

Place a sign in the area listing the shampoo and conditioners "we proudly use and recommend." I know of a few salons that put signs and posters on the ceiling so when clients are tipped back into the shampoo bowl they are faced with a sign hanging on the ceiling. If you try this, please make sure that it all looks polished and professional.

Manicure Stations

Keep your working products off to the side. Feature a product of the week. Have a tent card or small sign that stresses the product features and benefits. Select universal items the majority of nail clients would or could use. Paint nail tips with your techniques, mount them on a decorated board, and frame the collection. Put up posters of before and after nail makeovers. "You can have nails that look this great in one hour!" (Fig. 4.4)

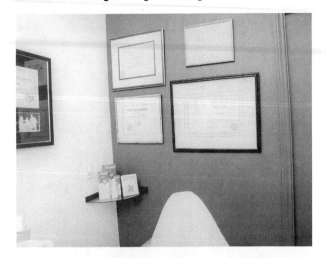

Fig. 4.5 Facial room, client's view. What do clients see when they are reclining back in the facial lounge chair? Here clients can see special educational certificates and crossover merchandise on the tiny corner display shelf. The salon has color coded each facial room by painting the end wall and added color-coded sheets and blankets. This sure helps take away that "medical" look. (Special thanks to Barbara Gauthier, Sherman Oaks, CA.) Photo by Frank Jackson.)

Facial Rooms

This is an area for peace and lack of clutter, but you have the chance for discreet displays in your treatment rooms. You can highlight skin care items or you might want to cross-merchandise products and put up items that are not skin related at all. A skin chart or graph works well as wall decoration and can lead the conversation to home care items. (Fig. 4.5)

Body Treatment Rooms

A cluster of Lucite shelves is a great place to start your displays in the body room. Carry out the salon theme or stress body care products. Body shots or photographs help to reinforce your home care message. If the room is used for multiple treatments, put up discreet posters highlighting four or five benefits from each treatment.

Reception Area

One key area is the place the client pays the bill. Leave room on the reception desk or cash out area for impulse displays.

These could be in a basket or displayed on a small mirror to get attention, even a plastic frame that can hold literature that announces the offer. Fashion color products, lips and nails, make great impulse items. Color sells so keep a display close at hand. (Figs. 4.6a, 4.6b)

This is a great area to use videos to help get your message across. Have a television monitor and recorder to play fashion, hair, skin care, even your own salon video commercial. Keep a video playing in the area with the sound off. Constant video audio can drive both you and your staff to distraction. Post a sign inviting your customer to turn up the sound to listen or provide earphones.

Bathroom

Yes, the bathroom. Some salons have a bigger bathroom than retail area. Frame product posters for the wall. Make sure you have sample products in the bathroom that you have for sale in the salon. If you sell hand and body lotion, you need to have one in the bathroom. Same is true for hand cleanser.

Designing Windows

There are three basic types of window displays.

- Closed background where the entire window is separated from the interior of the salon. There is a panel or wall blocking the view into the salon.

- Semiclosed background has a half partition that allows consumers to see into the salon and also a display set up in front of the partition.

- Open background gives consumers a full frontal view of the salon. They can see completely through the window into the interior.

Depending on your personal setup the window is a sales tool. Use your windows to create curb appeal. Windows need to have careful, professional displays for three reasons.

- Windows need to attract attention as cars drive by or consumers walk past the front door.

- Windows need to tell your salon story. They are clear billboards that show what you do, what products you carry, and why a potential consumer would want to walk into your salon.

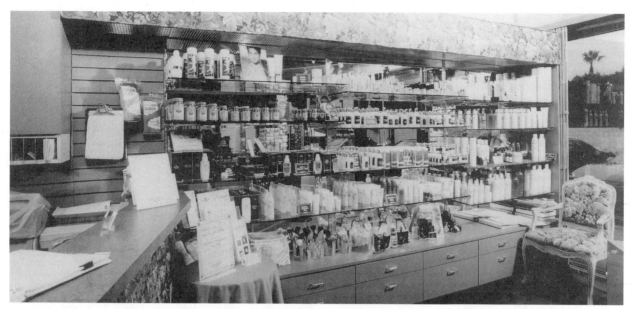

Fig. 4.6a Reception station—before. Even with limited space at a reception station you can still feature displays and promotions. (Photo by Frank Jackson.)

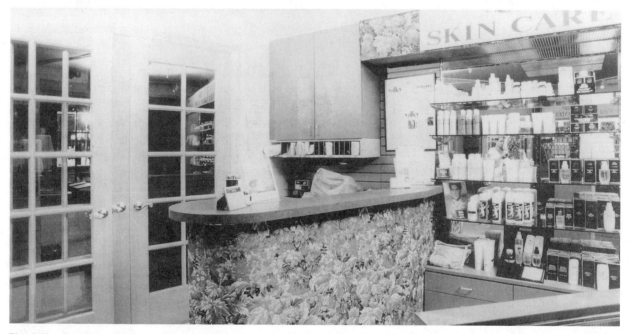

Fig. 4.6b Reception station—after. Notice the enlarged newspaper article behind the station to the client's right. This salon was listed in the "The Best of LA." So I took the article and had it blown up and dry mounted. It cost about $10 and every client cashing out will see this article. Keep appointment books out of sight. This appointment log was placed behind the counter and the product of the month was featured in a small display on the cash counter (third exposure of the special). (Special thanks to Barbara Gauthier, Sherman Oaks, CA.) (Photo by Frank Jackson.)

- Windows establish your salon image. Consumers will get an instant impression about your business based on what they see.

Go outside and stand on the curb or in the parking lot. What does your salon's window say to you? It should be clean, uncluttered, and match the flavor of the salon. Does the window make you want to walk in and find out what is going on in there? Or does it look like a typical salon with sun-faded posters and handmade "Help Wanted" signs gracing the glass?

The importance of window displays was illustrated for me one day when I was trying to locate a consulting client for a first appointment. I would have bet that it was a furniture store. The only items visible from the street were several chairs, a sofa, and a coffee table. No signage, no posters, and no product to tell me it was a salon. There was not a clue to tip me off that this location was a hair salon. I wonder how many other people overlooked this salon?

Display Theme Ideas

So now you have ideas for displaying hot spots. What do you display? Here is an idea list. There are different categories for displays. Use them or use the idea list as a launching pad for your own brilliant ideas.

Problem/Solution
Feature a common beauty problem that challenges your clients. Do you have a solution for dry fly-away hair? Bleeding lipstick? Nail polish chipping? Let your clients know! Tag the display with the beauty problem. Do you have a problem with. . . ? Here's the solution.

Seasonal
Capitalize on the seasonal changes and the need for product evaluation or updates. When the new seasonal clothes hit your local stores, start featuring "New Looks for Fall." Consumers will need different beauty products when the summer months are over and fall is blowing in. Fashion and beauty magazines traditionally detail the seasonal emphasis on eye, lip, hair, and color changes. Short quotes from these publications turned into professional signs might work well with appropriate product.

Vacation
Set up a vacation-directed display. Stock up and highlight travel sizes and products related to vacation hot spots—sun products for the ski-and-sea clients, swimmer's shampoo, eye masks and air-travel-specific products, high- or low-humidity products.

Change
Time for a change. How long has it been since you've had a new look? Watch and see if you service a high number of clients around their thirtieth or fortieth birthdays? How about class reunions? You bet! Place teasers throughout the salon highlighting these often traumatic life events. New jobs and a new career will require a new look and complementing products.

New and Improved
Three little words you see everywhere in the supermarket. Arrange a display and bring the client's attention to new products or products that have been improved. The word "new" is a hot button for many shoppers. Even tag the products on the shelf as "New," "Just Arrived," "Hot from the manufacturer."

Theme Related
Use holidays, special occasions, and community events as themes for promotions and displays—Mother's Day, Father's Day, graduation, a day at the beach, back to school. The possibilities are endless. Select a theme and carry it out throughout the salon. See chapter 21 for seventy different promotions. Tie in your external marketing with internal displays.

Sale
Everybody loves a bargain. Cluster a group of products together that are offered at a reduced price. They may be slow movers or a brand of products you were able to buy at reduced prices and want to pass the savings on to the consumer. Bargain baskets are a favorite for the budget conscious. Set up a Value Wall. Feature bulk items at a savings.

Line of Goods
A line of goods display is when you showcase one type of merchandise—all shampoo, all cleansers, all red nail enamel. You can mix brands, but not the product benefit.

Suggested Use

Cluster companion products. Display duos that are used together—shampoo and conditioner, nail enamel remover and color, day cream and night cream. Intensify the importance for use together. They may even be married together. Take a ribbon and tie the two married products together. Shrink-wrap beauty duos. Have a gift-with-purchase with an investment of two companion products—free brush with two styling aids, cleansing sponges with purchase of cleanser and toner.

Mass Mania

Warehouse type of display. Let's say your distributor has a supersale on firm-and-hold hair spray. You want to feature this product for the month. You buy like crazy and literally stock the merchandise in boxes in the salon. Think of the end aisles in your grocery store. They take one product and load up the end of the aisle to get your attention. You can use the same technique within the salon. Stack the actual cases as the foundation of your display. Decorate and open a few boxes for easy access.

Display Doctrine

Here are eleven rules to follow when creating sales driven displays.

1. 80/20 Rule. Eighty percent of the display should be product. Don't get carried away with tons of fillers and decorative doo-dads. They will take away from the featured product.
2. Make your display theme clear. When the clients look at the display they should be able to instantly decipher your retailing message. Place signs, cards, or brochures to support your message. Make your displays as easy to shop as possible.
3. Have a center point of the display. Select a visual hot spot to draw attention. This can be accomplished with color, shape of the product arrangement, or movement within the display. Look at adding a turntable or running lights, blinking lights, or strobe light to help attract attention. Do you remember the dancing soda cans and potted flowers? These crazy gimmicks literally stopped traffic in the store aisles. The movement and music definitely caught the attention of shoppers.
4. Product test-drive. Make sure you have a tester of the product featured for the client to open, smell, and try. Clearly mark the tester product. Place it out front and easily accessible.
5. Use color to create attention. Color is your primary way of attracting clients' attention. Use contrasting or harmonious colors to attract the clients toward the product. Primary colors work best, unless, of course, you are featuring bridal looks.
6. Fresh as a daisy. Keep displays looking fresh and brand new. Clean off used product, change items if color fades or consistency changes. Dusty product tells the client that this bottle or jar has been hanging around for a while.
7. Professional display signage. Use only the most professional lettering and have it checked for grammar and typos. Computer-generated type is usually easily obtained at the local print shop. Calligraphy is more expensive. Check the local art school for calligraphers. Resist using your own hand-lettered signs.
8. Display rotation. Change your displays frequently. Use your average client visit as your guide. If you see most of your clients every six weeks, your display may be changed every six weeks. The goal is to have these silent salespeople generating excitement.
9. Use display for staff training. Reinforce the message during staff meetings to continue talking up the featured items. Safeguard the staff from becoming bored if displays are left up too long.
10. Walk around the elephant. Walk around the display and make sure the theme can be seen from all sides the client can view it. Structure the display according to the client's panorama.
11. Face out. Position each product so that the front of the item is in full view for the client to see and read. Check periodically in case a product has been fiddled with and no longer faces out.

"Displayscapes"

Now you have display hot spots and display themes. You need to have a few ideas for arranging the bottles you selected. Here are five different "displayscapes." Think of it as landscaping a yard or summer garden. The placement of product adds to the beauty and profitability of the displays.

V-scape

Place your selected products in a V pattern. Think of a flock of geese flying south for the winter. There is a lead goose and all the others fly in formation. Put your first item in the front and line up two rows completing the V. The point of the V can be a tester bottle. (Fig. 4.7a)

W-scape

Arrange the cluster of products in a W shape. The tallest point of your display is the center point of the W. A variation on this theme is to turn the W-scape on its side and arrange the products to follow. This works great for a three-tiered etagere. (Fig. 4.7b)

M and M-scape

If your space is long enough create a product flow in the shape of two Ms. Center a tester product in the hollow of the M. (Fig. 4.7c)

Pyramid-scape

Take a volume of product and stack them up in the shape of a pyramid. Have your pyramid and a separate stock near it, because clients won't pull product from the pyramid for fear it will topple over. (Fig. 4.7d)

Magazine-scape

To magnify the product arrange items in a magazine format. Position the same item three across, then place two additional products in the same fashion. Look the next time you are at the airport magazine store. You'll see magazines displayed high on the wall and at least three across for impact. They are trying to get your attention to the cover of the magazine by repeating the visual statement. (Fig. 4.7e)

You are continuing to stage the retailing environment. Your design and flavor of the salon set the tone; the displays will add to the visual excitement. Now you are ready to evaluate your product lines and inventory mix. In the next chapter you will go shopping!

Display Scapes

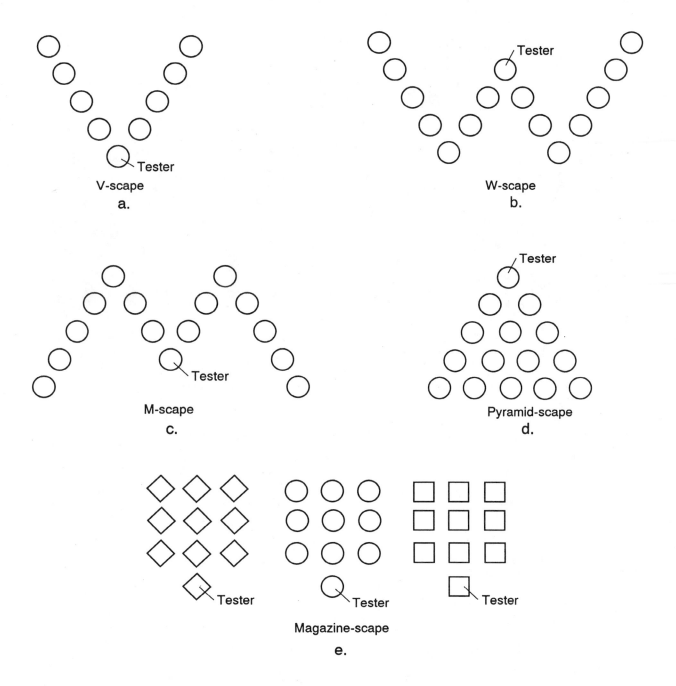

Fig. 4.7 Displayscapes—here are five "landscaping" designs for merchandising display.

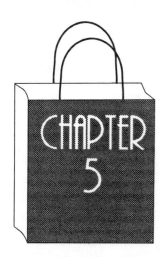

CHAPTER 5

SELECTING A PRODUCT LINE

I am frequently asked what product lines are best to carry in salons. I wish the answer could be a simple one, but it isn't. There are choices only you can make when selecting a product line, choices that will reflect you, your salon, and your clients. This chapter will help you make those decisions.

BRAND VERSUS PRIVATE LABEL

One of the very first topics often addressed by salon owners is the preference of selecting a brand-name line versus a private label line. Each product line has its place. Here are some options for you to consider if you are debating between the two product possibilities.

Brand Name Benefits

When I am talking of brand name I am referring to brand-name products sold to salons, not brand names available in drug and department stores. Selecting a brand-name line can offer your salon certain benefits.

Brand Name Identification

Many of the big hair companies spend millions each year on marketing. You and your clients can see their ads in magazines or on television. They sponsor sporting and environmental programs or health issues shows. The brand awareness is great. The exposure helps the name of the product penetrate the mind of the consumer. Those companies spending the big bucks on advertising are counting on the media exposure to strengthen the name and brand association of their products.

Marketing Support Material

The name brand companies usually offer ad slicks, posters, shelf talkers, mirror stickers, door decals, samples, consumer brochures, postcards, and videos. The companies provide you with marketing support materials to make the sale of the product easier.

Training and Education

This may be the biggest advantage in stocking a brand name. The big hair companies have several layers of training and educational support from top-name platform artists, to in-salon technical support staff. Look for a company that has an educational commitment not only to the artistic side but to the business side of the beauty business as well. Are they out there just offering classes in product knowledge or are they offering your training in business-building skills? It takes more than product knowledge to sell a product.

Image Association

When manufacturing companies are investing millions into an advertising campaign they are creating and strengthening the image of the product. When you decide to stock the line you are extending the image of the product manufacturing company to your salon. If the line is oriented to a young "happening" clientele then by adding it to your shelf you are saying to the consumer that your salon is young and happening too. The image of the product helps to support your overall salon image and identity.

The Down Side to Brand Names

Product Saturation

If you are considering a line, look and see how many of your immediate competitors also stock it. Yes, there can be strength in numbers and if tons of salons in your area carry the same line then it must be good, right? Well, the down side is if clients can buy the product in every salon on your block, why should they buy it from you? Well known is okay, but over-saturation is a sales killer. Look for a product with more exclusivity.

Markup

Brand-name products have several layers of pricing from the manufacturer, to the distributor, to the salesperson's commission, to your cost, to the end buyer's cost. I want you to be able to make some nice money. In order for you to do that, you will need to buy right and price your products right. Brand names may make that goal harder to achieve than private label markups.

Private Label Benefits

When you select a private label company you are buying products formulated, packaged and ready to be "branded."

Price

You will have greater flexibility in pricing a private label product. There are items you can buy for $1.25 and sell for $10, especially makeup. Private labeling eliminates the distributor. You can buy straight from the company—low cost to you. You make money because you have more room for profit.

Own Formulations

Depending on budget and commitment you can actually develop your own product line. You can formulate, package, and sell your own salon brand of products. Private labeling gives you the option of marketing your own product philosophy. You can create the story behind the bottles and jars. The salon becomes the star rather than it selling a brand-name star.

Many clothing stores do the very same thing. They stock brand name designers, and they have created a house line as

well. They have mixed the best of both worlds. You can do the same thing in your business.

The Down Side to Private Labeling

Marketing Support

When you select a private label line you will be responsible for marketing the product. That means you will need to produce your own sales literature—posters, prescription pads, point of purchase material. If you are capable of designing and producing the materials or have access to marketing help then private label may be one way to go. You will need to have a budget for promoting and marketing the line. If you don't have the budget, then stick with the brand name support. When you buy private label you open the box and you get the product with no sales support material.

Lack of Image or Story

A private label line can be a good product, but you will need to tell the consumer the product's story. The client will need to know the history of the product line. Did you design it? Did you work with leading chemists to formulate the product? Is it exclusive to your salon?

PRICE POINTS

A price point is the cost level of the product. There are three basic levels of pricing—low, middle, and high. The product you select will generally fall into one of the three categories.

If you have been car shopping recently you will obviously have seen price points in action. You probably saw the basic stripped-down auto version, the middle of the road car, and the luxurious model. Should you stock the equivalent of a Geo, Honda, or Jaguar? Product lines have as much diversity in price as each of these automakers.

Keep in mind which level(s) you need to satisfy your customer base. You should focus the majority of your product price points to fit the income and age demographics established in your chapter 2 survey. But don't forget to check their psychographic patterns. If your ten best customers profile shows a Jaguar-income woman who shops the discount drug store for makeup, it is wise to provide her with a convenient

Retail	Low	Middle	High
Hair			
Shampoo	$1–5	6–8	9+
Conditioner	$1–6	7–11	12+
Skin			
Cleanser	$1–8	9–18	19+
Moisturizer	$1–10	11–21	22+
Makeup			
Lipstick	$1–5	6–12	13+
Foundation	$1–8	9–14	15+
Nails			
Polish	$1–4	5–8	9+

Fig. 5.1   Product price points.

alternative in a low-end price. However, if price is not a problem for your Jaguar customer, high-end pricing will be the way to go.

In Figure 5.1 are some examples of average low, middle, and high price points for seven product classifications.

MULTIPLE LINES

In the beginning heyday of salon retailing, the concept was to stock one and only one brand of products. The salon was convinced that one line would be enough to carry for sales. Then in the mideighties the superstores hit. Giant supermarkets and stores covering tens of thousands of square feet of selling space opened their doors. They were selling everything under the sun and some were even slashing prices to rock bottom. They were giving consumers more bang for their hard-earned dollar. After the superstores emerged we started seeing a switch from single-line salons to salons that stocked many lines. What do you do now? How many lines of products do you really need?

There are four key elements to consider when adding retail lines.

Your USP

What is the Unique Selling Position of the salon? Is your salon designed to be small and exclusive? Do you offer specialized services or are you a one-stop shop? Do you want to offer every beauty product under the sun?

I'm seeing a split in stocking procedures. The two extremes are one-line salons and the full retail center. Is one better than another? It depends on the uniqueness of your salon. What type of business do you want? What is your commitment? And how much space do you have for retailing?

You will need to stock multiple lines if your goal is to be a one-stop shop for consumers, a place where they can purchase any conceivable beauty product. But make sure that if you stock it, you can turn the product over to make money.

On the flip side, let's say you have decided to align yourself with a product company. One full product line will give you the sales possibilities. You can get additional benefits from a one-line exclusive position.

Foot Traffic

How many clients walk through the front door of the salon a week? Your traffic count will help determine the number of product lines necessary. If you have more than two hundred clients in the salon in a week, you can have more than one full line. If you service less than two hundred per week, one well-rounded product line is sufficient.

Client Profile

Your client profile will determine product needs. Look at your client base. What percentage of your clients are under twenty? Under thirty? Under fifty? What percentage are men? Let's say that half your client base are mature, fifty-plus working women and half are teenagers. You will probably need two lines to satisfy the styling needs of these two diverse groups. If the majority of your clientele has chemically-relaxed hair, then you will definitely need an ethnically focused product line. Match your product line selection to your clients' needs.

Retail Space

The amount of actual retail space will determine the quantity of lines carried. You only have so much merchandising space, only so much shelf space. Every line, every product eats away at the space availability. If you only have twenty linear feet of shelf space, you cannot possibly stock two lines.

PRETTY PACKAGING

The ingredients and the product's benefits are important. But quite often the product will need to sell itself. Effective packaging packs the sale with punch. Pore over these five areas that relate to product packaging when you go to review a product line.

Get a Grip

Take a bottle and put it in the palm of your hand. How does it feel? Is it easy to grip? Is it too big and bulky for mature hands to use? The product will give you a "feel" while you're holding it. Is the bottle comfortable or awkward?

Size It Up

Look at the available sizes. Is it an appropriately sized container for the product? An eye cream in a 4-ounce jar is much too big. The client would never get through a jar before the product turned rancid. How many options does the line have? Are shampoos in 6, 8, 16, and 32 ounces? If so, do you need all the sizes available?

Able Application

Is the product easy to use? What type of lid is on the container? Is it appropriate for the product? Check and see the type of lid or closure the bottle has. Can you get the lid off the jar easily? Can you get the product out of the jar without hurting your wrist?

Easy to Read

The typeface of the product label needs to be easy to read. The layout of the name, directions, and ingredients need to be positioned for ease of reading, especially if clients are to use this product without their glasses or contacts. Stand back and scan a row of bottles. Can you read the labels? Can you decipher the differences between the items?

Eye Appeal

The product line needs to sparkle. When you look at a collection of the products are you visually attracted to the display? When you see the bottles and jars do you want to pick one up and check it out? How does the color of the packaging blend or detract from the salon? Does it visually jump off the shelf or does it die and blend into all the other products? This is especially important when working with private label products. Do they look like bare-bones generic or something special?

INGREDIENT FACT OR FICTION, HYPE OR HOPE

When you are selecting a product line you will be faced with evaluating product ingredients. Besides pricing and packaging, you will need to address the ingredients that make up the beautifying formulation. Two products may contain the very same ingredients, but the resulting product can be vastly different. Companies list in descending order the base ingredients that make up the product, but you have little way of knowing the percentage of ingredients used. This is one key area when you are forced to trust a manufacturers statement.

Ingredient Myths

There is an arsenal of information to plow through when selecting a product line. Please be aware of the many myths that have been born into the beauty business.

Natural or Organic

Especially with the green movement, natural and organic have resurfaced on the cosmetic scene. These two product styles can be misleading. A truly natural product would be unacceptable for retail. A truly natural item is made of ingredients in their natural state. This is impossible because you would have products molding and decomposing on the shelf.

Organic is frequently substituted for natural. This label still perpetuates the myth. Consumers and some professionals perceive an organic product to be better or safer than a synthetic one. In reality organic means the item is made from animal or vegetable products.

You can stock a natural and organic line, just make sure your product positioning and presentations are accurate and the product has consumer benefits.

Test Case

You have seen advertising claims stating that a product has been dermatologist tested, allergy tested, clinically tested, doctor tested. Investigate the nature of the test. Some companies label the products as tested, but you should find out what type of testing was done to support the claim.

Fragrance Free

Consumers have been lead down a primrose-scented path by the term *fragrance free*. This term simply means the product does not contain a synthetic fragrance that must be labeled "fragrance" on the container. Consumers may feel that being fragrance free will reduce the chances of irritation and sensitivity. Yet formulations may include essential oils or essences to enhance the smell of a product and still be sensitizing to the skin.

Hypoallergenic

This myth seems to be the best of them all. Back in the infancy stage of the beauty business, nonallergenic was used to distinguish milder, safer additives from harmful ones. Today hypo-actually means "less". So the term *hypoallergenic* really means "less likely to cause allergic reactions than products not labeled as such."

Wonder Formulas

Product ingredients go through phases. As hemlines go up and down and up again, ingredients fall in and out of vogue. If a new product is introduced and it fits your salon's product philosophy, by all means capitalize on the latest and greatest product development. Keep in mind that the fad product will run its course and at that time take it off the shelf.

Over the years, the major manufacturers of beauty preparations have developed a logical theme behind each product line or division. There are startup companies opening every day. I love to see the free enterprise system at work, but be cautious if you jump on their bandwagon immediately. Trust your gut and professional expertise when you are about to be seduced to buy a new miracle wonder product. If it is too good to be true, it probably is.

New Consumer Demands

The amount of information people are exposed to has never been greater. Consumers are better informed and better educated today than in any other period of time in the history of our country. This presents a buying challenge for salons. Not only will the product have to perform as promised, it may also have to go through environmental scrutiny. Your products may need to be ecofriendly.

Ecofriendly Products

When you are selecting a product line the product needs to match the salon's USP and product philosophy. Be careful if you are touting a "green" approach to your salon. You will need to make sure the products on the shelf and in the back match your verbal commitment to being ecofriendly. Here are a few areas to consider if this is your salon's approach.

Animal Testing

Check with the product supplier and manufacturer to determine whether any of the products under consideration have been tested on animals.

Human Safety Testing

Here's the catch to the no-animal testing. If the product was not tested on animals for safety, how was the product tested? If you are considering putting your reputation on the line for a product, it should have some backup of its safety record. Find out how or if the product line has been tested.

Animal By-products

Scrutinize the ingredients for animal-derived by-products. Check out the root source of the ingredients. There should be visible signs of plants and herbs listed on the ingredient label.

Petrochemicals

Investigate whether the product has mineral oil or any of its derivatives. If so, the product has petrochemicals in the formulation. If you want to shy away from these, be on the lookout for oil-laden formulations.

Packaging Properties

See if the plastics and glass used can be recycled. If one of your company goals is to reduce, reuse, and recycle, look for limited fluff packaging and recycling possibilities.

INVOLVING THE STAFF

If you have a staff, you will want to get their input on past product experiences with customers. You can also involve them in informal product testing. Getting the staff's interest and involvement is critical to your retailing success. Here's how to set up a testing program.

1. Test two lines of products.
2. Put samples of products into blank bottles. Mark the bottle with a number versus brand name, ie., shampoo for chemically treated hair—Number 1—Company A, dry skin mask—Number 3—Company C. When you compare two lines, this will help neutralize marketing and visual influences. You will test the product on results and quality before you test on marketability.
3. Assign each staff member one to three products to test from the line under consideration.
4. Half-head test. Instruct the staff to use the product on one-half of the head, face, or body. They can use their regular product on the other half. This gives them the perfect opportunity to comparison test the two, literally side by side.
5. Depending on the product, I would have them test for at least twenty-one days, during which time the staff members will record their impressions of the product. See Figure 5.2 for a form to use.

A word of caution about staff involvement. Quite often I've seen a new staff member go on board and declare, "I just love product XYZ and can't work without it." So the owner orders up the requested product or product line. The problem with this is that it diffuses display power and shrinks purchasing power. Hit-and-miss stocking confuses the client.

Once the testing has been completed, review the results. You will obviously be looking for products that work. If they fail at this level, you sure don't want them on the shelf. If the feed-

back has been good then you are ready to test for packaging, eye appeal, and price points.

GET YOUR CLIENTS IN ON THE ACT

Organize focus groups and client interviews and surveys to help you decide whether the product line is worth the investment. What better place to hear if the product is sellable than straight from the horse's (shopper's) mouth?

Focus Groups

Use professional help here for accurate results. There are marketing groups that will facilitate focus group sessions. If you have a large salon and high volume of gross sales, this may be a great outlet for information. The focus group may involve several of your good clients in a blind test.

Client Interviews

These can be as simple as calling a few of your best clients and asking for their input. People are more than willing to give you advice and their opinion. You will find a wealth of information sitting in your chair.

Surveys

Prepare a quick, multiple choice survey for your clients to fill out. Before they go back for their appointment have the salon receptionist ask the client to fill out the survey. "We are trying to improve our business and value your opinion. Please take a couple of minutes and fill this out for us. We would greatly appreciate your input." Hand out the surveys for three weeks to a month. Your customer base is the best source of information. They are already spending money in the salon. They already believe in you. Start here and see what you will discover.

A FORM FOR PRODUCT LINE SELECTION

In Figure 5.3 are twenty areas that need to be addressed before you take out your checkbook and designate shelf space.

PRODUCT QUALITY TEST

Product_____ Product Number_____

Company_____ Date_____

Staff Name_____

Rate the product 1 through 5. Five being the highest score.

Feel of the product	1	2	3	4	5
Smell	1	2	3	4	5
Results	1	2	3	4	5
Color	1	2	3	4	5
Texture	1	2	3	4	5
Easy to use	1	2	3	4	5
Easy to sell	1	2	3	4	5

Put in product-specific questions. (lather, cleanses, curls, holds, sets, etc.)

What beauty problem would this product solve?

Is there something we already stock that you like better?

What do you like most about the product?

What do you dislike about the product?

Would you buy this product for yourself?   Yes   No

Is this product needed in the salon?   Yes   No

Fig. 5.2   Salon product quality test.

First, star any feature that you think the line should have. There will be areas in which you are not willing to compromise. Keep those no-budge areas uppermost in your mind when selecting a line. Don't get swayed by emotion. Inventory is a commitment of time, money, and sales effort. Two of the three cannot be replaced. Use this shopping guide to help you through the decision-making process.

Don't get overwhelmed by the possibilities of products to stock in the salon. Evaluate and test. Shop around. These are silent salespeople that will be converted from inventory to cash.

Product Line Under Consideration

1. Key Consideration. Does the product line match the salon's unique selling position?

2. What market does this line target? (baby, child, teen, young adult, baby boomers, seniors, working women, men)

3. Whom do I want to purchase this product line?

4. What makes this product line different?

5. What is the story behind this product line?

6. How saturated is the product line in my area?

7. How complete or extensive is this product line?
   - Do they offer a chemical line?
   - Color line?
   - Back bar sizes?
   - Retail products?
   - Are all these areas necessary?

8. What services will this product line support?

9. What is the quality of the product?
   - Does the product philosophy match the salon's?
   - Does it live up to the claims?
   - Does it pass the staff evaluation?
   - Is there something in my current inventory that works better?
   - Is this a fad product?

10. What is the price point?
    - Low end
    - Middle
    - High end

11. How does the packaging fit the salon image?

12. What marketing support is available?
    - Is there co-op advertising?
    - Camera-ready ad slicks?
    - Samples of product?
    - Does the company provide consumer brochures?
    - If so, is there a cost to the salon?
    - Are display materials available?
    - Is there a point-of-purchase display?
    - Is there a floor-standing display?

13. What is the educational policy of the product company?
    - Do they offer in-salon training?
    - Do they offer training through the distributor?
    - If so, how often?
    - Do they offer educational videos?
    - Do they offer regional seminars?
    - Do they offer educational classes at major beauty shows?

14. Is there a product sampling kit to test the merchandise? If so, does the salon have to pay for it?

15. How often does the company release new products?

16. What is the availability of the product?
    - Do I get the product directly from the distributor?
    - Do I get the product directly from an independent sales representative?
    - Do I get the product directly from the importer?
    - What is the average delivery time from date of order?

17. What are the return policies?
    - Of the product line manufacturer?
    - Of the product line distributor?
    - Does the line have a product guarantee?

18. What is the minimum for ordering?
    - quantity?
    - dollar amount?
    - handling fee?
    - shipping fee?

19. Are there any special incentives for investing in the product line now?

20. Do I want to be a part of this product manufacturing company's family?

Fig. 5.3   Product line evaluation form.

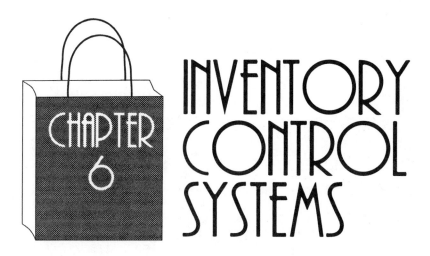

CHAPTER 6

INVENTORY CONTROL SYSTEMS

Plain and simple—inventory is money and product sales make money. The more product you sell the greater the profit. Inventory is not an expenditure, it is an investment. When you put money in your savings account you expect to earn interest. The longer you leave your money in the bank, the bigger the payoff. Well, inventory is exactly the opposite. The faster it moves off the shelf, the more money you make. The trick is to stock right, buy right, and price right. Monitoring your inventory can add up to 50 percent to your salon's revenue with the right sales system.

In this chapter we will go over what you need to stock, how much to stock, what to do once you get the bottles and jars in the salon, and how to price product for profit.

WHAT PRODUCTS TO STOCK

What you stock in the salon is determined by the services you offer. Are you a full service salon or do you just do nails? The service mix also governs your product mix. Here are some product categories to consider for your inventory mix.

- Cut and Style Salon: shampoo, conditioner, styling products, finishing tools, an assortment of brushes and combs.
- Cut, Color, Perm Salon: shampoo, color-enhancing shampoo, swimmer's shampoo, leave-in conditioner, intensive conditioner, styling products, mousse, gel, gloss, finishing tools, an assortment of brushes and combs, hair accessories, blowers, curling irons, hot brushes, diffusers.
- Skin Care Salon: collections for skin types (oily, dry, normal, acne), cleanser, toner, day cream, night cream, masks, exfoliants, hand and body lotions, body shampoo, eye makeup remover, eye cream, ampoules and serums, cleansing sponges, sun products.
- Make-up Center: foundation, loose powder, compact powder, concealers, eye shadow, eye pencils, mascara, lipstick, lip pencils, blush, nail polish, top coat, base coat, remover, makeup brushes.
- Nail Salon: Nail enamel, top coat, base coat, quick set, foot files, buffers, emery boards, nail polish remover, cuticle cream, hand and body lotions, body shampoo, body scrub, loofahs.

Also see Figure 6.1 for the results of a customer survey. These figures may help you determine what product categories you want to carry.

HOW MUCH TO STOCK

How much product you put on the shelf depends largely on how much space you have set aside for retailing. You can start with a small collection of products and keep adding as you successfully turn the merchandise. But you must make sure

**Customer survey of products purchased
in the last six months.**

Hand and body lotion	82%
Hair spray	75%
Perfume, cologne	69%
Eyeshadow	59%
Styling mousse	57%
Blusher	56%
Face foundation	54%
Scrubs and cleansers	44%
Makeup remover	26%
Sensitive skin products	22%
Haircoloring	18%
Home perms	16%
Facial masks	15%
Coloring for gray	14%
Antiaging products	12%

Fig. 6.1 Customer survey of products purchased in the last six months.

that even that small collection is large enough for the customer to trust that you are really serious about selling product. The absolute minimum is at least six pieces per product on the shelf. Twelve will work much better for creating a visual impact and consumer excitement.

As your retail business blossoms, you will be able to invest in more products and buy in larger volume. There is a lot to be said for volume. The more you have to sell, the bigger the return on your investment. And you will be given better prices and can take advantage of manufacturer's offers.

PRICING FOR PROFIT

There are two basic ways to figure the price of a product. You can set the price according to a percentage of markup on the cost of goods, or you can price the product as a percentage of retail.

If pricing for cost, you add X a set amount to the price of the item. Let's say the item costs you $1, and you can sell the product for $2. You are doubling your money.

If pricing for retail, you establish an acceptable percentage that will include both your retail business overhead and profit. Each product is marked up the designated percentage.

Let's say the target percentage is 40 percent. You buy an item for $1 and then add the 40 percent to charge $1.40. When you use this method you will have to be very careful when you put products on sale or special. If you put the item on sale for 50 percent off, you will then be selling the item for less than you paid for it, and that is not good.

Cost of Product	40%	50%	60%	100%	200%
1.00	**1.40**	**1.50**	**1.60**	**2.00**	**3.00**
1.25	1.75	1.88	2.00	2.50	3.75
1.50	2.10	2.25	2.40	3.00	4.50
1.75	2.45	2.63	2.80	3.50	5.25
2.00	**2.80**	**3.00**	**3.20**	**4.00**	**6.00**
2.25	3.15	3.38	3.60	4.50	6.75
2.50	3.50	3.88	4.00	5.00	7.50
2.75	3.85	4.13	4.40	5.50	8.25
3.00	**4.20**	**4.50**	**4.80**	**6.00**	**9.00**
3.25	4.55	4.88	5.20	6.50	9.75
3.50	4.65	5.25	5.60	7.00	10.50
3.75	5.25	5.63	6.00	7.50	11.25
4.00	**5.60**	**6.00**	**6.40**	**8.00**	**12.00**
4.25	5.95	6.38	6.80	8.50	12.75
4.50	6.30	6.75	7.20	9.00	13.50
4.75	6.65	7.13	7.60	9.50	14.25
5.00	**7.00**	**7.50**	**8.00**	**10.00**	**15.00**
5.25	7.35	7.88	8.40	10.50	15.75
5.50	7.70	8.25	8.80	11.00	16.50
5.75	8.05	8.63	9.20	11.50	17.25
6.00	**8.40**	**9.00**	**9.60**	**12.00**	**18.00**
6.25	8.75	9.88	10.00	12.50	18.75
6.50	9.10	9.75	10.40	13.00	19.50
6.75	9.45	10.13	10.80	13.50	20.25
7.00	**9.80**	**10.50**	**11.20**	**14.00**	**21.00**
7.25	10.15	10.88	11.60	14.50	21.75
7.50	10.50	11.25	12.00	15.00	22.50
7.75	10.85	11.63	12.40	15.50	23.25
8.00	**11.20**	**12.00**	**12.80**	**16.00**	**24.00**
8.25	11.55	12.88	13.20	16.50	24.75
8.50	11.90	12.75	13.60	17.00	25.50
8.75	12.25	13.13	14.00	17.50	26.25
9.00	**12.60**	**13.50**	**14.40**	**18.00**	**27.00**
9.25	12.95	13.88	14.80	18.50	27.75
9.50	13.30	14.25	15.20	19.00	28.50
9.75	13.65	14.63	15.60	19.50	29.25
10.00	**14.00**	**15.00**	**16.00**	**20.00**	**30.00**

Fig. 6.2   Price chart.

So when you are talking with a manufacturer's salesperson and he or she says you can make 50 percent on an item, make sure you ask if that is the markup on cost or on retail. The Price Chart in Figure 6.2 illustrates some markup percentages.

Psychology of Pricing

A jewelry store owner who was leaving for lunch one day told a sales associate to mark the jewelry in the front window 50 percent because the items weren't moving. The associate heard the instructions and altered the prices. By the time the owner came back from lunch, the window was sold out. She had been sitting on the merchandise for months and it just wouldn't move. She told the salesperson she was delighted the markdown items sold so fast. But the salesperson was astonished because she had raised the prices by 50 percent. The moral of the story is that pricing is a combination of science and psychology. In this case, the merchandise price was too low for the goods. The higher price made the jewelry more appealing to passing traffic.

Odd Pricing
One theory is to price items with odd dollars and cents—$5.93, $4.21, $22.75. The consumer perceives the product to be a real value because the odd pricing looks as if the merchant is figuring the product to the penny; $5.93 just sounds like a better value than $6.00. Odd pricing works better for your low- to middle-end products. Save your high dollar items for the next suggestion.

Even Up
In this pricing philosophy, you round the product to even dollars. Exclusive stores consistently round the merchandise up to even dollars—$10, $50, $120. Use this pricing option for your upscale product line in the salon. Use $5 denominations as your pricing guide—$5, $15, $25, and so on.

Cluster Pricing
With cluster pricing, items that are used together are the same price. This is one of my favorites if you are buying right. All lip items $6—lipstick, lip pencil, lip brush, each one is the same price. Same for eye products—$7.50 for eye shadows, mas-cara, liners. Base, powder compact, and concealer are one price.

Cluster pricing works well when you are closing with a format-style close. "Are you familiar with our pricing? No? Well the eye products are $7.50, the lip items are $6.00, and the basics like foundation are $12.50." This technique sounds much smoother than, "the eye shadow is $7.25 for the mattes, $6.75 for the frosted, pencils are $5.95, lipstick is $6.00, base is $15.25." The client (and the salesperson sometimes) can become overwhelmed with a barrage of numbers.

Discount Pricing
If you are a discount price salon this technique will work well for you. Here, you feature two prices on the bottle—theirs and yours. The competition sells theirs for $6.95, and you are selling the same thing for $6.25. You will make less money per bottle, but you can make up for it in volume by moving twice the amount of product at the discounted price.

Price Line
This is an easy technique for a three-tiered pricing structure. All of your inventory can be positioned into one of three price points—low, middle or high. All high-end shampoos are one price, no difference between brands as long as they are in the same price family.

Think of three different auto companies. Is there a price difference between a Honda, Ford, and Mercedes? You bet. The auto companies have price positioning down to a science.

Suggested Retail Price
This is the price the manufacturer suggests you use. This is only a suggestion, and you don't have to match it to the penny. If your salon is committed to customer service and offers home care lessons, product guarantees, client record-keeping systems, and follow-up courtesy calls, you have a right to charge more for the product to cover the overhead.

If you are a budget salon and you offer no-frills shopping, you may decide to price the product slightly under the suggested retail. If the only thing clients are getting when they buy the product from you is the product, then a good deal on the product is a must. Depending on the perceived value of the product and salon image you can get away with altering the suggested retail price. Clients are not going to drive across town to save 30 cents on a bottle of beauty goo.

STOCK MANAGEMENT

Your profit potential can be sabotaged by having too much stock on the shelf—or too little. If you have tons of bottles sitting on the shelf and the only thing they are doing is collecting dust, you are losing money. On the flip side, if you are out of stock on merchandise or don't carry goods your clients want to buy you can kiss those profits good-bye. The art comes when you balance the two.

Starting Point

Where is your retail business to date? Are you just starting or do you have some track record for your sales? The first thing we need to look at is what you have in stock right now.

SKUs

This is an abbreviation for Stock Keeping Units. Each item you carry in the salon is an SKU. If you carry one line with fifteen products you have fifteen SKUs. If the same line comes in two sizes and you stock both sizes, you now have thirty SKUs. Make a list of all the items you carry in the salon.

Stock Turns

A stock turn will tell us how the product is moving. If you buy three cases of Product XYZ and it lasts three days, you may not be buying enough product. On the other hand, if those same three cases last you six months, you are not getting your money's worth. The rule of thumb is to turn the inventory at least six to eight times a year.

On-Hand Minimums

These are your bare-bones, never-be-less-than minimums. This is the quantity of product you need in the salon for a given period of time. I prefer at least a three- to four-week supply. This can be shortened, depending on how fast you can get

products. As your guideline, figure out how long it takes to get products into the salon from the time you order to the time they are on the shelf. If you are dealing with a local supplier and you can get your order the next day, your on-hand minimums decrease. If you are looking at a couple of weeks from phone to delivery, your on-hand requirements increase.

Stock Rotation

When you are opening cases and stocking shelves, make sure the new merchandise is placed behind the current product on the shelf. Otherwise the product at the back of the shelf is old. Always rotate the product forward.

Never-Out List

Ever go to reach for a product and there is none on the shelf? Never-out lists will flag ordering levels. When you get down to a minimum amount, it is time to order. This is true in the dispensary as well as the retail stock. Post an order list in the dispensary and at the front desk. If you are on a computer system set your minimums so you will never be out due to lack of ordering.

Purchase List

Keep a running purchase order list. If anyone on staff pulls a product from the shelf or stock and the quantity is at the on-hand minimum stage, that product gets added to the purchase order. This is handy when you go to place your order. You are not relying solely on gray matter.

Stockroom Arrangement

Establish a permanent home for products that get placed in the stockroom. Set a pattern for product placement. Design a placement map for stock. Avoid the frustration of hunting for a product.

Counting House

Once you have established a routine for product inventory, you can go through three different styles of inventory.

1. Book inventory. Here, you reduce the product sales from existing inventory records.
2. Spot check. Select ten to fifteen items a month at random to spot check and actually do a physical inventory of those items. These numbers should match your book inventory.
3. The most extensive inventory practice is to administer a full physical count. Every product, every SKU, is counted. Check with your accountant for frequency, but if you are running a tight ship, you should be able to get away with one complete physical inventory every year.

If you have a computer inventory system, see if the system can read bar codes.

TO TAG OR NOT TO TAG? THAT IS THE QUESTION

There are several ways of handling the individual pricing of each item. The old saying, "If you have to ask the price, you can't afford it" has fallen by the wayside. Nobody wants to be surprised when checking out. Here are a few guidelines to inform the shopper of the investment price of the products.

Do you need to put price stickers on every bottle? Not necessarily. This will depend on how many products you stock and how fast you turn over the inventory. If you are just spreading your wings in retailing you probably will not need to price code each product.

Two techniques for informing shoppers are shelf clips or a price menu. A plastic clip can be attached to the lip of the shelf to hold the price card. Each product will have its own designated price clip. If you choose to post a price menu, I wouldn't make it billboard size, but a neat, typeset sign of all products displayed within the merchandising area.

If you have a high-traffic salon and many people ringing up sales, it will be necessary to code the products. The one rule I have here is do not use those little stick-on labels that have been written on with a ballpoint pen. If you have to price the product, do so with style and business savvy. Use pre-printed stickers or computer-generated price tags. You can purchase a pricing gun for a minimal investment. You can have sticky-tags printed and set the pricing gun per item.

NINE KNOCKOUT INVENTORY TIPS

Boss Buys Favorites

It is easy to get caught up in the fun and thrill of shopping for new products, especially makeup items. I can almost always tell the personal coloring of the inexperienced salon owner/buyer by the color mix in the product selection. It will be skewed toward warm or cool colors depending on the buyer's personal color palette. It is necessary to put personal preference aside when you are buying for the salon. The mix needs to match the salon's clients.

Blue Label Buying Patterns

When I worked for one product manufacturing company, I was astounded at the percentage of clients who ordered product to be sent overnight. They would place an average $198 order two to three times a month and then have it shipped overnight. The buying procedure was costing them. If they had planned their purchasing, they would have received free shipping on a $400 order.

Order Day

Once you have worked with your inventory to see patterns and needs developing you will then be able to establish an order day.

Once upon a time, my salon was ordering from more than thirty different suppliers. Some of the suppliers came into the salon, others offered telemarketing sales. After a while, I realized I was wasting time returning phone calls and sitting in appointments that didn't benefit the business. With some careful budgeting, I started ordering all products and supplies on the sixth day of the month. This gave accounting time to close out the month and prepare inventory orders. The office manager called in all orders on that day. This efficiency technique actually saved time and money by fine-tuning our ordering cycles.

Salesperson Appointments

If you are lucky enough to have a dynamite salesperson who offers you business advice and growth information by all means schedule appointment time for him or her. In my travels I have had the pleasure of meeting some wonderful sales consultants who offered business suggestions and moneymaking information to salon owners. These sales consultants are a gold mine of information, tap into their wealth of knowledge. If, on the other hand, salespeople just stop by to shoot the breeze and want to dig up dirt on your business, don't even waste your time. Don't give them your business.

Buying Incentives

Check with your suppliers to see if they offer buying incentives for volume orders. If you are making a financial commitment to increasing your retail business, see how they will help you in your endeavor. Be prepared to share you goals and commitment to retailing with your suppliers. They will need a little more reassurance than high hopes and promises. Tell them the budget and marketing efforts you will be expending over the next quarter. Ask them what they would be willing to do to help you achieve your goals.

- Talk to your suppliers and work out buying incentives, say special price breaks on multiple case lots.

- See if they will offer special educational classes for staff.

- See if there is a percentage volume discount on monthly specials. If it is substantial enough, you may want to stockpile a three-month supply of a fast-moving item.

- See what the supplier will do for a standing purchase order discount. Once you get your volume moving and have tracked the progress, look into a standing purchase order where you will guarantee to your supplier that you will purchase X amount of merchandise per month. What kind of discount will they offer if you are committed to buying $1,000 of retail product per month? A key account for one supply company I work with is $500 a month. You don't have to be Rockefeller to negotiate good deals.

Mammoth Sizing

Keep the inventory on the retail shelves to under sixteen ounces. You can stock a few of the liters and half gallons, but don't put them out for clients to see. There are two reasons for

downsizing the retail products. First, you will not make as much money with the jumbo bottles. Figure out how much clients would spend if they bought the equivalent in small sizes. What is the difference in price? The second reason, and perhaps more important, is styling options. Let's say you do Ms. Customer's hair today and she buys the jumbo bottle of shampoo and styling aid. Next month when she comes in, she decides she wants her hair colored and permed for the first time. The new look is great, but she needs new product to support the new look. But you sold her the lifetime supply last month. Now you're stuck. Increase your profits and styling options with smaller retail bottles and jars. By all means, you want to offer value-added product sizing, but I wouldn't focus on the jumbo sizes to build the ideal retail business.

Product Line Manager

Appoint a key person plus an assistant to be responsible for inventory. They are responsible for ordering, checking in orders, shipping documents, stocking, tagging, plus any function that you can delegate toward inventory control. This way you have two people keeping an eye on the shelves and merchandise.

Seasonal Ins and Outs

Once you have mastered your monthly inventory turn, look into adding hot seasonal items that go on the shelf for a limited time period. This holds especially true for seasonal makeup collections. If a color does surprisingly well you can add it to your permanent collection of colors. Other than that it has a very limited shelf life.

Add products that support the seasonal shifts your clients go through as they turn the pages of their calendar—sun care, back to school, winterizing your hair/skin/body, seeing red—a special for Valentine's Day.

Accounting System

Depending on where you are with your business you may be able to maintain your inventory records by using simple recipe cards and a box holder. When I first went into the salon business I was working for a full-service salon. They had never retailed much and I was forced to create my own record-keeping system. For a few dollars I was able to record all purchases. Today I can't imagine running a business without a computer. The investment will pay for itself in the long run. You'll have access to information you never dreamed possible. But whatever system you use, make sure you have some accounting for products sold and what clients are purchasing.

DEALING WITH DEAD INVENTORY

You've got stuff on the shelf that has been collecting dust for quite some time. What can you do? Discount, discard, or donate.

The first place to investigate is your supplier. What is their return policy? Can you ship merchandise back that doesn't move? Some companies will have a restocking fee, the average being 25 percent. If you don't have a return policy. . . .

Discount

Everybody loves a bargain. Set up a bargain bin or basket and reduce the prices. Try a buy-one, get-one-free offer. Try 50 percent off.

Donate

Let's say your salon image is such that you don't want to discount. Try donating your dead inventory. One of my personal favorites is to donate beauty products to a local women's shelter. Some will take the unused product and dispense it to the women and children in need. Others may have a thrift store whose proceeds go to fund the shelter. Check with your accountant, but you should be able to write off the cost of the products as charitable contributions.

Discard

As a last resort, you can always discard the product. Outdated, faded products look absolutely awful on the shelf. Get them off and out of sight. The outdated merchandise will visually mar your new product sales. It simply isn't worth the money to keep them on the shelf. Make room for products that will sell.

CHAPTER 7

CLIENT MANAGEMENT SYSTEMS

This chapter covers the best ways to maximize your sales by working your client base. Learning to work your record cards is like having your very own treasure map to fortunes. The clues you can find on your clients' history cards can lead you to the buried treasure chest of retail and service sales.

It is very unfortunate if your salon is missing the treasure map. Lots of salons have a handful of products on the shelf that they hope they can sell. When the item is finally sold it is the end of the story. A good record-keeping system will provide you opportunities for building sales and securing client loyalty to the salon.

SETTING THE STAGE

New Client Orientation

One of my favorite tips is to take every new client who comes into the salon through a New Client Orientation. The NCO is administered to give clients a firm understanding of your business. The orientation can be combined with a service consultation. Take fifteen minutes at the beginning of the session of the consultation. If necessary, ask clients to arrive before the scheduled appointment time—similar to the first visit to a doctor.

Depending on your setup the salon receptionist, manager, owner, or technician can take clients through the orien-

tation. The first contact a client has with the salon sets the whole stage for the rest of that day's service and strengthens the possibility of the new client returning to the salon for future services and products.

The main objective is to give the client a personal contact within the salon, one person who acts as the liaison through the maze of salon service and protocol. If the owner of the salon can be the contact so much the better. If you are trying to get out from behind the chair, doing the orientations will keep you in touch with salon clients.

- Introduce yourself and your position within the salon.

- Tell the client what you will be covering in the New Client Orientation.

- Establish why the client is in the salon and whether she is experiencing any specific beauty problems.

- Ask any questions you feel need to be answered before administering the service.

- Salon policies. If your salon has established salon policies as they relate to clients take this time to inform the client of them. This is the perfect time to stress your on-time, no tipping, stylist swapping, product guarantees, and/or no-smoking policies. Of course, you don't want a list of don'ts a mile long and they should not be phrased in a negative way, but use the time to set the client on a positive course for her salon adventure.

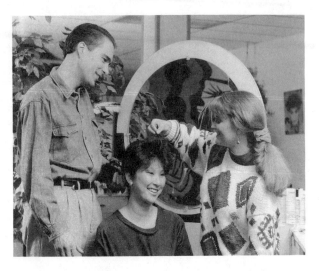

Fig. 7.1 Starting off on the right foot. (Photo by Michael A. Gallitelli on location at Rielms Hair Salon, Latham, NY.)

- Reinforce your job as the clients' salon contact. If clients have any questions or concerns or simply are not happy with a particular technician, have them come back to you. Salons lose clients when they want to change technicians. Clients know that their current stylist may have a fit in six weeks if the client is sitting in another chair. It is natural for the first stylist to take a desertion personally, but for the long-term peace and profit of the salon, it is essential for clients to be able to go to another stylist if they feel the urge. Be the salon's conductor. If clients want to catch another train, it's good for business to keep them from leaving the train station.

- Once you have covered all points, personally introduce the staff member responsible for the upcoming service to the client.

The New Client Orientation sets the selling stage. You are visually and verbally making a "We care" statement to the new client. See how New Client Orientation affects your long-term client retention numbers. (Fig. 7.1)

Client Record Card File

One of the key components to increasing your sales is to have access to the buying history of each client. One way to establish a history of your clients' purchases and services is to implement a record-keeping system.

I have seen salons take their client receipts and plop them into a manila folder. When the client wants to purchase an item she bought months ago, the staff member has to flip through the pile of receipts to hunt out the requested information. This setup is like having their treasure map torn up into tiny little pieces.

Record cards should have space for client personal information and space for recording product purchases in a spreadsheet format. (Fig. 7.2)

1. Personal information. Obviously you need the client's name, address, work and home phone numbers. If this is your only record card you may need to add space for allergies, contacts, referral, special notes, and service history. Use your discretion as to the amount of detailed information you want to know.

2. Product purchase history. The record card product area needs to be arranged in a spreadsheet format. I believe this is essential for increasing product sales. A spreadsheet style will allow you to look at the product history at a glance. You'll be able to spot heavy use products, favorites, and areas missing in their home care routine.

Down and Dirty

This may be as simple as a recipe card with margins and handwritten codes. I learned the value of record cards early on in my salon career. I was hired to set up a facial department in a hair salon. The salon had fifteen stylists and a very small retail business. One of my first missions was to increase retail sales. Much to my dismay this salon had never created a record-keeping system for retail products. They had chemical color cards, but that was it. The salon owner wasn't convinced she should go to the expense of producing cards for the limited volume of retail sales. At the time she couldn't see the value this effort could produce for the salon.

I remember purchasing a packet of recipe cards and a Lucite box to store them in (and still have them by the way). The little box of client record cards proved to be so valuable that it became the stepping stone for creating my own business. This is a very frugal way to begin building your sales.

Name _____

Address _____

City _____ **ST** ____ **Zip** _____

Day phone ( ) _____ **PM phone ( )** _____

	Mailings		Specials		Samples		Contacted	
YEAR	date	date	date	date	date	date	date	date
HAIR								
CUT								
COLOR								
PERM								
CONDITION								
Shampoo								
Conditioner								
Styling Aid								
Finishing								
Tools								
Misc.								
SKIN CARE								
FACIAL								
BODY TMT.								
Cleanser								
Toner								
Moisturizer								
Mask								
Body Care								
Eye Care								
Misc.								
MAKE UP								
LESSON								
APPLICATION								
Basics								
Powder								
Eye Products								
Lip Products								
Blush								
Tools								
Misc.								
NAILS								
MANICURE								
PEDICURE								
FILLS								
Enamel								
Hand & Body								
Misc.								

Fig. 7.2 Client record form.

Uptown Cards

If your salon has a growing column of retail sales you don't have the time to hand make your record cards. For pennies a piece you can design or use the sample provided to set up a record card system. As our retail sales grew the need for more administrative help increased as well. Manually filling in client records will work if you have a very efficient and dedicated person responsible for their upkeep. The next level is to have an office person post your daily client receipts to their respective client cards. If you have any volume at all you might want to pass this step and go directly to computers.

Commanding Computers

Quite honestly I can't imagine trying to run a salon, large or small, without the support of a good computer system. The investment can be substantial, but I have seen the investment pay for itself within weeks, and in some cases a few days.

A good computer system can assist you:

- As your inventory manager. A computer system can track on-hand inventory levels and on-hand minimum levels, print need-to-order reports, track fast moving items and slow sellers, monitor costs of goods, change prices, and help you avoid those costly out-of-stock situations.

- Advertising tracking. If you are investing your money you need to know how your investments are paying off. Computers can lead you to the buried treasure of marketing and advertising. The main clue is to determine your return on investment dollars. With the touch of a couple of keys you can find out how effective your marketing campaign is.

- Employee record keeping. Depending on the software you can keep track of payroll processing and evaluations and figure commissions and salaries.

- Point of sale. The system can act as your cash register, track methods of payment and gift certificates, and print receipts.

- A computer will show you your clients' purchasing history of both products and services. My only concern here is that the software allow you to see the product purchase history in a spreadsheet format.

- The system can keep tabs on client mailings, letters, cards, and statistics like birthdays and anniversaries, store chemical service records and haven't-seen-you-in-a-while reports.

- Prescription cards. Some of the systems have the capability of customizing prescription sheets. This unique technique can add hundreds of dollars in retail sales. Look at the amount of department stores that have gone high-tech with computer-assisted product recommendation.

Strengthening Business

I firmly believe that many salons across the country limit their success because they don't have a handle on their finances and client management programs. It's business as usual and it's the cigar box mentality. Your future success requires you to have a handle on the business side of the business. Many talented professionals go out of business after a short period of time because they aren't minding the dollars and cents side of the store. The strength of our industry lies in the firm foundation of our business practices. Record keeping and client management are instrumental in following the treasure map.

Working the Card File

Let's start when clients are coming in for repeat visits. Don't trust your memory on all the pertinent facts about every client you see. Even if you have an exceptional memory, don't risk guessing. Use the card to look for clues. (Fig. 7.3)

Date of Last Service
When were they into the salon last? What service did they have performed? Did they have multiple services? Does the amount of time that has passed between appointments affect the scheduled service?

Product Purchased
At a glance, you can see what products your clients favor. See if they are about due to be out of an item. Dates on the card will tell you the replacement cycle.

Cards Are Great Tools to Use as Maps
Especially for the client who has been using the same bottle of XYZ for a year when you know that if she were using the product

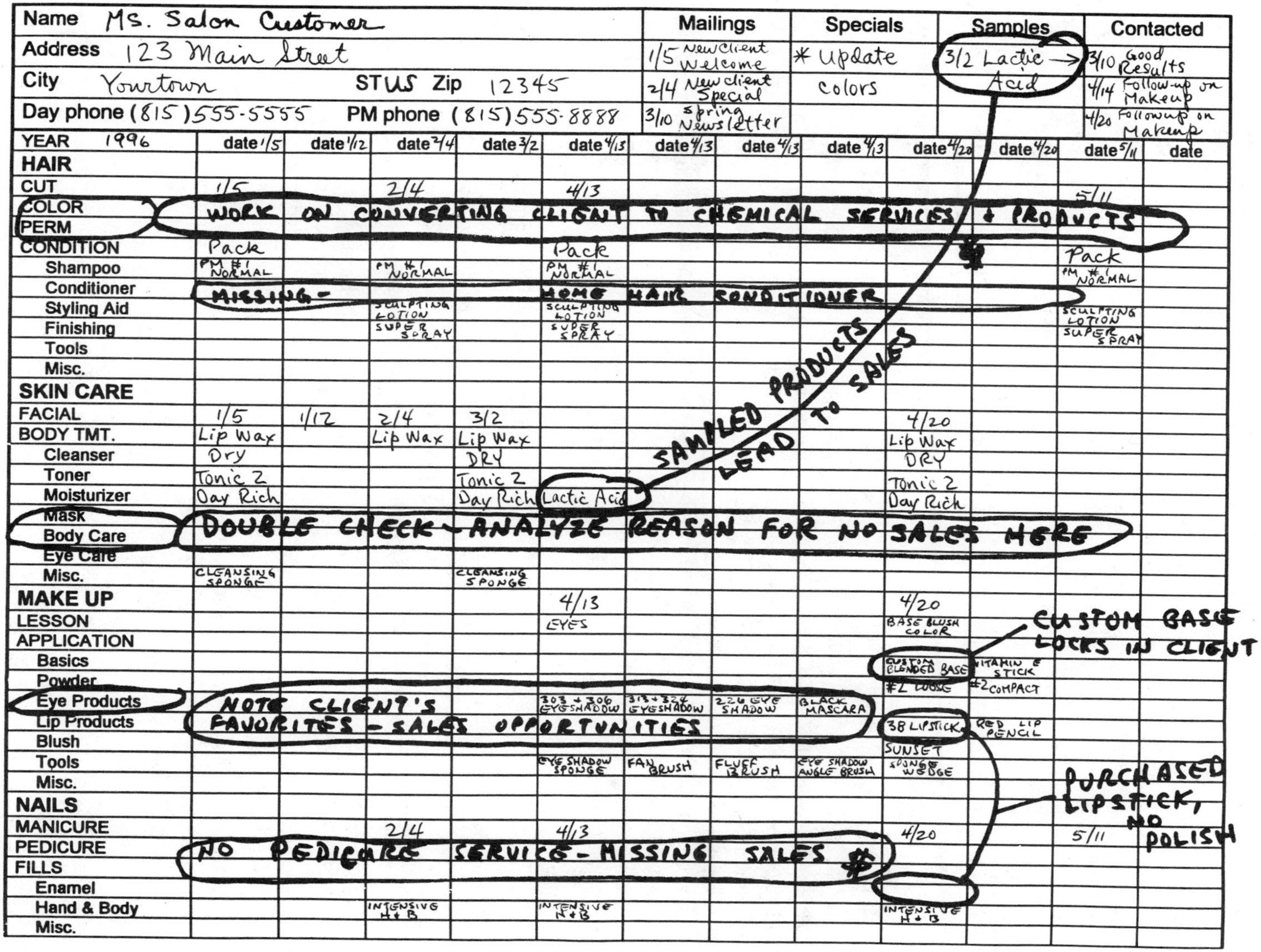

Name: Ms. Salon Customer
Address: 123 Main Street
City: Yourtown   State/US Zip: 12345
Day phone (815)555-5555   PM phone (815)555-8888

YEAR 1996	date 1/5	date 1/12	date 2/4	date 3/2	date 4/13	Mailings	Specials	Samples	Contacted
						1/5 New client Welcome	*Update Color		3/10 Good results
						2/4 New client Special	colors	3/2 Lactic Acid →	4/14 Follow up on Makeup
						3/10 Spring Newsletter			4/20 Follow up on Makeup
	date 1/5	date 1/12	date 2/4	date 3/2	date 4/13	date 4/3	date 4/3	date 4/20	date 5/11
HAIR									
CUT									
COLOR	1/5		2/4		4/13				
PERM									
CONDITION									
Shampoo	Pack				Pack			Pack	
Conditioner	PM# Normal		PM# Normal		PM# Normal			PM# Normal	
Styling Aid	Sculpting Lotion		Sculpting Lotion		Sculpting Lotion			Sculpting Lotion	
Finishing	Super Spray		Super Spray		Super Spray			Super Spray	
Tools									
Misc.									
SKIN CARE									
FACIAL	1/5	1/12	2/4	3/2	4/13				
BODY TMT.	Lip Wax	Lip Wax	Lip Wax	Lip Wax			Lip Wax		
Cleanser	Dry		Dry				Dry		
Toner	Tonic 2		Tonic 2	Tonic 2			Tonic 2		
Moisturizer	Day Rich		Day Rich	Day Rich			Day Rich		
Mask					Lactic Acid				
Body Care									
Eye Care	Cleansing Sponge		Cleansing Sponge	Cleansing Sponge					
Misc.									
MAKE UP									
LESSON					4/13		4/13		
APPLICATION					Eyes				
Basics									
Powder							Base Blush Color	Custom Blended Base #1 loose	
Eye Products					313+306 Eyeshadow		314+316 Eyeshadow	224 Eye Shadow	Ceramic Stick
Lip Products							Black Mascara	38 Lipstick Sunset	#2 Compact
Blush								Red Lip Pencil	
Tools					Eye Shadow Sponge		Fan Brush	Fluff Brush	Eye Shadow Angle Brush
Misc.								Sponge Wedge	
NAILS									
MANICURE									
PEDICURE			2/4		4/3		4/20		5/11
FILLS									
Enamel									
Hand & Body	Intensive H+B		Intensive H+B		Intensive H+B			Intensive H+B	
Misc.									

Handwritten callouts:
- WORK ON CONVERTING CLIENT TO CHEMICAL SERVICES & PRODUCTS
- HOME HAIR CONDITIONER
- SAMPLED OVER $100.00 OF PRODUCTS
- DOUBLE CHECK — ANALYZE REASON FOR NO SALES HERE
- NOTE CLIENT'S FAVORITES — SALES OPPORTUNITIES
- CUSTOM BASE LOCKS IN CLIENT
- PURCHASED LIPSTICK, NO POLISH
- NO PEDICARE SERVICE — MISSING SALES $

Fig. 7.3 Highlighted sales opportunities.

correctly it would have been gone months ago. Use the card to double-check results. If the client has only purchased shampoo and still complains about dry damaged hair, show her the card and say, "I see on your record card that you are only shampooing with Brand A. It is essential to follow that excellent shampoo with the daily conditioner for maximum results. Let's add this step and see what happens to the condition of your hair."

New Treatments or Techniques

Use the card to profile your treatments, especially chemical steps and color recommendations.

Samples or Product Introduction

Write on the card any samples you hand out to clients. The only logical reason to pass out samples is to introduce the product in anticipation of making a future sale. If you are making the effort make it pay off. Make a note on the card so when they come in the next time you can close the sale.

If you have introduced a product to clients and they didn't purchase it at the time, make a note on their card. You can also make a copy or carbon all prescription sheets to serve as reminders as to what you recommend.

Chatty Notes

People like doing business with people they like. One way to build rapport is to write a clue on the card to tickle your memory on a topic. "Last time when you were in you mentioned . . ." "I remember you were about to go back to school. How's it going?" You'll soon appear to have the best memory in town. All it takes is a little ink.

Lost Horizon

Look for sales clues in areas the clients have never purchased products. The spreadsheet tips you off right away to products clients may need to purchase or be introduced to.

Specials

Use the card to see if the clients have used the product on special. If so, they may want to take advantage of a sale. "You might like to know that this week we have a 50 percent off on your favorite shampoo. If you want to take advantage of the offer, just let me know and I'll pull a bottle or two for you before you leave." If they haven't tried the special item now is the time to bring it up.

Goals

When you begin to work with clients determine their beauty goals. Length of hair. Condition. Color. Overall appearance. How they would like their skin to look in six months. How long they want their natural nails to grow. Whatever their goal, write it down in quotations. All of your treatments and product recommendations will follow suit to support the beauty goals. This technique also plants a long-term commitment and relationship in clients' minds. It tells them you want to help them meet their desire, that you are in for the long haul, not just concerned for the thirty minutes they are in your chair.

Use their goals to support your product sales and services. Let's say you suggested a product they really need to achieve their goal, and they say, "no" or "I want to think it over." You have the perfect opportunity to stress the fact that "earlier you shared with me your goal to do X. This product is key in helping you achieve your goal. Do you really want to put off achieving results?"

Telemarketing off the Card File

Personal contact is important. Here are five ways to go treasure hunting using your card file.

Update the Data Base

If you are switching from a manual card system to a computer you can give clients a courtesy call to verify their information. My very first task working in a cosmetic store (besides dusting) was to call the entire card system and update the information. They had more than three thousand clients who had been into the store at one time or another. For weeks I had to call each client to update the records. We were doing it because the store was being sold and the new owner wanted a current crop of cards. At first it was tough to call these strangers, until I told them who I was and that the call was a brief courtesy call to verify the information on file and then share a special or mail them a coupon as a thank-you.

Follow Up

Every new client should receive a courtesy call seventy-two hours after their visit. The call is to thank clients for selecting your salon and to see how they enjoyed their visit. This is a great time to follow up on the products they purchased. Do they have any questions? How are the products working? You can also confirm their next appointment.

Special Announcement

Use your card file to notify clients of special services and limited offer specials. If you're computerized, you can even pull up all clients that have purchased, let's say, custom-blended base and notify these shoppers when you add custom-blended powder. Maybe the promotion of the month is exceptional for a limited section of your client base. Send out a special mailing or flyer to announce the offer. Save money by targeting limited offers and announcements.

Celebrations

Use your card file to send birthday, anniversary, or holiday mailings. Birthdays are one of my favorite times to contact clients. Besides, what other personal holiday sends clients to the mirror?

Newsletters

Telephone marketing can increase the response rate to the specials in your newsletters. Consider making two computer mailing lists: one for label printing, the other with phone numbers for follow-through. Send a newsletter to your own home to test the delivery date. When you know the letters are in-home, call customers to confirm that they have received them and verbally highlight advertised specials.

Monitoring Sales

I wouldn't begin to run a salon without an established record-keeping system for monitoring sales. You have too many bodies passing through the salon to remember who bought what. A little ink and some think time will add volume to your daily sales.

The other reason to expend the effort is to support your customer service direction. When Ms. Customer brings in the empty tube of lipstick and the color has vanished and the name on the bottom of the tube is blurred all you have to do to make the sale is turn to your trusty card system. An effective client management system is a win all the way around.

CHAPTER 8

SERVICE, SERVICE, SERVICE

Customer service has been the buzzword for a while. Yet when you talk of offering exceptional customer service what you are actually doing is setting your salon apart from the competition.

In this chapter we will be going over twenty-eight ways you can institute exceptional customer service policies, techniques and actions that will give the client a warm, comfortable feeling about your salon, but that will also make the cash register ring. The goal of this chapter is to design policies and standard operating procedures that make it as easy as possible for people to shop in your salon. The motto is, "easy to shop, easy to spend money."

GOOD OLD-FASHIONED SERVICE OR BYE-BYE CLIENTS

For many of us, customer service ended when self-serve gasoline pumps were turned on. Up until that dreadful point, consumers from all walks of life expected and anticipated honest, hard-working, loyal, client-satisfied service. Let's see if you and I can bring a little of that back into today's business.

There are two reasons to promote exceptional service: The competition is tough out there, and some of today's clients leave the salon, don't come back, and never tell you why. I have heard that

- One percent of your clients quit coming because of death.
- Three percent move away.
- Five percent switch to do business with a friend.
- Seven percent feel the prices are too high or too low.

- Fourteen percent leave because someone on staff didn't handle a grievance or complaint to the client's satisfaction.
- Sixty-eight percent stop coming because of the indifference of attitude on the part of the staff.

Just think if you could save over 60 percent of your current client base and add new clients and add additional sales. That would be business heaven.

Customer service shouldn't be lip service. Here are some key ways to increase your current level of service in the salon. Make it easy for the client to shop with you.

Store Hours

Take a look at the hours your salon is open. Do you cater to working women? Do your hours of operation reflect the desire to service women who are on tight time constraints? Now, I'm not advocating that you keep the salon open twenty-four hours, although some do, but to make sure you are open for business when your clients are free to come to the salon.

I am constantly amazed when I see retail places that close at 6:00 P.M. Unless you are located in an area that becomes deserted after 5:00, you may need to be open until at least 7:00 P.M.

Early Birds
Evaluate your morning hours. Some salons are open for business before clients' work hours. This may be an untapped market for you. For those early birds, a stop off at the salon

may be the ticket. Poll your clients to see if they would take advantage of early bird hours. Even a skeletal staff could take care of the early risers.

Night Owls

For the night owls, look at your closing hours. If you have enough clients requesting late hours, consider staying open later, even if it's one or two nights a week. The first retail beauty store I worked in stayed open two nights a week until 9:00 P.M. Quite often we did more sales from 5:00 to 9:00 than during the rest of the day.

Preferred Appointments

If you have the opportunity to schedule your own work day, look at offering preferred appointments. These are times when the client would need to come in that conflict with your normal hours of operation. For the luxury and your inconvenience, charge more for the appointment. You could price the time with a percentage surcharge, say 20 percent for the preferred time. You might find some customers more than willing to absorb additional expenses for the luxury and convenience of scheduling appointments that fit their lifestyles versus a store's schedule.

Punctuality Plus

Today's clients will not be kept waiting in salon reception areas. To set your salon apart from the competition, establish an on-time policy. Guarantee your appointment times. If the stylist is more than fifteen minutes late starting the appointment offer $5 off for every five minutes after that. This is a radical move but think of how you could surpass your competition by such a policy. The one commodity today's consumer doesn't have enough of is time. Over 85 percent of the women in the United States are expected to work outside of the home by 1995. Will these women give up their leisure time waiting in the salon while someone is playing catchup? I don't think so.

If by chance you are going to be late for your scheduled appointment, give clients a courtesy call and let them know how much you are off schedule. Be realistic and tell them the truth. Give them an option to keep the appointment or re-

schedule. And remember, time is money, for you and your clients.

The Big Squeeze

There will be many occasions for you to suggest additional services and treatments for your clients. Feel free to squeeze them in if it doesn't make you run behind. Select a buddy from your staff and pair up with him or her for team work. Work with each other to service the necessary squeezes. Split the money if need be if one has the time to take an additional sale. Half the pie is definitely better than an empty plate.

Hire Friendly, Knowledgeable People

It should almost go without saying that the staff needs to be friendly and courteous. I know it can be difficult to stay up and positive all the time, but when it comes to face-to-face contact, nothing less is even remotely acceptable. Clients coming into the salon expect and deserve exceptional personal relations. You can't afford having someone on staff who is grumpy, mean, cold, or indifferent toward clients.

There are no job boundaries when it comes to sales. Stamp out "not my job" from the salon vocabulary. An attitude of "not my job" will instantly snuff out the flame of service. If you personally can't handle a client's request, inform the client that "you'd be glad to get the perfect person to help her."

Staff Arrivals

Arrive fifteen to twenty minutes before your first appointment or opening hours. Rushing in after the client has been sitting in the reception area is bad for business. The station or treatment area should be prepped the night before so when you arrive you are ready to work. Reduce the morning tension by preparing your work area in advance.

Arrive for work groomed for the day. You never know when clients may be early. Your primping should have been completed at home. You are the measuring stick for looking good. Always be prepared to set the example.

Prompt, Efficient Service

When it comes to establishing the ultimate salon with an emphasis on retail, prompt and efficient service is a must. The front desk person in the salon is key to increasing sales. He or she quite often is the first and last contact the client will have with the salon.

I am writing this a few days after checking into a hotel for a seminar. The employee on the front desk argued with me about hotel procedure. I was clear on what needed to happen, yet he didn't listen. Finally, in desperation I requested the manager to settle the issue. Within two seconds my dilemma was cleared up. The manager declared, "Of course she is right. Why in the world would you do it the way you were trying?" Not only was the beginning of my stay tainted, but when the bellhop took me to my room, he told me that every client he had waited on that day had problems checking in with that particular desk clerk. My question was, "Why even give him access to customers when he repeatedly caused problems?"

The Greeting

Remember that the sale starts as soon as clients walk through the front door. Greet clients as soon as they enter the salon. My personal goal is to have three staff members acknowledge a client, even if the person isn't "theirs." (Fig. 8.1)

Some greetings can be:

- "Hi, how are you today?"
- "Good to see you."
- "Hello, Ms./Mr. So and So."

Watch the flattery technique that clothing stores have unfortunately adopted. Have you walked into a store and within seconds been complimented by a salesperson? They seem to reference your shoes, jewelry, clothes, bag, whatever. Then seconds later another clone from Camp Compliment showers you again. You know your clients well enough to notice if something is new or particularly flattering. At that point, go ahead and make a reference to it if you feel inclined.

Honor the Appointment Time

This is an important sales commandment. If a client arrives late and you can still proficiently perform the service, by all means start. The one thing that can hurt your professionalism and sales is to run behind and keep your other clients waiting. If a client is too late for you to accomplish the service see if someone on staff has the time to take care of her. If so, shift her over. It's better to keep the money in the salon than to send a client down the street; she might not come back.

If you have flexibility in the treatment, firmly ask your client this question: "I see that you are unfortunately fifteen minutes late for your appointment. I must honor the appointment times that follow you. What do you want me to leave out of the treatment today?" Now I realize you can't just cut one side of her head, but you might have to turn her over to someone else for finish work. In a facial, you will regrettably have to shorten the wonderful massage. For nail service, your assistant will have to polish.

If a client is habitually late, take her aside the first time and stress the importance of honoring the designated appointment time. The second time, you will have to reschedule. The third time, tell her you like her as a person, but you can't afford her as a client. She will have to go somewhere else. Now, this may sound drastic coming from me when I am telling you how

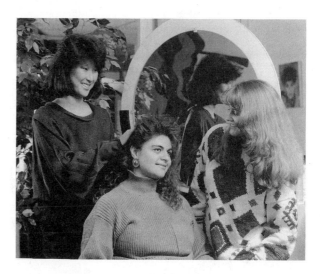

Fig. 8.1 Greeting the client. (Photo by Michael A. Gallitelli on location at Rielms Hair Salon, Latham, NY.)

to increase your sales, but trust me when I say you can't afford them. The late offenders are upsetting your punctual clients. The five, ten, or twenty customers that follow Tina Tardy should not be penalized for her lateness.

"Here's My Card"

When a client is leaving the salon after a service, hand her one of your personal business cards. "Here's my personal card. I have written down my hours on the back. If you have any questions feel free to call me here at the salon." This simple and cost-free technique shows that you are concerned about your clients. Don't wait for the receptionist to fill out a card for you. Have a business card holder on your station.

A Pleasant Environment

At the beginning of the book, we went over in detail the importance of creating a positive environment for your clients. Sell through the senses of sight, sound, taste, touch, and smell.

When it comes down to customer service, pay close attention to the tension in the salon. There will naturally be up days and goofy days when everyone has the giggles, but watch out for tense undercurrents in the salon. No one wants to shop or stay in a place of business when you could cut the tension with a butter knife.

Establish the rule that when staff hits the front door, all their emotional baggage is left outside. They may claim it after hours. I have made staff go back out the front door and reenter the salon if they walked through with an attitude.

If there are problems to be hammered out, do them one on one or during your regular staff meetings. Never discuss salon problems on the selling floor.

You are to be the gatekeeper of harmony and happy sales. Guard the salon environment at all costs. A client will be able to pick up emotional undercurrents quicker than you think. Don't jeopardize your sales. Who wants to hang around a place for an hour or more if it isn't fun or at least enjoyable?

Ban Pricing Surprises

Make sure your clients know up front the investment for the service or product. If you are recommending an add-on ser-

vice, tell the client exactly how much extra it will be. "Mrs Carlin, I am going to strongly suggest that we do an intensive conditioning treatment today. Your hair is showing signs of extreme dryness. The treatment will take an extra fifteen minutes and will be $15. Let's give it a try."

Scheduling multiple services is like money in the bank. When you perform different services keep an accurate record of charges. I've seen clients repeatedly get upset and leave salons when they are charged one price this month and a different price next month for the exact same service. Be consistent. Be credible for your clients. If you're not set up on a computer system, keep accurate client files, even if you have to use recipe cards. Don't jeopardize your relationship by sloppy book work.

Ticket Ticklers

"Thank you" is a powerful statement. Make sure you verbally thank your clients for their business, but also put it in writing. When you write up the client's ticket, turn it over and boldly write thank you on the back. Skip the smiley face some waitresses put on the bottom of their restaurant checks.

The AnnTaylor fashion store chain does a neat trick with its receipts. They are folded up and tucked into a company envelope with a special thank-you printed on the outside. This technique makes the receipt look like a note or letter versus a bill. Nice added customer benefit.

Sacking It Up

When a client buys product from you, how does it look when it leaves the salon? I know a lot of women who like to shop. Part of the fun for them is that when they get their new goodies home they get to unwrap them. The purchases aren't just new items, they are new gifts for themselves. They are little personal treasures. Make clients want to purchase your products by decoratively wrapping them up.

The only limitation to wrapping creatively is your budget. At least have a shopping bag to put the product into. Wrap each item in tissue and place it in the bag.

When I made the salon's commitment to retailing, new shopping bags were a must. Taking a cue from the department stores, I looked for a paper-handled bag and tissue. The sacks became part of the salon image. They even had their own name—The Foo Bags. At the time I couldn't afford to have 50,000 sacks custom-screened, so I found plain bags and personally signed each one with a metallic magic marker. They were then stuffed with two sheets of salon-coordinated colored tissue and ready for product. I knew we hit a nerve when clients would tell us they kept the bags and used them again because they were so pretty. A twist on recycling and maximum marketing.

It's a Wrap

Keep an assortment of wrapping paper on hand. Offer to gift wrap any purchase for your clients. Stock holiday-inspired themes as well as ribbons and gift tags. Save your clients time and hassle if they purchase gifts from the salon by offering to wrap their goodies free of charge. (Fig. 8.2)

Conquering Client Complaints

Learn to handle client complaints and you will increase your sales. There is no way around it, at some point some client is

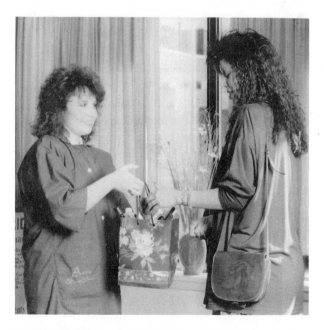

Fig. 8.2   It's a wrap. (Photo by Michael A. Gallitelli on location at The Austin Beauty School, Albany, NY.)

going to voice a complaint. How you handle it will determine if you keep the client or send her shouting to her friends.

There are six steps in handling complaints successfully. When clients comes into the salon and start to express concern:

1. Take them aside for privacy. You want them out of earshot of other clients. "Let's go over here where we can talk."
2. Express your concern for their situation. Stress that you are here to help rectify the problem. "I'm sorry you are unhappy. Let's work this out."
3. Ask clients to explain the nature of the problem. Hear them out completely without interruptions. "Please explain the nature of your dissatisfaction. I want to be able to solve this for you."
4. Ask clients what they would like for you to do to solve the complaint. Don't leap to conclusions. They may just want you to know of their particular quirk or situation. "I'd be glad to rectify this for you. What would you like for me to do?"
5. Don't argue with clients. It isn't worth it. Even if you feel their complaint isn't justified, try to negotiate. As a last resort, do what you can to meet their request. If it's money back, you can give them the money back. The few dollars you might lose on the service or product isn't worth the amount of bad mouthing a disgruntled client can and will do. "Here's what I'll do for you."
6. After you have handled the complaint make sure you follow up with clients, either by phone or by mail. You need to check and see if they are still happy with the results.

Now, I know the hair on the back of your neck may be standing on end, but the one or two complaints you will need to handle aren't worth getting upset over. Returns, requests for redos, product sensitivities are a fact of doing business. Even if you know you are absolutely, positively in the right, don't haggle with clients. If clients are a real pain in the neck, you don't have to service them again. There is always that one client that's never satisfied. Just be thankful you've got tons of great clients.

There are three types of complaints you will see in the salon—dissatisfaction with a product's results, unhappy with a service, sensitivity to a product.

If a client is unhappy with product results, find out how it didn't meet the expectation. "What specifically didn't you like about the product? I'll be glad to solve the dilemma." Try and switch the product for one that better matches the client's expectation. Maybe there was a communication gap during the recommendation stage, and the product didn't live up to the expectations because the beauty goal wasn't clear.

If a client is unhappy with a service find out why. "Tell me specifically what you don't like about the perm." Remember to hear the client out and don't interrupt.

If a client is unhappy because a product caused sensitivity, take it back immediately. There will be a handful of clients who are truly sensitive to ingredients in products. A few have found that if they claim to have sensitive skin, they are perceived as sensitive human beings. Either way don't mess with the sale. Politely refund the money. Take the product back and check the formula. If the product looks suspicious, send it back to the supplier or manufacturer. Sensitivities are always touchy issues. Don't play up the problem, just offer to refund the money.

The golden rule here is that most clients will continue to do business with you if you satisfy the complaint on the spot. If you show good faith and super customer service, they will continue to patronize your salon. The trouble begins when dissatisfied clients leave mad or they feel unsatisfied. These are the clients who will tell anyone who will listen the horror story about your salon. The rule is that unhappy customers will tell at least nine other people their sad tale. The problem magnifies because those nine will tell nine others and so the story goes.

Give everyone on staff the authority to handle client complaints immediately. The first person the client talks to can solve the problem. The more times she has to tell the story, the more time she has to get angry and hostile.

Your Salon Pledge

Guarantee your products and services. Take a stand and stand behind your work and professional products. Have you ever purchased products only to get them home and find they don't work, they are the wrong color, you just don't like them? You've made purchase errors before and you're in the business. Think of the money your clients have wasted. Ease the pain and stress of shopping in your salon by guaranteeing every product and service for ultimate client satisfaction.

Cash In on Credit Cards

Make shopping easier by offering credit card charging privileges in your salon. Many salons shy away from accepting plastic because of the percentage points you pay to credit companies. If you seriously want to increase your retail sales you should allow clients to pay with plastic.

Right now, the typical cards are Visa, MasterCard, and American Express, but that list may grow or change within the next five years. Do you need all three? It depends on your client base. If you are trying to attract the upscale, affluent client, then all three are a must. Visa and MasterCard have floor limits. American Express allows its clients to charge without a ceiling on the bill. Your bigger retail clients will use American Express.

Shop around for business rates. I've seen them as low as 1.8 percent for Visa and MasterCard. With American Express you have several options for depositing the charges—same-day credit, three-day direct deposit, or if you mail it in you receive a deposit check within ten days. If you can live without the money for a few days, the percentage rate drops dramatically. Shop around for rates, but do set up the service to take credit cards. The results are in the bank.

The main reason for accepting credit cards is the convenience for your clients. Allow them to spend money with your salon by cash, check, credit card, even debit cards. Before too long, if you are set up to accept cards you'll be able to offer the convenience of debit bank cards. The ATM debit will work through your electronic processing equipment. No one can afford to turn away a sale. Accept all types of payment, for service and for increasing sales. (Fig. 8.3)

Mail Order Madness

If you have exclusive products that no one else in the city has, set up a mail order department. Who says your clients have to grace the salon to buy products? Just make sure you have a budget for promotion and personnel to take care of billing and packaging. If customers can shop on television for everything from soup to nuts, your clients can pick up the phone to order products from you.

Establish a corporate account from United Parcel Service. They can come to the salon daily or upon a phone call

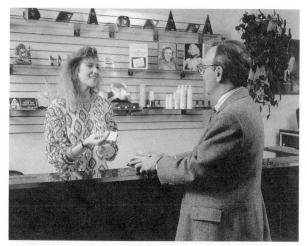

Fig. 8.3 Cash in on credit cards. (Photo by Michael A. Gallitelli on location at Rielms Hair Salon, Latham, NY.)

after you have established an account. With some boxes, packing materials, and mailing labels you will be all set to ship out products.

This mail order service is exceptionally good for out-of-town clients. If they live far from the salon, or simply can't make it in, have them call in free with a minimum purchase. Make it as easy to get products from you as possible.

Deliver the Goods

Contract with a delivery company. If the purchase has to be there in a narrow gap of time, have the products delivered. You might even have someone on staff personally make the delivery and contact. Even if your requests for this service are minimal, have a delivery service company contact. Depending on your cost, you can offer free delivery with a minimum retail purchase or for a nominal charge.

Preferred Parking

When a new client is scheduled for an appointment, make sure she knows how to find the salon and where to park. Check to see if your shopping center will allow you to offer special salon client designated parking. Keep staff autos and motorcycles

out of the prime parking spots. If you are lucky enough to have street-front parking, save those precious spots for clients. Make staff park in a different area.

House Calls

Take your services to the streets. Pack your beauty tool bag. Clients are requesting in-home services. Make sure you check with state and local authorities first, but if it's okay offering house calls may add another notch in your customer service belt. Make sure you price your services accordingly. Take into account your travel time, product costs, time for service, parking, cabs, gas, and set your prices accordingly.

You may just want to offer this unique service at the holidays when everyone's schedule gets crazy or you may add house calls as part of your salon repertoire. VIP clients enjoy the privacy and convenience. Even for those less blessed than the Rockefellers, a house call can make them feel like a queen for a day. Plus, if you physically get into their bathrooms, you can see for yourself the brands and types of products they are using. I've even charged clients to go through their cosmetic drawers and cabinets to clean out the old stuff. What a great way to add both service and retail sales.

Blooming Beauties

Blooming beauties can be sprinkled through the salon, but don't lose sight of the fact that you are there to sell services and products. Too many flowers and plants may overdecorate the environment. Place a beautiful bouquet in the reception area, one by the seating area if needed, and one on the cash-and-wrap station. Make sure the one for the front desk doesn't take up too much space. You'll need to have counter space for point of purchase and impulse items.

Pillow Notes

I like to present a client with a single stem flower if it happens to be her birthday or anniversary. If you offer facial or body treatments leave the flower with a brief note for the occasion.

Southern Hospitality

Good old-fashioned southern hospitality is hard to forget. I fondly remember summer visits to my grandparents' house in Alabama. It was always a treat to go down there. Even as a youngster, I realized that their kindness and eagerness to see to your comfort seemed to be instinctive. When the kids were excused from the table, every aunt who had her hand in the cooking would always state, "Hope you enjoyed it." It wasn't really a question, but more of a matter-of-fact statement. What a glorious thing to say. Think of applying it to your salon.

Your customers are your guests, paying guests. Think of treating everybody entering your salon as you would treat a guest in your home. I want them to feel comfortable, treated with respect, and catered to. My southern aunts always made me feel cared for and they went out of their way, a practice I carry with me today. Hope you add a little southern hospitality to your salon.

Add on a Lagniappe

Lagniappe is an old Louisiana custom where you give clients more than they paid for. In the old days, a merchant would throw in a little something extra with purchases. I guess you could say that lagniappe may have been the original gift with purchase. When a client bought a dozen eggs, the merchant would throw in an extra one. If the purchase was for a pound of hand-milled flour, an extra handful would be added to the bag. Try adding a little lagniappe when a client buys something from you.

1. Give the client a unique comb or brush with a new look.
2. Brow shaping with facial.
3. Clean clients' rings with every manicure.
4. Give cleansing sponges after each facial.
5. Give the client an informational brochure—summer sun care, changing day to night hair looks, long-lasting makeup techniques, stress busters, save your nails.
6. Travel-size product with any full-size purchase.

What could you do in your salon to add a little lagniappe in your daily practices?

The 72-Hour Golden Rule

The first 72 hours after a client leaves the salon are critical for client contact. Every new customer and any client who changes her look or buys new products should receive a courtesy contact.

Contact by Mail

Drop the client a welcome-to-the-salon card, a personal note from you reiterating your pleasure to do business with her. Stress the importance of home maintenance. Think of how impressive it would be to you if you received a personal note from someone you just did business with.

Contact by Phone

"Hi, this is Jane from SuperService Salon. This is just a quick courtesy call to see how you are doing with your new haircut." Or, "I was just calling to see how you like the new color. When you left the salon you were looking great. How are you doing with it?" The important thing to stress is that it is a quick courtesy call, that you aren't going to take up her time. This is the most efficient tool for following up with a client who had a complaint or needed to switch products for some reason.

Reach Out and Touch Your Clients

In reality, many of your clients work. You can leave your message on their answering machine. The important goal is to let clients know you are thinking of them and you appreciate their business.

If you are swamped during the day, take a few minutes at the end and call your clients. It's easier to keep a client than to go out and scrounge for new ones. One plastic surgeon I know calls every patient the night they had surgery to see how they are doing. Now, if he can perform surgery at 5:00 A.M., see patients all day, and still call his surgical patients after 7:00 P.M. you can too.

Thank You, Thank You, Thank You

The power of the written word is amazing. A personal note from you to your clients can and will produce outstanding results and tons of goodwill. If you have a small operation, print blank cards that you can fill in. If you are swamped, you may prefer to have cards preprinted to save time, but make sure you add a personal note to the bottom of a preprinted card to add that personal touch.

Here is a collection of sample thank-yous. Use them as is, or rewrite them to suit your style and personal flare.

Long-Term Client

This is the client that is sometimes easy to overlook. She is constantly there, a warm smiling face even on bad days. Take a few minutes to say thanks for that client's continued loyal support.

- Your name ranks high on the list of our loyal and distinguished "repeat" clients. It's special people like you who year after year give us proof that we are setting the pace for beauty technology here in our hometown. It is to friends like you, (client's name), that we owe our continued success.

- I want to express my sincere appreciation and continued dedication to offering you the best possible service and products. Thanks so much.

- So many times we go through life and overlook telling those people that we care about how much we value them. Thank you for your business and please know that I do appreciate your continued support. Thanks a million.

Happy Birthday

- Best wishes on this special day. All of us at (your salon name) look forward to helping you through the beautiful years ahead. Thinking of you.

- Happy Birthday to a beautiful person.

- Everybody here (your salon name) wants to wish you a beautiful and glorious birthday. We hope your day is filled with love, sunshine, and surprises. Happy B-Day.

Customers after Purchase

- Thanks for letting me help you on Tuesday. I know that selecting a new look can be overwhelming; I hope I helped ease the stress. I'm here Tuesday through Saturday so if you have any questions, don't hesitate to call. I'm here to help. Let me know how you like your new look.

Customers When They Don't Purchase

Yes, I want you to send a note to the client that didn't buy your recommendation. This gives you the opportunity to contact the client without pushing the service or product directly. They may have had many reasons for not buying today. The timing or the stars may not have been right. This little note plants the seed for the client to contact you when the need arises again.

- Thank you for allowing me to show you the new home care program for permed hair. I enjoyed meeting you and I appreciated the opportunity to cut and perm your hair. We couldn't get together on your home care needs this time, but I hope that when you think of (your salon name) you'll remember me. Please feel free to call or stop into the salon if there is any way I can be of help with your beauty needs. See you soon.

Referral

- Thank you for suggesting to Ms. Royce that she try (your salon name). Your referral is the best compliment I could receive. I promise that your friend will receive the best service we have to offer. Special people like you make being in business a pleasure. Look forward to seeing you soon. Have a beautiful day,

When a Mix-Up Occurs

- We regret any inconvenience our lack of communication may have caused you this week. We sincerely do our best to give you the quality service you deserve and want to know immediately when our clients feel our efforts are not all they could be, as well as when you feel we are doing our best for you. Thank you for being patient with us on Monday.

Above and Beyond the Call

There are times when someone crosses your daily path and exhibits an outstanding performance. Those people that go beyond the call of duty should receive a note of appreciation (and a business card).

- Thank you. It is gratifying to meet someone dedicated to doing a good job. Your efforts were sincerely appreciated on Saturday when you (fill in). It's not every day you meet someone who can efficiently get the job done and with style and grace. You can and did. If I can be of any service to you, please don't hesitate to call. Have a great day.

New Customers

When a potential person becomes a money-spending client send a thank-you note. Think back and try to recall if anyone you have done business with has ever called you or dropped a note in the mail for a minor purchase. How about after a major outlay of cash?

- Thank you for becoming our customer. I was pleased to serve you and offer you our most sincere welcome. You can be assured that we will do our best to merit your continued confidence and goodwill shown by joining our family of satisfied customers. Welcome to the beautiful family of (your salon's name).

- A friendly thank-you for your business. Everyone on staff takes great pride in providing you with the best possible service and techniques. We will always do everything we can to assure your complete satisfaction. We look forward to many opportunities to service you in the future. With dedication and excellence.

Haven't Seen You in a While

- It seems like a long time since you have taken advantage of our services. We've missed you and want you to know that it has always been our genuine pleasure to serve you. Your friendship and goodwill are important to us. We want you to know that we are here to do all we can to ensure your complete satisfaction. Hope to see you soon.

- I realize that we haven't seen you in the salon in a while. Hope all is great with you. You are missed and I truly hope to see you soon.

Gift Certificate When Purchased by Client

Acknowledge your good clients when they purchase a gift certificate for a friend or colleague. This client is a gold mine. If they like your service so much that they are willing to buy gift certificates for others, jot off a note.

- Thank you for treating (Alexis Montgomery) to a pedicure. When she comes in for her treat I will give her the special treatment, the one you have delightfully received in the past.

- I really appreciate your many referrals. They are the best compliment anyone could give me and the salon. You are a special friend to the salon and to me. See you next week.

CASHING IN ON CUSTOMER SERVICE

When it comes to Service, service, service just ask yourself what you can do to be of better service to your client. There is never a traffic jam when you go the extra mile.

Every action in the salon creates one of two impressions—a negative one or a positive one. Which one do you want your client leaving with? Take action today to plant the seeds of super customer service with every client you see. Treat your clients with as much attention and service after you've sold them as before.

PART TWO
DEVELOPING YOUR SELLING SKILLS

CHAPTER 9 PERSONAL REFLECTIONS

I'd like to say we do not judge people strictly on appearances, but every human being is guilty, even if they claim differently. I understand that within the first five to seven seconds opinions are formed; the mind races, judging likes and dislikes. It's a natural, intuitive action to quickly assess other people, to size them up, to look them over, to judge them based on appearances. And most of this sizing up is done before one word is spoken.

This may be a difficult chapter to face; it will challenge you to be brutally honest with yourself about yourself. This chapter plays a critical role in your success. (Maybe even more importantly than your technical skills.) I hope you are ready for a little change. If you are not selling to your potential or desires you may want to implement many ideas outlined in this chapter.

Why are personal reflections important to your success? Successful selling begins and ends with you. Your level of success is directly related to who you are, what you look like, how you sound, and what you say. These components are the foundation for making the sale easier.

Powerful and effective communication skills will be the number one talent to possess in this decade. The goal of this chapter is to make sure all your communication skills—verbal and nonverbal—are working together. Your verbal and non-verbal communication must support your technical expertise.

This chapter is divided into three sections. The first section will deal with your image and the perception the client forms about you. The second area will address how you sound to your customers. The final section will give you tips and tools for building a strong dialogue with the person in your chair.

Each section is designed to support your desire to be the best you can be, to be the success you desire. Of course, you'll sell more in the process.

PERSONAL REACTIONS

When people see you for the first time, their minds automatically calculate eight factors. Not all behavioral scientists can agree on the order of importance, but all eight areas are evaluated. They are: gender, skin color, age, appearance, facial expressions, eye contact, movement, and personal space.

Gender

Male or female. Dominant versus submissive, strong versus weak, powerful versus gentle. Think back on what you heard as a child. "Wait until your father gets home." Mom may have been screaming at the kids all day, but as soon as dad walked in what happened? Yes, you guessed it. The kids instantly straightened up. It's a conditioned reflex.

I feel there is a slight advantage to being a male technician or stylist working in the beauty business. The first salon I worked in had a fantastic designer. Eric's appointment book was filled every day and had a waiting list longer than Rapunzel's hair. He invested a lot of time and money into developing his craft and it seemed that all Eric had to do was barely recommend something to his client and it was sold. Now, there were other good stylists in this salon, but his authority and maleness just seemed to make the cash register ring.

Some women put more weight on a man's opinion about their looks and appearance than on another woman's. Some women don't trust other women to tell them the truth regarding their attractiveness and sex appeal. If you're caught in this cultural trap, you will need to present yourself in a confident and knowledgeable light.

Like Attracts Like

It's a natural human condition to be intuitively comfortable with someone similar to yourself. When you meet someone similar to yourself, you don't have a physical communication gap to hurdle. People form a natural acceptance, a commonality of life. People are more comfortable around others very similar to themselves. Please don't misunderstand me. It's not prejudice, it's just observation, a quick calculation, a flash of an image registering in the brain.

Fortunately the walls of restriction and narrow-mindedness are crumbling before our very eyes. Companies are doing business around the corner and around the world. People are learning to deal with other nationalities and backgrounds as the global economy develops. Hopefully, the difference in our skin colors will fade into oblivion and everyone will recognize and accept the fact that all people are created equal.

Age

For decades, society has been gravitating toward a youth-oriented environment. Fortunately, with the onset of the aging baby boomers, those born between 1945 and 1964, less emphasis has been placed on mature people trying to look and act eighteen again.

People are reading your face. You can hide your body with clothing. Put a wig or hat on to hide your hair. Slipping on gloves, socks and shoes can cover up a multitude of sins. But your face is always exposed. What does it reveal? How old? How young? What have you done with yourself? Do you look tired? Hassled? Energetic? Full of life? Worn out? In need of a vacation? Tanned and toned? Based on your assumed age can you do the job?

Age can be a deterrent. Being either too young or too old

can have its drawbacks. When I first started selling skin care and makeup, I kept getting, "What do you know about wrinkles? You're too young." My response was either, "I'm actually sixty-three and the products really do work" (which usually got a chuckle) or "I know enough. I'm not planning on getting any wrinkles." My responses deflated their questions about age.

Former President Reagan in his presidential debate with Democratic candidate Walter Mondale was concerned that his age would be against him in his bid for reelection. Roger Alles was the only political advisor to Reagan who felt his age issue should be confronted head on. Seconds before the debate began, Alles whisked away the president and worked out a strategy.

During the broadcast, the dreaded age issue did surface and Reagan's response was brilliant. "I want you to know that I will not make age an issue of this campaign. I am not going to exploit, for political purposes, my opponent's youth and inexperience."

Appearance

What does your appearance reveal about you? Are you appropriately attired for the salon and its clientele? People look for visual signs of success, signs that tell them you've made it and you must know what you are talking about.

You never get a second chance to make a good first impression. Have you been out on the town and someone comes across and asks, "Are you a hairdresser? You must be in the beauty business by the way you are dressed." Is it a compliment or a double-edged sword? Do they make the statement because your attire screams of fad-funk-trendy? Do you look so pulled together that you have to be in the business because the average person couldn't pull a look like that together?

Years ago, a man called my office to schedule a business appointment. When asked what the appointment was concerning, he acknowledged he was an accountant and wanted to talk to me about handling my business bookkeeping and accounting needs. That was fine with me as it was my least favorite area of the business.

As soon as he put one foot in the front door, I knew a business relationship was doomed. He had greasy hair, dirt under his nails, scuffed shoes, no watch, wrinkled suit, and an armful of papers stuffed into a manila folder. There was absolutely no visual sign of success to be found. I was not convinced in the least that this man should or could advise me regarding the success of my business. Then during the brief meeting he rattled on about needing new clients, his lack of funds, and his organization's disorganization. The total of his impressions unfortunately left me with a negative attitude. He may have been the world's most brilliant accountant but based on his inappropriate appearance I would never know. He lost my business. To this day I wonder how much additional business he has lost due to his appearance.

Facial Expressions

It is estimated that the eighty muscles of the face are capable of making more than seven thousand different facial expressions. Using a full-view mirror express the following emotions (watch your facial features, body language, hand gestures, every action): confusion, elation, sadness, timidity, sincerity, anger, happiness. Are many of the expressions similar? Could your expressions be misinterpreted or mistaken for another reaction?

Many beauty-industry people forget that they are surrounded by mirrors in the salon, mirrors that reflect the slightest movements. A shrug, wrinkled nose, snarl, or huff that you think is hidden from others may be reflecting in another mirror in the salon. Be extremely careful and always present your best face forward.

Eye Contact

The eyes are the windows of the soul. Clients look deeply into your eyes. Do they show signs of vitality and excitement? Do your eyes need soothing drops to wipe out the red road maps? Do you make direct eye contact and really look into your clients' eyes, or are you darting around the room?

Movement

Actions speak louder than words. Is your body language supporting or undermining your spoken word? Are you fidgeting, tapping your fingers, or bouncing your knee? Do you walk with a purpose or a poor-me shuffle? Watch your body language at all times because your movements reflect your thoughts and subconscious activity.

Personal Space

Do you respect the person's private physical space, not necessarily the work station, but the invisible, private bubble that surrounds each person? Depending on the person, the bubble may allow you to get very close or hold you at bay. Do others feel safe if you are keeping your distance? Does your energy and vitality radiate to the client? Or do you hold everything in and make it difficult for others to get close to you?

FIRST IMPRESSIONS——NONVERBAL

On the next page you will find a few photos. Take the next few seconds and assess each one individually. Write down at least five impressions you receive from the photos. What do you see? What type of people are they? What's their job or occupation? What is your general impression of the people? Is this someone you want to get to know? What do you read in their facial expression? What type of life do they have? What is their level of income? Are they loveable? Approachable? Afraid? Shy? Confident?

Customers are reading your appearance and making assumptions based on their immediate impressions. Within just a few minutes you were able to come up with all kinds of assumptions, simply by glancing at each photo. Remember that every client is doing the same assessment of you.

Personal reflections are:

- fifty-five percent nonverbal
- thirty percent verbal
- seven percent words and phrases

When clients meet you for the first time, 55 percent of their reaction to you, positive or negative, is based on your nonverbal cues. They are looking at your clothes, body language, style, presence, charisma, attitude, facial features, hairstyle, makeup, accessories. Once clients have accepted your nonverbal cues, the next 38 percent of their response is based on your verbal skills and how you sound. The remaining 7 percent of their reaction to you is based on

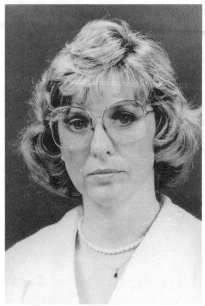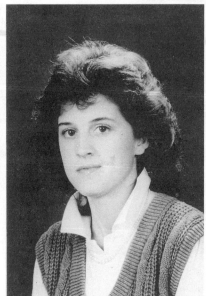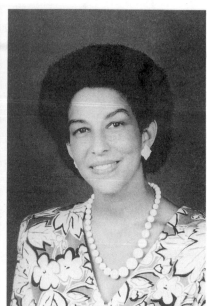

First Impressions.

your chosen words and phrases. Clients must feel comfortable and mentally accept the first two areas before a positive relationship can develop.

PERSONAL PACKAGING

Describe the image and impression you wish to transmit. If you are female, do you want to look: Sassy? Classy? Contemporary? Upbeat? Cute? Sexy? Casual? Regal? Romantic? Feminine? If you are male how do you want someone to describe your image? Sharp? Conservative? Hunky? Upper crust? Elegant? Trendy? Fashion forward? Country? Preppie?

My salon used to do referrals to an outstanding progressive salon in our town. Every time we would send new clients to the salon we would have to warn them. "Don't panic when you see the way they look. They won't do that to you unless you request it. Once you get past the initial impression you will see that any of the stylists can do a super job." The entire staff was talented, unique, and creative. The drawback at the time was that their appearance frequently shocked new clients. Their image erected invisible barriers. Why overcome more

obstacles than you have to? Why make business any harder than it has to be to begin with?

What is the first thing that flashes through your clients' minds as they sit in your chair and see you standing behind them? The panic question is, "Is the stylist going to make me look like he or she does?"

Have you ever had a day when you knew that you looked great? Good for you! Did the day seem to run smoother? Was it filled with energy and excitement? Did it feel as if you were hitting on all cylinders? The next section will uncover your personal packaging potential.

Ladies' Boutique

Clothes
The first goal for maximizing your personal packaging is to figure out what style, texture, shape, and color of clothing works best for your lifestyle and body type. If you are like most women, you are your own worst critic, practiced at picking apart the good and shredding the negative. Across the country you will find image and fashion consultants who specialize in creating a look and image that is perfect for you. Turn to a

professional for his or her well-trained eye and objectivity when designing your makeover and update. Many private consultations include clothing selection, defining body silhouettes, ideal textures and weights, color charting, even personal shopping. I know you may be saying to yourself that you know what you like and live to shop, but keep an open mind for the possibilities of someone helping pull your look together. It never hurts to have an objective opinion.

Wardrobe Building

Once you have the image direction, it's time to invest in building a suitable wardrobe. Using your budget and conscience as your guide you can start with a few basics and add to your new and improved wardrobe over the weeks and months ahead. Quality garments last from season to season. It is better to invest in a few pieces that will wear from year to year.

Correct Fit

Select clothing in your true size or even a little larger. Better-made clothing is more forgiving and generous in its sizing. Even expensive clothes that are too tight will look cheap and inexpensive. Don't read the labels for sizes if it hurts. Go for the proper fit and even beautiful bargains will look costly.

Comfy Casual Catastrophes

Clothes that are too casual weaken your visual authoritative position. Dressing overcasually will cut into your selling potential. If you are teasing tresses on the terrace of the Tropicana, modified casual clothes are not taboo. Other than that, save the shorts, T-shirts, sandals, beach wear, and barer-than-bare for vacations, not the store!

Solid Foundation

Match undergarments to your skin tone or clothing. Watch out for panty lines and patterned prints revealing a little too much. A properly fitting bra can take years off a body and make pounds disappear (almost as easily as shoulder pads). If necessary, secure bra straps to keep them from falling down on your shoulder.

Leg Up On the Competition

Legs should always be covered with stockings. Never show up on the floor with bare legs. If you live in a hot, humid climate, tote your hose to work with you and put them on when you arrive. Bare legs are great on the French Riviera, but if you plan to sell a lot of merchandise wear hose. Select hosiery colors in your exact skin tone or one matching the hemline of your skirt or slacks. Shy away from the suntan colors except for an exact match to your skin tone. Hose that are too dark or off tone will attract unwanted attention to your legs and feet.

A run in the hose leaves a sloppy impression and indicates that you are not paying attention to details. Clients can spot a run a mile off. If you are particularly hard on hose stash a few extra pairs in your tote bag or locker.

Set yourself up positively for the day from the inside out. Avoid grabbing hose with holes and little runs that may decide to creep down your leg inch by inch—that's better than spending the day wondering if the little run is traveling down your leg in view of others.

Fancy Footwear

If you work in the main salon and are around haircut leftovers, always wear closed-toe shoes. Hair clippings can work their way under the skin and cause serious and uncomfortable irritations. Keep shoes polished and looking their best. A simple trip to your favorite cobbler can add months and maybe even years of life to your shoes. Keep an ear out for "clickers." Clickers are the noise shoes make when the tiny, plastic heels have worn off and the metal rod in the heel is clicking and scraping on the concrete. For a couple of dollars a cobbler can eliminate the grating, irritating noise.

All That Glitters

Jewelry can be your trademark or statement maker. If your job requires that you lean over your customers, avoid any pieces that might clink and clank your client on the head. Pay attention to bracelets and earrings that make too much noise. Clinky jewelry might be fun for you to wear, but it is incredibly irritating to your client. Keep all jewelry sparkling clean and free of rough edges and pieces that could catch in the hair or scratch the skin.

Hygiene Highlights

After you complete your normal morning routine, don't forget to spritz on the deodorant, gargle with mouthwash, and dab on the cologne. Don't get carried away with the perfume; spritz low on the body around the ankles, knees, and waist. This allows the fragrance to travel up around the body instead of saturating the cologne at chest and neck level. Fragrance is a subtle finishing touch to your look, but be careful that you don't douse yourself in cologne.

Double check clothes for spots and if they need to be pressed or ironed. Linen may be fashionable wrinkled, but everything else needs a good pressing.

Coiffure Dos for You

I'm sure you have heard the old fable about the cobbler's kids never having shoes. How long has it been since you've had a makeover? Do you remember suffering from beauty school hair? Were all your friends trying out their new trade on your locks? You must set the example for your clients. They look to you for guidance. And they look at you to see if you follow your own advice. If you've been locked into one style for years, you can't expect your clients to be advocates of change, now can you? You must be the perfect example for healthy, shiny, stylish hair.

Skin Care

The skin is the largest organ of the body and often the most neglected. A monthly facial will brighten the skin, remove dead skin cell buildup, and help makeup go on smoother. And you deserve a little TLC too. Let someone else take care of you. Have your esthetician shape your eyebrows and remove any traces of facial hair.

Makeup

Over the years, the beauty business has bagged on a few celebrities who packed it all on, trying to hide a multitude of sins. Don't cover up, clear up any minor skin imperfection with a skin treatment. Schedule an appointment with a makeup artist to keep abreast of the latest face fashions. Get help selecting the best look for you. Face your clients knowing you look your absolute best.

Darling Digits

First select the length of nail that is comfortable and appropriate for your work. Keep the cuticles in condition so the rough edges don't get caught in the hair. No polish is better than chipped nail color any day of the week. The favorite of the rich

and famous is the French manicure for hassle-free nails. Try the French manicure for no fuss and no color-to-clothes matching.

Mirror, Mirror on the Wall

Before you walk out of the house every morning scrutinize your appearance. If any piece of clothing or jewelry jumps out at you as not quite right, take it off. As with everything in this life, the attention to the tiny, minute details will set you apart from your competition. Your challenge is to feel and dress like a ten every day. If you have on something that is making you uncomfortable and self-conscious take it off. Don't let your appearance sabotage your chance of making the sale. Remember that 55 percent of the client's reaction to you is based on your nonverbal signals.

Tales from the Dark Side

Years ago, a young girl about to graduate from beauty school called and scheduled an interview. I was finishing in the back of the salon while she filled out the application. When she completed the form, the salon coordinator informed me the applicant was ready and that I was in for a surprise. I was shocked when I walked into my office. She arrived for the interview wearing blue jeans; hiking boots; leg warmers; corduroy jacket with a heavy, furry lining; dirty, stringy hair; makeup that had to have been applied with a putty knife; and blue daggerlike nails.

My second thought after the shock wore off was that she had never had an interviewing class in school. But, upon questioning her, I discovered that just that week the entire class had gone through an interviewing and image workshop. She had? Not only was her attire inappropriate for the beauty business, but the salon's clientele would never react positively to her as an employee. Clients could not trust her for beauty tips based on her appearance. Maybe there is a salon she would have fit into, maybe in the rugged wilderness of Timbuktu, but even then the blue nails would have to go.

The Well-Dressed Man

Men have it easier than women in the morning. The ten-minute morning dash is common for men. Ten minutes from the time their feet hit the floor they can be showered, shaved, dressed, and heading for the door. Oh, to be so lucky. Here are a few powerful pointers for the well-dressed man.

Clothes

Select clothing appropriate for your age and body shape. Invest the time to assure you have properly fitting garments, if that means hemming, seaming, and tucking then by all means do so. One area to watch your waistband. Avoid the construction-worker syndrome where the drawers droop a little too far south.

A Wonderful World Full of Color

The color spectrum of men's clothing has widened over the past few years. Don't be afraid to add color to your wardrobe. If you feel you need some coaching hire the service of a professional color consultant. Invest in a color charting session. Properly charted, you are then armed with a wide array of wonderful colors to build into your life. Wearing the perfect color helps to brighten the eyes and skin. Color can be used to spice up a conservative collection of clothes.

Fit To Be Tied

Neck wear is a man's trademark. Ties can be statement makers, similar to the impact women's jewelry can make. Have fun with ties and try out new colors and patterns. By all means pack away ties that are too extreme or out of fashion.

Feet Beat

Shoes say a lot about the man. After a quick glance, many women scrutinize the condition of a man's shoes. Keep shoes polished and looking their best at all times. The style and condition of shoes reveal secrets and passions about the owner. You can always tell the characteristic and quality of a man by the condition of his shoes. A well-dressed man pays attention to his shoes.

Diamond Jim

Whether you're a man of simple pleasures or you prefer to emulate Diamond Jim Brady, select simple and smooth-around-the-edges jewelry. Keep a watchful eye for abrasive or rough edges that might get caught in the hair or scratch the skin.

Hair-Raising Tale

If you are sporting a beard or mustache, here is one critical rule: keep it trimmed so that you can see the faint trace of your lip edge. If your hair grows down and covers the lip edge, your communication is weakened. Many people read lips to reinforce what they are hearing. The power of your words and phrases is dramatically decreased if your lips are hidden. Keep the beard or mustache, but keep it trimmed and tidy.

Get Some Respect

People in the beauty business are always crying, "We need some respect. We are not taken seriously as professionals." Could the industry be sending mixed messages by saying one thing and dressing completely in the opposite manner? Keep in mind that you are in the beauty business, not the bizarre business. Look to the top leaders in this field. The really heavy hitters dress fashionably classic in a style that reveals taste and quality. The career you have chosen is selling hope, self-confidence, and image. You can't expect your clients to look great if you don't.

If you feel I am belaboring the image issue, take a good look around the next trade show you attend. How many attendants would you let style your hair or give you a facial, teach you makeup or do your nails based on their appearance?

The Morning After

Remember the photos you analyzed back on page 98? If you need a little inspiration, here's what an updated hairstyle, makeup, and image consultation can create. (Figs. 9.1–9.3)

Your image is a silent language. It has the power to communicate to everyone around you. Your image will speak louder than your words. Your potential is catapulted if your image reveals a polished, confident and capable professional who practices what you preach.

THIRTY-EIGHT PERCENT VERBAL SKILLS

In the last section, we covered the effects your appearance has on your level of success. In this section, you and I will concentrate on the next 38 percent of the image pie—your voice and sound quality. (Fig. 9.4, p. 104)

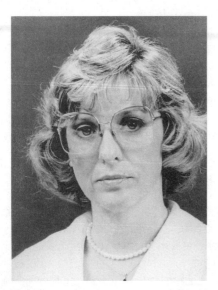

Fig. 9.1a Before. "Wanted to get rid of the frumpy look." When she came into the salon she looked at the carpet the entire time with one hand on the front door, just in case she had to bolt.

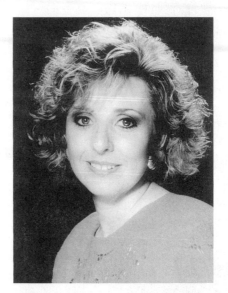

Fig. 9.1b After. What a transformation. This shy, insecure woman went to work for me in the salon. Her confidence sprang forth and she handled herself beautifully. She glowed. What a jewel.

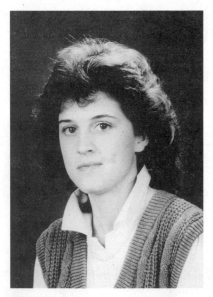

Fig. 9.2a Before. She came to us because she was having trouble at work. She was not taken seriously. At twenty-four, her school-girl image deflated her authority faster than a pin in a balloon.

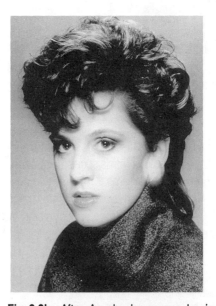

Fig. 9.2b After. As a bank manager, her image needed to carry some weight. By the way, she became engaged after the "After," but I won't take total credit for that development.

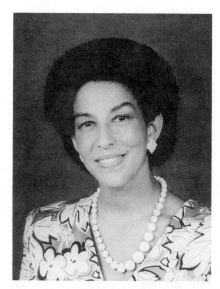

Fig. 9.3a Before. Typical look, plagued with round lines. Her bubble hairstyle hid her beautiful features and dramatic personality.

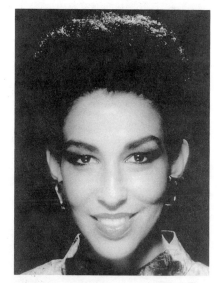

Fig. 9.3b After. Her husband was extremely stylish. When we completed her makeover, he didn't talk to her for a few days. Finally, he came around and admitted he was used to receiving all the attention and he didn't know how to deal with his wife's new look.

If you were a fan of the *Family Ties* television sitcom, you may have seen the episode where Mike Sievers was at a high school dance. A cute, young blonde caught his roving eye. He worked up his courage to ask her to dance. As he was holding her close and basking in the moment, she decided to talk to him. Out of her perfectly made-up mouth burst forth a most amazing voice. It was high-pitched, whiny, shrill, incredibly irritating, and shredded Mike's perception of the perfect woman. Poor Mikey and anyone else within earshot.

The client's window of information grows as you speak. When you open your mouth to speak you either confirm or deny your nonverbal language. Your image pie has a hundred pieces. You are adding to or subtracting from their impressions of you as soon as your words flow forth. You either support or undermine the client's perception of you. How do you sound? Is your voice weak? Loud? Hard? Tense? Monotonous? Nasal? Shrill? Colorless? Irritating? Pleasant and easy to listen to? Do you have a voice someone could listen to all day?

If your voice sounds soft and timid, the client's perception is naturally one of timidity and passivity. If your voice is hoarse and rough they may be taken aback at the roughness of your image. If your voice is authoritative, knowledgeable, and commanding it will then be easier to build trust and rapport with your clients.

The first piece of information to digest is that you hear a different voice than the one your clients, friends, and loved ones listen to every day. You are hearing your voice as it echoes through your head. Others have the advantage of hearing the tone and quality as it is directly transmitted to them, through the air and through their ears. Have you ever heard yourself on a tape recorder? My guess is that you proudly announced, "That doesn't sound like me." And everyone else listening to the tape swore: "You sound just like that."

A very important building block in your selling success sequence is how you sound to your clients. Many people take their speech and voice for granted. Many actually abuse their

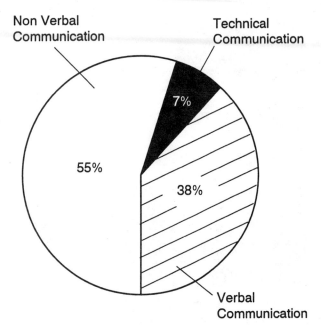

Non Verbal Communication

Technical Communication

7%

55%

38%

Verbal Communication

Fig. 9.4   Image pie.

vocal apparatuses. Irritants such as cigarettes, alcohol, caffeine, and poor nutrition can take their toll on your voice.

As a communicator, you must be aware that the sound of your voice can produce a physical effect and response in the listener.

- The chances of increasing their adrenaline flow increase in direct proportion to the rate of speech.
- Notice the subtle changes if you are talking softly and calmly. You can see the body physically responding as it slows and calms down.
- Yelling at someone may cause their blood pressure to rise.
- Talking rapidly can make the customer's respiration quicken. Their breathing will become shallow and high in the chest.

Your voice indicates your overall emotional state. Your voice will mirror your levels of fatigue. And your voice will reflect your stress levels. Many of these physical changes will be noticeable in the voice before they surface anywhere else in the body.

Breath of Life

You can go days without food and water, but only seconds without oxygen. All too often we overlook the natural rhythm of life, the invisible life support system. You do not need much air to speak well, but what you do with the air is critical to your speaking voice.

You must begin by learning proper breathing techniques to build a strong voice. Before developing a powerful voice you must evaluate your breathing techniques. Don't chuckle and say, "I must be doing it right, I'm still alive." A multitude of factors inhibit proper breathing, putting a strain on the body and, subsequently, on the voice.

Breath Observation Challenge

Sit on the floor with your legs straight in front of you or in a full or half lotus yoga position. The goal of this exercise is to concentrate on your breathing. First, block out all intruding thoughts and simply concentrate on the flow of oxygen. Feel the air flow through your nose and imagine a single molecule of air traveling down inside you into the lungs and diaphragm. Imagine every cell of your body filling with needed life-giving particles. As you exhale, allow the carbon dioxide and all the impurities to leave your body.

The real challenge is to focus on your breathing for one full minute. Inhale and exhale at your normal pace. Concentrate on the flow of air. If a barrage of intruding thoughts crashes in on your exercise, reset the clock and begin again. The challenge is to concentrate on your breathing for a full, uninterrupted sixty seconds.

Is it tough to do? You bet! Awareness is half the battle, and you have spent a few minutes focusing your energy on proper breathing. Congratulations! If you couldn't keep the focus, don't despair. Keep trying over the next few days and feel your progress. Focus on blocking out those intruding thoughts. Investing a few minutes each day will payoff in strengthening proper breathing practices.

NOTE: If you are having difficulty tuning out the thoughts try this exercise. Imagine your thoughts are a parade and you are merely an observer. You are sitting on the shady side of the street and simply watching the parade pass you by. This allows you to remove yourself from the barrage of thoughts. Once you see yourself on the sidelines watching the parade, physically turn away from the parade so you are facing another direction. With this subtle shift, you are in control of your thoughts. So, instead of totally tuning them out and struggling, you are allowing them to pass without being involved. Now, you can return your focus to your breathing.

Wave of Relaxation
Stress takes its toll on the body in many ways. It may be zapping you of much-needed energy and fuel for facing the day. Try this tense-and-hold technique for relieving tension and stress in the body.

Lie flat on the floor on a blanket or exercise mat. Wiggle out and take ownership of the spot. Take a few seconds to get comfortable. Place your hands alongside your torso with palms up. Make sure your legs or ankles are not crossed. Imagine your body is pure liquid and it is being poured onto the floor.

Now, tense up your entire body and remain in that position for five seconds. Scrunch and contract every muscle possible. Feel the tightness and compacted energy as you intentionally tense up your body. Scrunch and relax. Notice the wave of relaxation as you uncurl. Repeat the scrunch for eight seconds and relax five times in total.

Second Wave
Now that you are lying flat on the floor start by concentrating on your feet and toes. Just tense up the feet and toes and hold for five seconds, then relax. Moving up the body repeat this process traveling to the calves, thighs, stomach, buttocks, chest, shoulders, arms, hands and, finally, the face. Repeat the full-body tense, hold for eight seconds, and relax. Take five and lie there a few minutes longer and sink into the floor. Allow your body to feel as if it weighs a ton. Remain in the dead man's pose for as long as your schedule permits. You should be feeling the wave of relaxation wash across your body. Learn to let go of the stress and tension that is harboring itself in your physical temple.

Relaxing is critical to your general health and well-being. Another benefit is that your voice will relax too.

Breathing and Posture
Through the course of time, men and women have been forced to constrict, contract, and suck in every muscle. The result is bad breathing practices due to fashion and grooming dictums. Young women are coached to stand up straight, shoulders back but tucked under, the stomach held in. Young military men are drilled to perfect ramrod straight posture. Shoulder level, chest out, head straight, eyes forward. I get tired just thinking about the drills. Proper breathing techniques lead to good posture, which leads to good speech, which results in great communication. Remember, selling is communication and communication is selling.

To breathe properly while standing, your feet should be shoulder-width apart and your weight distributed evenly. Keep your head raised to eye level. Elongate the expanse from your clavicle to your stomach. If you are in a sitting position, sit up straight. The only part of your back that should touch the chair is the lower part. Sit with feet planted firmly on the floor, leaving your hands free to gesture.

The Posture Challenge: Book Walk
Remember watching *Romper Room* as a child? The best exercise was when the children placed a book or basket on their heads and marched around the room to the music. The tune went something like, "See me walk so straight and tall. I won't let my basket fall." So take out a hardback book. Place it on the flat of your head and see how long you can parade around keeping the book from crashing to the floor.

Voice Communication

Proper breathing and positive posturing are the support network for powerful voice communication. Before we get into the how tos and what to dos for excellent voice communication, you will need to make a tape recording of your voice. You will use this audio tape frequently throughout this section. Take a few minutes and follow the guideline for making your tape.

Sound Checks
Begin by making three samples of your voice, approximately two to three minutes in length. The samples are to be recorded at different times during the day.

1. Sound Check One. Tape your voice first thing in the morning. This early-bird tape registers your voice when you are relaxed and fresh from a good night's sleep.

2. Sound Check Two. Record early afternoon. Many factors by now will influence your natural speaking voice.
3. Sound Check Three. This session is to be scheduled in the late evening when you're relaxed, but not too sleepy.

Record normal conversations, phone calls, treatment procedures, talking yourself through your morning makeup. Any comfortable dialogue is fine.

Once you have captured your three sound checks go back over the tape and tune into the subtle differences between the three times of day. Is there a dramatic difference between them? Do they all sound close in range? Good!

Now that you have gotten used to hearing your true voice it's time to add to your sound check tape. Read the following samples. Don't try to change your voice for this exercise. Speak as you normally do at this time. Don't force yourself to project a "speaking voice." To receive the maximum benefit from this challenge simply be yourself and experience each Sound Check.

Questioning

- What type of look do you desire?
- What can I do for you today?
- How did you find out about our salon?
- What is your favorite color?
- Do you prefer a cream or frost lipstick?
- Do you like dark or light colors?
- What kind of change did you have in mind?
- What problem are you having with your hair?

Self-Pep Talk

Today is the perfect day to capture all my possibilities. This day is filled with golden opportunities to service my clients. I will be abundantly rewarded for my talents and knowledge. I will not waste a single minute of today. I will use my gifts and talents to help people explore their image, needs and desires.

Dialogue Directions

"The easiest way to find the salon is to take First Avenue to Third Street. At the stop light, make a right onto Third and proceed one and a half miles. Turn left on Beauty Lane and make an immediate right into our driveway. Parking is in the back. Our address is 333 Beauty Lane."

Now, hold on to the tape. You will be referring back to it shortly.

Power Voicing

Quality Control

Monitor your voice quality. Your voice is as unique as your fingerprints. No one sounds like you do. Millions of Americans engage in what speech pathologists call "voice suicide" by striving to throw their voice. They are trying to sound macho, sexy, authoritative, provocative, unnatural. Throwing your voice can cause severe, sometimes irreparable, damage. The quality control goal is to polish your natural voice. The remaining sections will give you pointers for polishing the true voice.

Five components of a great voice are:

1. Vocal structure. Your speaking mechanisms make up the natural voice. These include the size of your larynx and length and width of your vocal cords.
2. Sound chamber. As you speak, the sound bounces through your throat and sinus cavities and then out of the mouth. Proper breathing, remaining relaxed and open allows the sound a freer and expanded area to bounce around in.
3. Breath supply. Earlier in the section, we covered several breathing techniques. It is a natural reflex to tighten up, tense up, and even hold your breath if you become nervous or upset. Don't signal to your customer you are nervous by holding your breath. You should guard against holding your breath for obvious reasons, but also because it constricts your riverlike flow of emotions and words. You may not even be aware of when you are holding your breath; ask friends and family members to point it out to you.
4. Stressful stranglers. Stress affects the body in a multitude of ways, one being your voice. Stress constricts and prohibits clear open sounds from coming forth. If you hold your stress inward you are cutting off an easy and open flow of words and phrases. Words stem from thoughts. Thoughts stem from emotion. Stress puts a damper on the smooth and natural flow. Your voice will tip you off when under simple or exaggerated levels of stress.

5. General well-being. A powerful and healthy body can produce a powerful voice. Your total health and well-being will support your effort to enhance the quality of your voice.

Six Quality Killers

1. Speed. Talking too fast or too slowly for the listener will hinder the perceived quality of your communication.
2. Dullsville. Monitor your voice for dull, lifeless sound. Pay particular attention when you frequently have to repeat phrases. Avoid the "Attention, K-Mart Shoppers" syndrome. When your job requires repetitive phrases make sure your voice reveals your enthusiasm, even if you've had to say the same thing twenty times that day. You may be tired of saying something, but the information is new to your client. A dull, lifeless voice doesn't carry passion or conviction.
3. Monotone. Johnny One Note sounds as if most of his vocabulary went through the take-me-to-your-leader school of communication. Listen to your tape to hear any colorless, monotonous projections. Keep an ear out for flat lines in your presentation. People want to hear a range of sound and syllables.
4. Rigid Reflex. Guard against holding your neck and shoulders in a rigid, inflexible posture. Relax your neck and shoulders and allow the sounds to move up and out.
5. Nasality. Talking through your nose instead of allowing the sounds to come clearly and openly through the mouth. Remember Ernestine the telephone operator? Lily Tomlin played this character with a nasal sound.

   To find out if you have a problem with nasality pinch your nose with the thumb and index finger and repeat this sentence: "I am mining for gold in Madagascar." If you felt a slight twinge on the N, M, or NG sounds that is okay. You will have a slight degree of nasal tones on words that contain N, M, or NG. Now try, "I am a success magnet." You should have only felt the tingle on *magnet*. Nasality is easy to correct. Simply open your mouth and allow the complete sound to travel from the emotion center, up your throat, and out of the mouth. Don't pinch the sound off at the nose. Speak clearly and articulate the sounds.
6. Breathiness. Long ago, someone stressed the fact that if your voice had a "whisper" tone to it, it was considered sexy. I was attending a convention when a beautifully attired woman stood to make a presentation. Everything was in place; her hair, makeup, nails, suit, Cartier lapel pin, briefcase, everything. She had a dramatic, powerful image. She must have been extremely successful in her company. Then she opened her mouth. She had commanded the group's attention with her nonverbal appearance, but when she "whooooosed" out her first few words the crowd was completely taken aback. Her breathy approach to relating her report left us all dismayed and confused. Due to the mixed signal the group did not know if they could accept her information.

   If you catch yourself sounding breathy, merely cast the sound forward, forcing it past your teeth.

   In Figure 9.5 you'll find some names. Can you hear the voices that go with them?

Perfect Pitch

Pitch is the natural highness or lowness of sound. Clients and coworkers will form judgments and opinions about you, based on your voice, with startling accuracy. Speech researchers claim that your socioeconomic background, status, age, attitude, and trustworthiness are detected in your pitch.

1. Voice Inflections. When you want to signal to the listener that you have completed your thought, your voice should come down at the end of the sentence. "This color looks great." Period. End of sentence. You are making a declaration or statement. Raising your voice at the end of a sentence signals that you are posing a question. "This color looks great?" You are now signaling your indecisiveness and lack of authority.

   In the selling chapter, you will learn the strategy for asking proper questions. At this time, I just want you to monitor your voice for rising inflections. When you do leave the sentence lofting in the air, it's as if you are waiting for the listener to grab hold and validate your statement, as if you were not sure of your statement before you began.
2. Singsong Voices. Hum a few bars of Neil Diamond's classic hit "Song Sung Blue."

   As you were singing, did you feel your voice shift up and down with the melody? Singsong voices travel up and down the scale as if they were dancing along instead of

---

Famous Great Voices

Katherine Hepburn	Sir Lawrence Olivier
Lauren Bacall	Ronald Coleman
Franklin Roosevelt	Frank Sinatra

Distinctive Voices

Robin Leach	Cary Grant
Jimmy Durante	Bing Crosby
W.C. Fields.	Mae West
Paul Harvey	

Fig. 9.5   Voices you remember.

trying to communicate effectively with the client. Keep your voice from playing connect the dots or follow the bouncing ball. It may be lyrical, but a singsong voice is difficult to take for a long period.

3. Monotonous. The opposite of singsong is monotony. This is where every word comes out at the same pitch. Flash back to a teacher, preacher, or professor who had one tone and level of voice. Boring! The voice reflects the inner being. It is as if there is no passion or life force stroking the flames of communication.

Find Your Perfect Pitch

CHALLENGE: Go back to your sound-check audio tape and listen to the section on questioning. Listen to your rate of speech. Are you zipping along? Is your voice rising at the end of each question? Are you suffering from monotony murder?

You will have a natural range. As the voice becomes stressed and filled with tension the vocal cords tighten up. This causes the vocal cords to vibrate faster than normal. As you work in your natural rhythm, your relaxed state allows the vocal cords to be relaxed too. The less strain on your voice produces a lower, more comfortable sound.

Prime Rate

Listen to the speed of your speech. Does it zip along quickly? Do you run out of air before finishing a thought? Is your speed slow and predictable? Do your words run together? Can you clearly understand every word? Do you pause for emphasis or to punctuate a point?

The average person speaks at 130 to 160 words per minute (wpm). Fast talkers average 160 to 200 wpm or as one of my favorite presenters, Zig Zigler, exuberantly declared, "I can talk with gusts up to 200 miles per hour." Someone just dragging along will average 110 to 130 wpm.

CHALLENGE: Get out your sound-check tape and listen to the questions and self-pep talk—in total around 120 words. Can you understand each word? Do you get a rhythm from listening? Is the voice level acceptable and clear? Time yourself against the averages I have given.

Also remember that the speed of your speech is often determined by geographical factors and personality. The best test is your observation of the listener. Are you boring the client (too slow)? Are you hard to understand (too fast)?

Eloquent Enunciation

Power voices practice sharpening their articulation. They practice the distinctiveness of individual sounds. As you listen to yourself on tape do you hear sloppy diction? Words like "gonna," "didchawanna," "warsh?" Sloppy or lazy diction can lead to one or more of the following problems.

Substitution. Listen for instances where you may have altered the real word.

- "gonna" for "going to"
- "jest" for "just"
- "warsh" for "wash"
- "git" for "get"

Subtraction. Sounds or syllables left out.

- "suprise" for "surprise"
- "probbly" for "probably"

Addition. Adding letters and syllables.

- "ath-a-lete" instead of "athlete"
- "bee-yoo-tee-full" for "beautiful"
- "seg-a-ment" for "segment"

Role Reversal. Transposing sounds.

- "preform" for "perform"
- "interduce" for "introduce"

Now I am sure you do not wish to sound stuffy and pompous, but don't let lazy lips sink your selling ship. Learn to enunciate your words clearly. Leave no room for missed communication.

CHALLENGE: Go back to the tape, and this time listen to the direction section. Could you find a salon simply by listening to your voice? Are you clear and succinct? Do your words run together and sound like mush? Have you sufficiently paused for emphasis?

Repeat the Dialogue Direction with Emphasis

"The easiest way to find the salon is to take First Avenue/ to/ Third Street. At the stop light make a right/ onto/ Third/ and proceed one and a half miles. Turn left/ on Beauty Lane and make an immediate/ right/ into our driveway. Parking is in the back. Our address is 333 Beauty Lane."

Volume Control

Monitor your volume. Do people seem to lean forward as you speak as if they can't hear you? Or do they lean way back to put some distance between you and their eardrums? Are you frequently asked to speak up or repeat what you said?

You must learn to control the volume. Ignoring the volume of your voice may force clients to switch you off, tune you out, and turn their attentions to something or someone else. Manipulate the environment for maximizing the conversation.

- Shut open doors to block out excess noise.
- Turn off any machine not in use.
- Physically move closer to the client.
- Talk directly to the client.
- Channel your voice purposefully into the telephone receiver.

CHALLENGE: Time to listen to your sound checks. This time listen to the overall clarity, quality, pitch, rate of speech, and volume.

A strong, powerful voice is a valuable asset. It is essential to match your voice with your nonverbal communication sig-

nals. Remember your personal communication success formula— 55/ 38/ 7 equals 100 percent success opportunities.

Power Voicing Do's and Don'ts

So far we have covered what your image and voice represent. Now is the perfect time to tackle the remaining 7 percent in the communication formula—your words and phrases. In this section you will receive fine-tuning tips for packing your presentation with added punch.

The words and phrases you choose to use will sustain and hold the client's previous image perceptions. The client has already formed 93 percent of his/her impression about you, even before tuning into what you are saying. Good communication attracts clients to you.

Burning with Emotions

Imagine, if you will, that you are an old-fashioned potbellied stove, the kind where you have to throw logs of firewood into the belly of the stove. The logs ignite from the still embers and catch fire. The smoke then rises through the pipe chimney and puffs out of the top.

Your words travel in the same path as our burning logs. The stomach is considered the center of emotions. The force then sends the energy or the sounds up through the throat. Then out of the mouth the spoken word flows.

Pick a subject you are really passionate about—food, travel, cars, clothes, whatever. Notice how exciting and easy it is to talk about your passion. The passion or conviction of your words fans the flames of emotion. An open, free-flowing channel of communication is formed. Don't allow the garbage of negative emotions to cloud up the signals.

Now, think of a really difficult topic to discuss. The death of a loved one, a broken heart, an employee confrontation. Do you instantly feel your stomach beginning to churn? Notice how constricted you feel on the inside just thinking about this difficult topic. Notice how much harder it is to get the words out. The passion and conviction are significantly weaker than when speaking about your favorite subject.

Good communication is keeping the emotional source open and uncluttered. The entire channel must have the energy and clarity to put forth your words and feelings.

True, honest communication comes from deep within the soul. Have you ever talked with someone and you just knew they were blowing smoke? This is the basis for people believing in you, your image, and your advice.

CHALLENGE: Take out the sound-check tape again and this time listen to the self-pep talk. You should be able to hear the conviction of your words as you read the copy. Do you believe what you hear? Do the words come from the soul? Would you believe the person you are listening to is sincere?

Don'ts

1. Offensive comments. Guard against stereotypical phrases and offensive language. You will alienate your listener as fast as the words leave your mouth. This rule goes for potentially touchy jokes too.
2. Overkill on the apology meter. Listen to yourself. Do you apologize for every little thing? Does your body withdraw so you physically appear to take up less space? The next time you are in a restaurant and are waited on by someone in the fifteen to eighteen age range, tune in and listen to their apologies. I am truly concerned for these youths as they try to fit into their career fields in the next couple of years. They are easy prey for someone to walk all over them, due to their verbal insecurities.
3. Smiles. Of course you want to smile but constantly grinning and looking like the cat that swallowed the canary plants seeds of deception and insecurity in the client's mind. Women naturally smile easier than men. Unfortunately they have a tendency to smile more frequently when under stress. Men, however, smile defensively, as an act of separation. Genuine heartwarming smiles are great, but be cautious in overproducing the cheesy grins.
4. Hedging. Hedges are waving the flag of insecurity. "I don't want to make waves but..." "You may not agree with me, but...." "I'm not certain." "I may be wrong." "Gee, I'm not sure." If you are not sure, shut up. Get the facts first. Believe in what you are saying as you make your statement. When you preface your statement with a hedge, the client will automatically discount whatever you have to say.

5. Fillers. Well, people are guilty, you know, of puffing their phrases, uh, when they feel, like you know, they have to talk all the time or fill space. Use pauses, but don't fill your sentences with uh, you know, like fillers.
6. Tie downs. Tie downs resemble a caboose on a train; they bring an end to the sentence. Tags or tie downs are questions added to a statement. "Your skin looks great, doesn't it?" You are seeking an affirmation to your statement. This is good when used to close a sale.

   Women tend to use tags for validation in conversation. "The sky is blue, don't you think?" As if you can't look up into the sky and figure this one out all by yourself. The voice will go up the scale and slide into a high pitch to make sure the listener knows it's a question. This power voicing glitch is a killer to the true professional and will appear to make you sound dumb and insecure.
7. Cluttered communication. Don't be a rambling Rose or Roy. If necessary jot down a few notes to keep you on track with your presentation, dialogue, speech, whatever. Remain focused on the topic at hand and lead the customer through the process.
8. "I'll try." Does that mean you will or won't? I'll try is weak. Either you will or you won't. It's either yes or no.
9. Do not take it upon yourself to reduce a client's name—Suzanne to Suzy to Suz, Christine to Christy to Chris, James to Jimmy to Jim, Charles to Chuck.
10. No endearments. Do not use any of the following: honey, hon, toots, babe, doll, dear, dearie, handsome, sweetie, cutie pie. Save the flowery words of endearment for your loved ones not your clients.
11. Avoid insider's jargon. Keep your language simple, direct, and to the point. Select well-chosen words, free of industry lingo. Keep your language from becoming too complicated when explaining service and products.

Do's

1. Avoid gender-based pronouns. Eliminate gender phrases from your vocabulary. "Okay guys lets get down to work." "Now guys, you know it's time to get serious about sales quotas." Don't exclude staff and clients by using male directives.

Old Lingo	New Lingo
Businessman	Business People
Chairman	Chairperson, Chair
Fellow Worker	Coworker
Employees and their Wives	Employees and Spouses
Housewives	Homemakers
Man-hours	Work Hours
Manpower	Work Force
Salesman	Salespeople

2. Use parallel words. Men/women. Ladies/gentlemen. Boys/girls. Guys/gals.

3. Call others by the name they offer you. If the client tells you her name is Mrs. Smith, then by all means call her Mrs. Smith until she acknowledges any differently. She has indicated a formal greeting until she feels comfortable with you or maybe she prefers to be called by her married name.

4. Powerful communication is inclusive. Add others into your conversation as appropriate. Don't ignore the person sitting next to you pretending not to listen; include them in the activity.

5. Talk directly to the client. Refrain from looking at the floor or to the left or right of the client. Focus all your attention directly to the client. They are the most important person in your life at that time.

6. Pack your presentation with punch. Learn to add punch and power to your words. Try this exercise. Read the following sentence normally. Then read it again punching the one word underlined.

> The man robbed the bank.
> The man robbed the bank.
> The man robbed the bank.
> The man robbed the bank.
> The man robbed the bank.
> The man robbed the bank.

What message was conveyed as you read the sentence the first time? Did you hear the different meaning as you read and punched each sentence? Carefully place your punch to emphasize a point.

7. Pause for the cause. I remember a close friend's mother commenting on how late her boyfriend stayed one evening. "Gee, Mom, I'm sorry. Did the noise keep you up?" Her mom chuckled and replied, "It wasn't the noise. It was the silence that bothered me."

Silence generally makes most people uncomfortable. Yet, used in selling, silence can be a valuable asset. Make your statement or declaration, share your advice, then pause. Allow the client to digest the information before you launch into more dialogue. Use pauses to accentuate your statement.

8. Practice and rehearse. You must be organized and comfortably prepared. Tape record your sales presentation before you try it out on a client. Don't rely on just thinking on your feet lest you get caught with your foot in your mouth.

If after going through this complete chapter and listening to your tapes, you feel you would like additional help in the voice department, hire a voice coach. Look in your Yellow Pages or call the speech and performing arts department at your local university or college and ask for voice coach referrals. You may not need years or even months of voice therapy but a well-trained ear can design a personal program for building a powerful voice.

It may be hard to imagine that your image and what you say can have such an impact on your success and the way clients respect you, but they do. This was a hard chapter for me to write because I didn't want to offend you or make you uncomfortable, but I want you to be able to accomplish all you desire. If your image, voice, and vocabulary are holding you back, I hope you have the courage to make some changes. The rewards will speak for themselves.

You are the most important element in your success formula. When you invest in yourself you can't go wrong. Ben Franklin is noted for his sage advice that "If you empty the coins of your pocketbook into knowledge, they never go wasted."

CHAPTER 10
PERSONALITY SELLING

Have you ever been in a conversation with someone and things just clicked? Were you so in tune with each other that you could practically finish each other's sentences? Similarly, have there been times when you struggled to establish some kind of connection with a person and there was no way you could get through?

This chapter is the foundation for understanding yourself as well as your customers. You may learn every sales dialogue in this book, but if you fail to understand what makes people tick, your success will fall short of your true potential. Learning to build rapport with your customers is essential to your success.

The biggest mistake you can make in communication is to assume that other people think the way you do. Personality selling is taking the responsibility for understanding and learning about others—how they think, feel, and project themselves. Once you build your understanding you can then respond to other people in their "language." The best compliment a client can give you is to say, "My stylist really understands me. He talks my language!"

I am not trying to lump people into a few categories. Over the last twelve years, I have relied heavily on personality selling to build my success. Have fun with this section of the book. I have presented this information all across America and I always get the same response from the audience: "Where has this information been all my life?" "If I only knew this stuff sooner, I would have known how to handle Mrs. So and So." "Finally, a system for selling and dealing with the public."

Imagine one hundred finely tuned baby grand pianos neatly lined up in a huge empty auditorium. You slowly walk up to one of the pianos and with the skill of a true virtuoso strike a note, any note. Within seconds the other ninety-nine pianos start to reverberate as a result of the energy. The ninety-nine pianos tune in with the first one.

The goal of this chapter is to broaden your people skills, to provide you with the ability to tune into other people's personalities. Of course, you will sell more product and service after internalizing and incorporating the information into your daily life. These skills will make you a better salesperson, friend, spouse, parent because you have made the effort to understand and get to know the people around you.

OBSERVING BODY LANGUAGE

The door swung open and into the salon walked a young woman. She inched her way in, took two steps, and made a beeline straight for the chair in the reception area. Her shoulders were hunched. Her head was drooping so low that her chin touched her chest. Her eyes were cast downward. Within a few seconds her arms wrapped around her waist, clutching herself as if to hold on for dear life. I didn't recognize her and she didn't have an appointment. She apparently had never been into my salon.

I approached her cautiously and gently. Her body language told me that I had to treat her with kid gloves. She resembled a scared, skittish doe in the thick of the forest. This client sought out the salon to help her hirsutism problem. The excessive hair growth on her chin and throat triggered the young woman's body movement and expressions.

Reading body language is the ability to observe and translate body movements. Body language should be read as a series of actions; it should not be dissected movement by movement. It should be read like an entire sentence for human animation, not word for word or action for action.

Four Areas of Personal Space

Everyone has a comfort zone or personal territory, an instinctive distance we allow others.

The big top helps to paint the picture of personal space. The lion tamer understands its importance. Flash back to a time when you have seen the daring man enter the cage with six roaring, hungry lions staring directly at him. The lion tamer can control the situation by respecting the lions' personal space.

The lion tamer cracks the whip, and the lion, on cue, advances toward the tamer. He cracks the whip again and the lion stops. The lion retreats when the tamer starts walking toward it, reversing the action. As if by instinct the lion backs up just until it feels threatened due to the invasion of its personal space. The lion then starts to lunge forward. As soon as the lion tamer backs out of the lion's space, the lion stops in its tracks. The lion stops because the tamer has removed himself from the lion's personal space.

Due to the very intimate nature of the beauty and fashion goods and service business, you will be dancing through personal space with every customer you meet. Understanding, respecting, and learning how to maneuver through it can and will make your customer feel more at ease.

Dr. Edward T. Hall, a professor of anthropology, in his book *Silent Language* stated that there are four defined areas of personal space: public, social, personal, and intimate. Each area has a far and close range.

Public Space

Far public space is when you are twenty-five feet or more from others. Notice the Secret Service and the distance they put between their charges and the public. Notice the distance between the professional public speaker and the rest of the people on the platform. (Fig. 10.1a)

Zoos and animal parks have observed the far public space theory, mostly for the safety of the animals and the public. Have you noticed what happens when you get a little too close to the cages at the zoo? The animals usually back up, retreat, and then hightail it to a remote area of the cage.

Close public space is twelve to twenty-five feet. Close public space guidelines are utilized when you give formal speeches and make presentations from a designated platform. Speakers position themselves twelve to twenty-five feet from the first row of the audience.

Social Space

Far social space is seven to twelve feet. That's the big boss's desk or work area. They say you can judge the boss's ego by the size of the office or work space. Big bosses never want to get too close. They like to keep their distance, maintain their objectiveness. Have you ever heard one say that they needed to back away from something to get a better view of the problem? (Fig. 10.1b)

Close social space is four to seven feet, which is the general "business" distance we keep from someone. This is the acceptable business distance. Unfortunately most salons are set up so that the stations are practically overlapping each other. At this safe business distance we are already crowding the client, by minimizing the social space.

Personal Space

Your far personal space is two and a half to four feet. Here, you "keep someone at arm's length." A perfect example of far personal space is when two men meet on the street. They'll shake hands or maybe even embrace, then automatically step back two feet or more as if to be free. (Fig. 10.1c)

Close personal space is one and a half to two and a half feet. This is when you're still close enough to hold or grasp your partner's hand. Picture a couple huddled over dinner.

Intimate Space

Most beauty services are conducted within this range. If you jump directly to this level of closeness you jeopardize making your client feel uncomfortable and possibly squeamish. Take a few minutes to warm up to the client, especially new customers. Many clients are insecure and self-conscious visiting a beauty salon. Forcing the client into close physical space can be threatening (like the lion) and intimidating to some customers. (Fig. 10.1d)

Warm clients up with general conversation while they are seated in the reception area. Spend a few minutes consulting with the client before caping and draping. It's best to take a

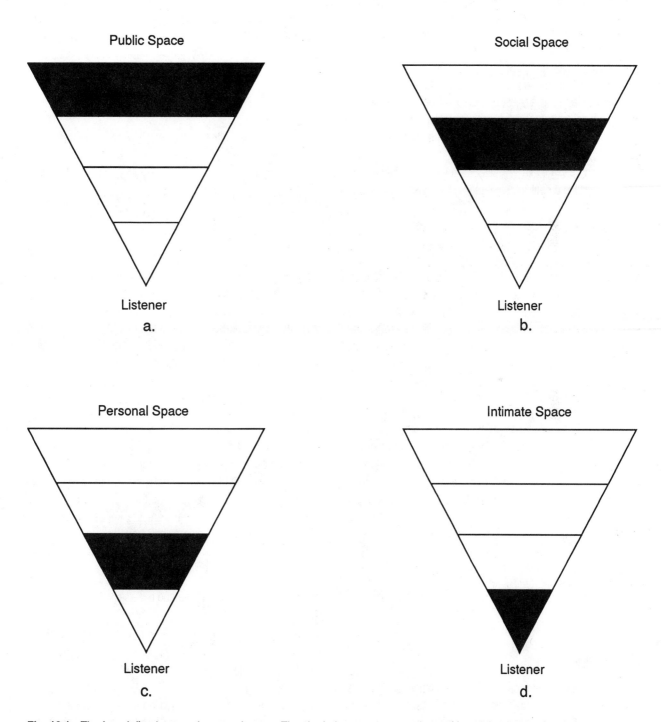

Fig. 10.1 The four defined areas of personal space. The shaded area represents the position of the speaker in relation to the listener.

new client to a private consultation room to maneuver through the personal space boundaries.

Far intimate space is six to eighteen inches. You notice the closeness, but you are not touching. Picture an elevator. At every floor the elevator stops and people get on. As the elevator fills up with people, do you feel yourself tensing up, standing straighter and more rigid? As the elevator jams with people your personal space shrinks and becomes restricted. Your body posture becomes more rigid so as not to invade other people's space.

Notice how clients will select alternating chairs in the lobby. They skip a seat to avoid getting too close to someone already seated.

Close intimate space is about as close as you can get because it is actual physical contact. For example: a kiss on the hand, peck on the cheek, or big bear hug. Every salon service requires some form of physical contact. Be cautious about lunging right in there. Beauty industry people are naturally caring and expressive people. Give the client time to ease into the togetherness. Your ability to ease clients through the personal space boundaries will help them to feel comfortable, which results in a positive reaction to the salon visit.

Universal Expressions

In any culture, in any language, there are similar ways of expressing emotions strictly through body language—universal languages of love, excitement, fear, sadness, shame, respect, joy, surprise, distress, and disgust. You could express these emotions without speaking the native tongue. Take a moment, stand in front of a mirror, and act out each of the universal expressions. The objective is to notice the subtleties, mannerisms, and gestures you use to express yourself without saying a single word. Of course, every culture has its own set of acceptable nonverbal behaviors, but these ten are universal.

Body Moves

Remember earlier when you read that body languages are like sentences and not like single words? Well, let's take a look at the different body regions that speak volumes on their own, starting from top to bottom.

Head

Is it sitting square on the shoulders ready to face the world? Is it slightly tilted to the left or to the right (as if questioning or pondering)? Is it dropped forward as in hopelessness or thrown back as in disgust?

Torso

Are the shoulders straight (good posture), slumped (burdened), angled like a seesaw (back may be out), rounded forward (given up hope), or are they being shrugged (I don't know)? Is the torso leaning in toward you (eager, ready), or is the torso leaning away (are you talking too loudly, putting distance between you)?

Arms

Are they hanging loose and down to the side (at ease, carefree) or resting on the armrest of the chair (comfortable, bracing)? Are they folded across the torso (bored, holding in their stomach) or are they folded behind the head like wings (suggesting power)? Are they holding the chin up (contemplative, restful)?

Legs

Are they crossed? If so, at the ankles (etiquette training) or the knees (number four position, bold, masculine)? Is it left over right or right over left (European fashion)? Are the knees close together (apprehension, uptight) and the feet firmly planted on the floor (okay with the world)? Are the knees spread wide apart (protecting space) or are they bounding up and down (nervous habit, irritated, impatient)? Are the knees curled up in the fetal position (afraid, childlike)?

Eyes

Are they closed (refusing to look at the situation)? Are they blinking frequently (lying, nerves)? Are they hidden behind dark sunglasses (what do they have to hide, eye irritation)? Is there rapid eye movement, darting all around (usually visual dominant)? Are they staring (concentrating or just plain rude), fluttering (feminine gesture), winking (playful), or squinting (can't see, or forced to look at a situation)?

Hands

Are they fidgeting (stress), gripping (tense), playing (bored), tapping (impatient)? Are the palms open (willingness, openness) or closed (not ready to handle the situation or rejecting)? Are they intertwined (prayerful, introspective) or are they tented (pondering the possibilities)? Are the hands hiding the mouth (hiding their words)?

Sitting

Notice how people sit. Are they sitting on the edge of the chair (anticipation, eager) or are they slumped back (careless and sloppy)? Are they constantly changing and shifting (indecisive)?

Standing

Notice how people stand. Do they appear to take up a lot of personal space (I'm important attitude)? Do they keep alternating their weight from foot to foot (restless)? Do they rest their hands on the hips in a notice-me attitude?

Walking

Notice how people walk. Is their pace brisk (busy, efficient) or do they saunter in (lackadaisical)? Do they take big strides (places to go, lot of ground to cover)?

What do all these signals mean? They could represent a million and one different things. My intention is to point out body language possibilities. Remember that body language reflects inner feelings and attitudes. Become an astute observer of how people consciously and subconsciously use their bodies as an extension of their words.

Visual Buying Cues

There are four definite "I'm ready to buy!" cues to look for when you are dealing with customers.

1. Pupils dilate. The acceptance of your offer will show in the windows of the soul. The pupils will dilate and the eyes take on a wide-eyed and eager look.
2. Respiration quickens. The customer's breathing pattern speeds up. Now, he/she is not going to hyperventilate but, as the person becomes excited, the adrenaline kicks in and the breathing gets faster.

3. Leaning toward you. When the client has sold him- or herself, there will be a natural leaning in toward you, closing the gap you share. Notice the action of the torso and shoulders. When the shoulders move toward you stop selling; the client is already sold.
4. Blotching. That's right. Some of your customers will even get a mild case of the hives. Some may turn splotchy from the excitement.

Do the physical buying cues remind you of anything else? The physical buying cues resemble the symptoms of being in love. I bet you are thinking back to a time when you got really excited over a special date. So hopefully the physical buying cues will be easy for you to remember. Remember that people purchase products emotionally and support their decision with logic. So if they are not excited they are not going to buy.

Just as you can jump in your car and drive off without thinking through every step, you too will "tune into" other's actions, verbal and otherwise. Now when you get into the car to go somewhere, you don't have to go through the mental checklist of how to drive a car. You instinctively follow the natural pattern that you've learned over the years. Reading body language can be exactly the same way with just a little practice.

One day my friend BJ and I were out shopping. BJ wanted to purchase some new perfume but no salesperson was in sight. We waited and waited until BJ spotted a salesperson in another department halfway across the store. She turned to me with a twinkle in her eye and asked if I would like to make a bet that she could get that salesperson to come over and help her. Of course, I took the bet. I knew the store's service record. "Watch this," she announced.

BJ turned away from the counter, scanned the store and locked eyes with the salesperson. She held her look for what seemed like an eternity but in reality was about three seconds. She looked him over quickly, from head to toe, as if questioning his ability to handle the transaction. Then she quickly turned away and faced back toward the counter. "Don't look, but in about two seconds he'll be over here," she proudly announced. And sure enough, he was. "Excuse me, my name is Joseph, and I've noticed you've been waiting a while. How can I help you?" BJ purchased her new perfume and I got a first class lesson in reading and understanding the powerful use of body language.

LISTENING SKILLS

By the time you are twenty years old, your ears have been registering sounds for over 36 million hours. It's been estimated that in one eight-hour work day:

- You spend four hours listening.

- You hear two hours.

- You actually listen one hour.

- You understand thirty minutes.

- You believe fifteen minutes.

- You remember just under eight minutes.

The first time I heard those startling statistics, I was positively exasperated. I felt I had a pretty good memory. Then I stopped to really listen to what was happening around me. "Excuse me, would you repeat that?" "I'm sorry, I don't understand. I missed the first part." "Oh my, I can barely hear you." "I can't listen to her, she's so annoying." As I concentrated on conversations around me, I reluctantly had to admit that maybe people really don't listen as they should.

To be a great listener requires effort and action on your part. Why should you extend yourself to be a good listener? You listen for opportunities. You should actively listen for nuggets of information, clues your clients reveal about themselves, their needs, desires, fears, and wishes—cues that will help you establish a solid foundation for building rapport. Listen for statements that can help you close the sale.

Developing your listening skills will pay off. One day, while I was giving a quick lip wax ($5 service), the client and I started to chat. We started talking about how she discovered the salon and what results she expected. She then casually mentioned she was getting married in a few months. She started to talk about her wedding plans, the parties, and the honeymoon. The result of our casual conversation led to the bride-to-be to schedule over $600 in services. The bridesmaids purchased a full-day pamper package. We did the makeup for the bridal photos and the wedding day makeup for the bride, mother of the bride, and mother of the groom. She booked four pre-wedding facials, two full-leg waxing sessions (they were spending their honeymoon in Hawaii), and a manicure and pedicure prior to the big day.

It is definitely easier to be a good talker than a good listener. It is just plain harder to listen. Most people can listen four times faster than the average person speaks. The average speech speed is 130 to 160 words per minute. No wonder it's so easy to fall into listening lethargy, with your brain processing words four times faster.

Good listening is not a passive activity. Opportunity sits in your chair every hour. Assume the responsibility for making the most of your listening/selling possibilities.

Opportunity Trigger Number 1: Two to One

The true balance to conversation and listening is simple: the formula two to one. You have two ears and one mouth. It makes perfect sense that you should be listening twice as much as you are talking.

Recently a friend was in a salon having his hair cut. Halfway through his service he overheard the stylist at the next station say, "Oh my, we have been talking so much here, I've finished half your haircut and I haven't even asked you how you wanted it styled." Boy, is that dangerous!

Opportunity Trigger Number 2: Hear with More Than Your Ears

You transmit sound through your natural hearing instrument, your ears, but you will weigh the words with all your senses. Your eyes will make an assessment based on the other person's body language or nonverbal cues. You can select your words but your natural body movements will either support or undermine them.

A while back, I was working a trade show when an attractive, smartly dressed woman walked up to the booth and stopped in the center of the front display. She grabbed my hand and eagerly asked, "Was that Mrs. So-and-so? I just admire all she's done. I am such a fan." The entire time she was touting the accolades of someone she admired, her head physically was shifting from left to right, side to side, similar to a "no-no" type gesture. Under the scrutiny of my watchful eye the interaction continued.

She stopped by the booth to inquire about an audio cassette program called "Whole-Brain Success" an associate and

I produced. The tapes relate to being more, giving more, and having more. "So share with me one of your success goals," I naturally inquired. She responded, "Well, I really want to be rich. I really, really want to improve my financial situation." Her response was encouraging.

My desire was to help her open up and share more information. It struck me as incongruent that during her entire explanation her head kept turning left to right. Her mouth was saying "Yes," but her body language was screaming "No way," as if she hadn't convinced herself yet.

Opportunity Trigger Number 3: Read My Lips

If you're easily distracted and your attention span flutters in and out, focus your attention on the speaker's lips. Now, I know you may be thinking, what about eye contact? I thought I was supposed to always look at the eyes. Yes, you do need to make eye contact, but when I really need to connect I focus on a person's mouth. Reading the lips reinforces the verbal sounds and the physical cues, and focusing on the lips helps to keep your eyes from wandering.

Opportunity Trigger Number 4: Set the Stage

Stage your business to minimize environmental distractions and maximize listening opportunities. Chances are the client will be physically coming into your place of business to do business with you. You have the advantage of being in the driver's seat where you can control the environment.

Observe the noise levels in your business. Are there culprits hindering your communication? Investigate the following: air conditioner, volume of the telephone, the music selection and volume, traffic noises, doors slamming, surrounding workstations, washer/dryer areas, bathroom noises, voice levels, computers, printer, copiers, fax, and the overall acoustics of the building. Your business doesn't have to resemble the hallowed halls of your local library, but be ultrasensitive to the noise pollutants that may be cluttering up your communications.

I was assisting an enterprising salon owner who desired to move and expand his business. We were conducting site selections and one place we visited was automatically knocked out of consideration. We went to the salon during a weekday. Due to the horrible acoustics of the building, we discovered we could not carry on a conversation in the tone and level that would be necessary for servicing a client. The business identity matched, the staff was great, the location was even excellent, but the decision not to move there was loud and clear. If you cannot talk to your client, you certainly cannot make the sale.

Opportunity Trigger Number 5: Concentrate

Focus all your energies and attention on the speaker. Channel your senses to hone in on what the speaker is saying. Read between the lines. Observe their words and actions.

Put yourself in the other person's chair, shoes, and thoughts. Establish rapport. Build a connection. Give the other person your respect and general courtesy by hearing him or her out completely. Give the person your undivided attention. Many customers will patronize your fashion and beauty business, not just for products and service but for human contact and compassion.

Opportunity Trigger Number 6: Clarify

Others may not be good at clear communication of their thoughts, desires, and needs. Try to help clients clarify their words and meanings. If you are not sure what clients mean, where they're headed, or what their point is, speak up and ask for clarification. "Toni, I'm sorry, I'm not clear on what exactly you want me to do." "Mrs. Paterson, would you give me a detailed description of what you're looking for?" "I'm not clear on what you specifically want me to do, would you list out the duties?" Words and phrases have different meanings to different people. Make sure you're both on the same track.

NOTE: "Do you want your hair cut over the ear?" Be careful! This question can mean different things to different people. Does it mean that the client wants their hair cut over the ear? Or does it mean the hair is to be left long to cover over the ear? One sentence can have two dramatically different meanings. Cover yourself and clarify.

Opportunity Busters

Five errors to resist when listening are:

1. Resist interrupting. Slam on the brakes if you catch yourself jumping in midsentence, interrupting the other person. Interruptions can be interpreted as a power struggle or the need for creating dominance in the conversation. Constantly interrupting the other person is rude, and it is going to greatly hinder your sales success. If you are talking you are not listening.

2. Resist finishing their thoughts. You want to achieve optimum rapport, but resist chiming in and finishing off the other person's thoughts. Don't assume you know exactly what they're going to say next.

3. Resist internal dialogues. Stop the wheels from turning; silence those little voices whispering or shouting in your head. They may be trying to get your attention for things to do, places to go, projects left unfinished, last night's arguments, even flashbacks to your last client. Millions of dialogue surges will try to get to the head of your thoughts. Turn the volume down on internal dialogues. One dialogue at a time, one conversation at a time, one client at a time.

4. Resist fast forwarding to your next response. All too often you ask a question, then, before the other person has a chance to respond, you are off thinking. "What do I need to say next?" "What am I going to ask?" You ask a question and then while they're responding you're off racking your brain deciding what your next move should be. Avoid the temptation.

   Effective listening has the same actions/reactions as tennis. Your action is based on the other person's reaction or response to your question. You must wait for your opponent to hit the tennis ball back to your side of the net before you make a move on the court. Listen to the entire response to your question, before you ask the next question.

5. Resist listening to surrounding activities. When you are involved with another person direct your energies and attention toward that person. Block surrounding activities, other conversations, other shoppers, and other clients.

   NOTE: If you are chief cook and bottle washer (namely, the boss), wearing multiple hats while you're servicing the client can prove to be hazardous to the health of your business. It's an entrepreneurial instinct to want to know every single thing that is happening, every second of the day in your business. I've observed other business owners and I, myself, have been guilty of dividing my attention between the clients and business activities. Clients can feel neglected, short-changed, or, worse, not important. Resist the temptation to pull double duty. Focus on your client.

CEREBRAL DOMINANCE

Several years ago I became involved with the information I am about to share with you because of a desperate need to understand my staff and customers. Out of sheer frustration I became fanatical about trying to figure out what makes people tick. Dealing with the public can be trying and testing on days.

I pored over books and magazines in my quest for human understanding. I sat through hundreds of classroom hours. The inner lightbulb finally illuminated when I was introduced to the principles of cerebral dominance and neuro-linguistic programming (NLP). Don't panic. They're big words for two life-changing ways we look and relate to other human beings.

Left/Right Brain Dominance

In the 1860s a French neurologist named Paul Broca and a German neurologist named Karl Wernike made some key discoveries about the brain. These neurologists were studying patients with brain damage and discovered that when certain areas of the brain were damaged, the patient lost the ability to speak intelligibly. One hundred years later Roger Sperry and coworkers at the California Institute of Technology designed a series of experiments that determined the characteristics of the two sides of the brain. Sperry's work ultimately won him a Nobel Prize.

What does this have to do with selling? Cerebral dominance tells you that every person has predominant tendencies and characteristics. Once you learn the differences, relating to your customers becomes a snap.

Let's take a look at the brain. First, clench your hands and make a fist. Then put your hands side by side in front of you, knuckles touching. You now have the basic shape of your

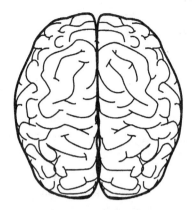

Fig. 10.2 Right and left hemispheres of the brain.

brain. Picture a walnut with its texture and crevices and you have the outside appearance of the brain. The cerebrum, which is the largest area of the brain, is divided into two hemispheres, the left and the right.(Fig. 10.2)

The human body has nine body systems. Each system is dependent on the other systems to coordinate the body's millions of activities. The brain coordinates and controls every single bodily function.

Each side of the brain operates independently and simultaneously. Every person has a dominant or a more comfortable side of the brain they exercise, whether it's the left or the right side. If you were to exercise your right arm by physically doing one hundred arm curls with a five-pound weight every single day which arm would be more developed, the left arm or the right? Obviously, the right arm. The same thing is true with cerebral dominance.

Every person has a dominant side, developed through genetics, education, and intuitive behavior. You and your clients have a dominant operating side. The comfort zone expresses itself in the way you talk, think, feel, and even dress. The more you know about yourself and your clients the smoother your daily interactions will be.

Self-quiz

Take the next few minutes for the following quiz, before you go any further in this chapter. Don't try to guess what your an-swers should be, just be honest and true to yourself. Doing so allows for uncovering your left and right dominant side.

1. You have just left the theater. Do you
   a) remember the lyrics?
   b) hum the tune?
2. You're asked to give directions to a location. Do you
   a) write them out?
   b) draw a map?
   c) both?
3. When faced with a problem, do you
   a) think about it, write down the possibilities, prioritize the answers, and then select what's best?
   b) wait and see if it solves itself?
   c) mull it over for a while, then discuss it with someone close to you?
   d) flash back on past events, remember the outcomes, and then make a decision?
4. When you buy a new car, do you
   a) do your homework, read the brochure, find out the consumer rating reports?
   b) pick what color and model you'd like to drive around in?
   c) check into specification and standard equipment and what's available for options?
   d) physically sit in the car first to see if you feel right behind the wheel?
5. Are you sold on an idea
   a) after you've carefully analyzed the details, step by step?
   b) if you can see the end picture or if the idea feels right to you?
6. Do you like to change the decor of your office or home frequently?
   a) no
   b) yes
7. How would you best describe your work space, desk, closet and/or garage?
   a) It's a mess but I can find what I need.
   b) Everything is in its proper designated place.
   c) You need a map to find anything.
   d) Needs a little picking up but other than that it's in order.

8. When you go on vacation, do you
   a) take plenty of reading material, just so you won't get bored?
   b) cut loose and forget about work and responsibilities?
   c) I never take vacations. It's a waste of time.

9. When it comes to watching the clock, are you
   a) extremely punctual.
   b) within a few minutes of the designated time.
   c) close but no cigar.
   d) always late.

10. Do you remember faces easily?
    a) yes
    b) no

11. In social situations do you prefer
    a) to be spontaneous?
    b) to be planned in advance?

12. Are your goals
    a) clearly defined?
    b) written out and divided into action steps?
    c) thought about?
    d) you don't have any.

13. Circle the activities you enjoy.

Swimming	Dancing	Playing chess
Writing	Gardening	Playing an instrument
Traveling	Sewing	Photography
Doing nothing	Collecting	Drawing
Shopping	Reading	Arts and Crafts
Cooking	Kissing	Hugging
Bicycling	Fishing	Golfing
Playing tennis	Walking	Debating
Running		

14. When you hold a pen or pencil, it is in your
    a) right hand straight with the page.
    b) right hand hooked fingers facing body.
    c) left hand straight with page.
    d) left hand hooked fingers facing body.

15. Hold a pencil horizontal to the ground. At arms' length, frame, the pencil with a straight line, frame or door. Keep that position and close your left eye. Did the pencil move?
    a) yes
       Now close your right eye. Did the pencil move?
    b) yes

16. When you make notes do you
    a always print.
    b) always write.
    c) both.

17. When you've obtained a new piece of equipment (stereo, VCR, computer), do you
    a) read the directions carefully before installing?
    b) jump in and then if it gets difficult you'll reach for the directions?
    c) I wouldn't even think about hooking it up.

Scoring

Now that you have completed the quiz, add up your total points scored.

1. a) 1
   b) 9
2. a) 1
   b) 9
   c) 5
3. a) 1
   b) 9
   c) 6
   d) 3
4. a) 1
   b) 9
   c) 4
   d) 6
5. a) 1
   b) 9
6. a) 1
   b) 2
7. a) 6
   b) 1
   c) 9
   d) 5
8. a) 3
   b) 9
   c) 1

9. a) 1
   b) 3
   c) 6
   d) 9
10. a) 7
    b) 1
11. a) 9
    b) 1
12. a) 4
    b) 1
    c) 7
    d) 9

13.
Swimming	9	Dancing	7
Writing	2	Gardening	5
Traveling	5	Sewing	3
Doing nothing	9	Collecting	1
Shopping	7	Reading	3
Cooking	5	Kissing	9
Bicycling	8	Fishing	8
Playing tennis	4	Walking	8
Running	8	Debating	2
Playing chess	2	Playing an instrument	4
Photography	3	Drawing	9
Arts and Crafts	5	Hugging	9
Golfing	4		

14. a) 1
    b) 7
    c) 9
    d) 3
15. a) 8
    b) 2
16. a) 9
    b) 1
    c) 5
17. a) 1
    b) 4
    c) 9

Totaling Your Score

Now total up all the points you have scored for each question. Divide the total by the number of questions answered. (The number of questions answered will vary due to question 13.)

For example: if your total is 125 for 25 questions, your dominant number would be 5.

Left_____Right

| 1 | 3 | 5 | 7 | 9 |

There are no right or wrong answers in the self-quiz. The closer you are to the middle of the graph the easier it will be for you to deal with a wider range of personalities.

Left and Right Brain Dominant Characteristics

Now that you have figured out where you fall in the left/right dominant pattern, let's take a detailed look at the characteristics of each side of the brain. As you read the descriptions, clients will come to mind. Write down their names in the margins. You may say to yourself as you read through the list that you favor characteristics that are on both the left and the right side. That's great. Very few people are completely one side or the other.

The following describes the opposite characteristics of the left and right side. Each section will give you two descriptions that detail how people use their brains. Many of the descriptions will paint a picture of the person's attitude or actions.

Linear Thinkers/Visual Thinkers

LEFT—Linear thinkers process in terms of lines and structures. Think back to your childhood. How were you taught to take notes in grammar school? I bet you were instructed to write your lessons on a big sheet, wide line, yellow note pad. Also in your kit of school supplies were number 2 hard lead pencils. Your first and last name had to appear in the upper right hand corner, printed neatly. Notes were to be taken in outline form. Our early childhood experiences in school have contributed to the linear left-brain-dominant characteristics.

A linear thinker might say something like, "Jim, I have three items I need to discuss with you. Now for Item 1 . . . Item 2 . . . Item 3. . . ." They have a tendency to express themselves in list form.

RIGHT—Visual. Patterns, colors, phrases, and descriptive words keep the visual dominant person occupied. They can see things in the "mind's eye." "Don't just tell me, show me." If asked to describe the weather a visual person might respond, "Today is going to be another outstanding radiant day. It appears the sun is highlighting the azure-blue sky with flecks of powder-soft, white, billowy clods." Visual personalities have the artistic ability to paint pictures with their words and phrases.

Analytical/Imaginative

LEFT—Analytical. When faced with a decision or problem to solve an analytical personality will tend to break down the problem into manageable components. Once the problem has been categorized, they can think it through. Analytical personalities want to think things over. "Gee, I need to think about it."

Frequently you can catch these people mulling over things in their heads. They can think so hard you swear you hear the wheels turning. These people do come to decisions and can make up their minds. Just don't expect them to make snap decisions.

RIGHT—Imaginative. Right dominants can see things the way they are or the way they could be. Pictures pop into their imaginations. They can release a mental picture and grab the concept, idea, or impression. It's easiest for this group to "see" the makeover before physically subjecting to any of the alterations. Say "Picture this . . ." Then watch their eyes light up!

Language/Color

LEFT—Language. Left-brain-dominant personalities are fluid and articulate in their manner of speech. This group has the ability to master foreign languages both in written form and verbally.

Left brain dominants have a commanding presence when they speak. Words seem to float off the tongue and dance right into the ears. The flip side to the eloquent orator is the person who throws fourteen-syllable words into conversations just to impress people.

RIGHT—Color. Color stimulates the right side of the brain. The impact of color can be positive or negative, appealing or offensive. Colors can represent symbols, feelings, or moods. The world is not black and white to this group. Listen for colorful words and phrases. Their natural speech sounds like a box of crayons that has sprung to life; sea-foam blue, fields of per-

iwinkles, neon lights dancing in the gray horizon, nothing could match the dazzling brilliance of the ruby and emerald ring.

Reading and Writing/Depth

LEFT—Reading and Writing. This group will not leave home without reading material. Panic can strike the moment this group runs out of things to read. The next time you are in the airport gift shop watch this person frantically searching for reading material to purchase before the plane takes off. Notes, lists, and to-do sheets are as natural as breathing for this group. Casually observe the number of pens and pencils they may have in their pocket, purse, or briefcase. Chances are they've kept the stationery store in business.

RIGHT—Depth. While their counterpart is reading about life's issues, causes, and concerns, the right brain dominant is diving heart first into the real depth of the issue. If you were "hanging out" in the sixties, you experienced depth with statements like, "Man, why are we really here?" "What's the true meaning of life?" This group tends to look deep inside themselves for the answers. They are not willing to totally accept someone else's views and beliefs on issues that run close to the heart.

Math/Rhythm

LEFT—Math. Mathematics, equations, and formulas add up easily for the left side of the brain. Adding, subtracting, dividing, and figuring percentages are easy and natural. This next question will separate the left and the right. Do you balance your checkbook to the penny? Do you tolerate being close or even a few cents off? Does it drive you nuts until every penny is accounted for? If so, chances are you're a dominant left. If your response was, "Huh, why I can't be overdrawn, I still have checks left." You favor the right hemisphere of the brain. That's okay, just have your accountant keep the books.

RIGHT—Rhythm. If the left side is for balancing the checkbook, the right side is for rocking with the rhythm. Music and rhythm massage the brain. If you prefer to boogie to the beat and dance until dawn, watch for toe tapping, hips swaying for Rhythm and Blues personality cues. When you're strolling through the mall, notice people when they get close to the music store. Many customers may not walk into the store, but Bebop their way down the aisles. Subtle music can have a natural, almost primal response for this group. The right brain subconsciously responds to music and rhythm. Pay particular attention to the music selection you have playing in your business. Watch the rhythm of your voice. Vary the speed and pitch to keep your right brain dominants in sync with your presentation.

Reason/Imagination

LEFT—Reason. "What's the purpose?" "I need an explanation." "What's the justification?" Left brain dominants will have a very definite reason or purpose for their actions. This group is easy to sell once you've uncovered their reason or motive for buying. Ask questions that help to pinpoint their reason. "Share with me how I can help you today." "Clarify for me the problem you are having with. . . ."

RIGHT—Imagination.The Wonderful World of Disney hires imagineers, people who can imagine and bring things to life. Disney succeeds in an uncanny way by using the imagination as a launching pad.

The right side has the ability to create mental images of what's not actually present. The right side is broad minded in the possibilities of what's not "in the natural." This side loosens up to explore uncharted waters, unusual works of art and literature.

Logic and Facts/Creativity

LEFT—Logic and Facts. Left brain dominants will tend to stick to the straight and narrow path with logical processes. Forget flowering up the conversation. Keep it short, to the point, and factual. This side is notorious for wanting or needing to know the who, what, where, when, how, and why.

RIGHT—Creativity. Free flowing. No boundaries. Unlimited possibilities. Creating. Designing. The right brain needs to operate with the freedom and luxury of creativity. They allow things to bloom and take shape. Ideas and projects can then emerge forth as great works of art, literature, fashion, movies, beauty, and inventions.

Organized/Cluttered

LEFT—Organized. The left side coordinates and organizes everything. A place for everything and everything in its place. Simple, clear, clean, tabbed, dated, and in triplicate.

RIGHT—Cluttered. This group feels comfortable surrounded by "organized" clutter. They have piles of stuff, but just give them a few minutes and they know exactly where everything is located. They can find it, even if it looks a little messy to the left brainer.

Strong/Gentle

LEFT—Strong. Look for cues in the personality, attitude, and overall demeanor. This side comes off as being strong, not just physically but also in relation to personal space. They have broad shoulders and appear as if they can carry the weight of the world.

RIGHT—Gentle. Don't assume the opposite of strong is weak. It's gentle, soft, more feminine. You can sense with the right brain dominant that it's okay to get close, to approach them, to get more intimate. But do not overwhelm them by being too outspoken or intimidating.

Details/Big Picture

LEFT—Details. Read the fine print. Cover every angle from A to Z. One of their great strengths is their ability to follow through with projects and their attention to detail. They're the people you want to have on your team if you want things done without supervision. Their attention to filling in the details is a real asset.

RIGHT—Big Picture. The right side imagination can run wild with childlike excitement, planning, scheming, and uncovering the big picture of possibilities. They have the ability to conceptualize the idea and formulate the desired end results. They can see the big picture but fall short in taking all the necessary detailed steps for achieving the results. The right side loves step A and step Z, but feels pressured and confined if forced to fill in the details of B to Y.

Critical/Appreciative

LEFT—Critical. The left side is quick to find fault or question everything that you say. This group's not rude, but they can be a tad quick on the negative trigger. If you have a client who is constantly critical, keep in mind the person may be locked in to operating on the left side. Notice the lips on the strong left-brained person. Critical people tend to appear as if they have been sucking on lemons for days. It's hard to be open and loving if your lips are puckered up.

RIGHT—Appreciative. "Thank you." "I appreciate what you've done." "You're so kind." The right side reminds us to be appreciative of others' actions, kind words, and services well done.

Serious/Humor

LEFT—Serious. Left brain dominants have a very serious side. They wear a down-to-business expression on their faces. Every situation has a serious undertone.

RIGHT—Humor. The right side sees life through light-hearted eyes, and they are able to find humor in most of life's events. Watch for the twinkle in the eye, the lightness in the step, and that big heartwarming smile. This group will be the first to tell you a new joke. They love to laugh.

Experience/New

LEFT—Experience. Dominant left personalities tend to base today's decisions on what has happened in the past. Some people take root in previous experiences so deeply their tentacles reach into today's actions and overshadow the outcome. Of course, we should all learn from past events, positive or negative, but beware of the person who lives completely in the past.

A new client came into the salon and during the course of her New Customer Orientation she repeatedly stated she had an allergy to lanolin. The salon coordinator, efficiently, boldly, and in a bright red magic marker highlighted the top of her chart, "Don't use lanolin, allergic." As I started the treatment, I proceeded with my usual line of questioning and the subject of skin sensitivity crept in. I was curious how this client determined she was allergic. Had she gone through the battery of tests for allergies? No. Had her doctor declared her allergic to lanolin? No. How did she discover the problem? She noticed it. How long had she been avoiding lanolin-based products? Sheepishly she admitted that it had been over twenty years. What spurred the allergy? She finally admitted that when she was in high school she had broken out one time from wearing a wool sweater. Therefore she must be allergic to lanolin. Locked into the past? Absolutely! Would I have ever been able to convince her otherwise? Probably not. Did I try? Definitely no. She had chosen to be locked into the left side and all the convincing in the world would not have changed her perception.

RIGHT—New. Every six months or so it seems that manufacturers are introducing new and improved products. The word new is a stimulant for the right side of the brain. Mention to a customer that a new shipment has just arrived and watch her eyes light up. New trends. New fashions. New products. New colors. New packaging. Hot off the press. Be the first to own the newest. Gets your blood racing, doesn't it?

Thinks/Feels

Left—Thinks. Right—Feels. The major difference between the two hemispheres can be easily summed up. The left dominant hemisphere thinks things through. The right side operates on feelings.

Left and Right Recap List

LEFT	RIGHT
Linear	Visual
Analytical	Imaginative
Language	Color
Reading and Writing	Depth
Math	Rhythm
Reason	Imagination
Logic and Facts	Creativity
Organized	Cluttered
Strong	Gentle
Details	Big Picture
Critical	Appreciative
Serious	Humor
Experience	New
Thinks	Feels

Visual Cues for Left/Right Brain Dominance

Left brain people wear clothes that are of a straight cut with squared-off shoulders, necklines, and lapels. If the clothes have a pattern it will be in stripes—horizontal, vertical, or geometric.

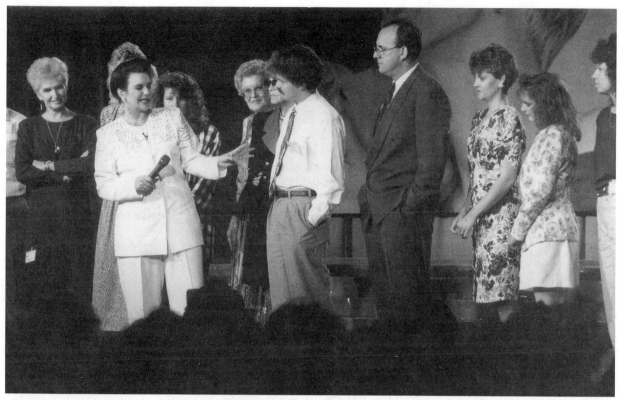

Fig. 10.3   Look at left brain characteristics. (Special thanks to Redken Regional Program, Corpus Christi, Texas. Photo by George Orsatti.)

Colors tend to fall into black, white, navy, gray, brown, and occasionally red. (Fig. 10.3)

Hairstyles will be geometric, straight, bi-level, no-fuss, no-fluff, trimmed, tidy, dramatic, or dull.

Jewelry will be kept to a minimum but will be classic and expensive. Shoes, handbags, and briefcases are basic and well cared for. Socks will almost always match the shoe color.

Right brain people will wear clothes with more flare and fun and lots color. This group will put together the most unlikely color combinations that look great. The clothing lines will have more movement and a rounded, softer silhouette. (Fig. 10.4)

Hairstyles will run the gamut from funky to trendy to fluffy to bizarre. Remember this group gravitates toward new and fun trends. Right brainers do not want to be confined to a corporate look or dictum.

They tend to favor big purses, the everything-plus-the-

kitchen-sink type bag. Look for patterns, flowers, and prints on their clothing, shoes, bags, jewelry. You may even see this group sporting only one earring or three or more or some that don't match.

Helpful Hint: If you want to see a dramatic representation of the left/right visual cues observe the left-brained contestant on *Jeopardy* versus the right-brained contestants on *The Price is Right*. Also see figure 10.5.

Cerebral Options

If you are a right or left dominant, can you change? Of course you can. There may be days, weeks, months, even minutes when you feel completely right or left. There may be certain circumstances when you need to be more left brained, such as when you go to see your local banker for a loan. If you are taking a day off and will be experiencing a museum you may

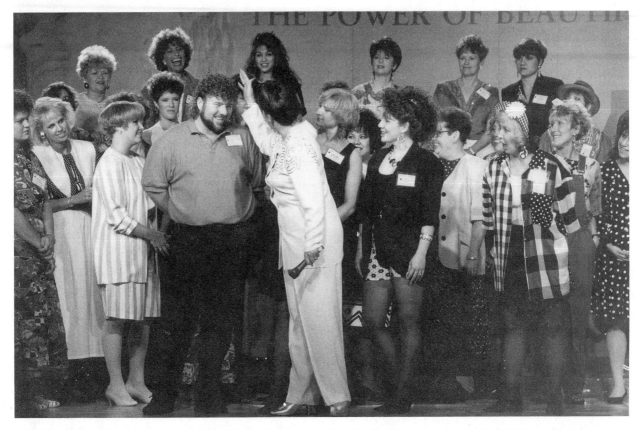

Fig. 10.4   Look at right brain characteristics. (Special thanks to Redken Regional Program, Corpus Christi, Texas. Photo by George Orsatti.)

want to throw caution and logic to the wind and be in a right-brain frame of mind. There may be periods in your life where your natural tendency is to operate more left or right. The goal here is to understand the differences and be able to relate to someone that is different from you.

Some friends of mine were sitting around the dinner table when one of them, Susan, decided it would be fun to catch a movie. After she announced her brainstorm, her husband, Mark, became upset. "We can't go to the movies. It's already seven o'clock and the movie starts in thirty minutes. We have a fifteen minute drive, and we need to get a baby-sitter. I have to be up early in the morning for work."

Does that sound frighteningly familiar? Who was right, Susan, Mark, or both? This is a classic case of miscommunication. Susan is right brain and Mark is left brain. Understand-

ing how to deal with the other person is paramount to good rapport.

The next time Susan could still be fun, lighthearted, and spontaneous. She would just have to give Mark a little notice or preplan his logical approach to the evening.

Can you now see how difficult communication can be? Can you now see how you should, as a successful professional, step aside from yourself and put yourself in the other's mind set?

Whole Brain Selling

A male (very handsome, left brain) colleague of mine was teaching a seminar on whole brain marketing. He asked the

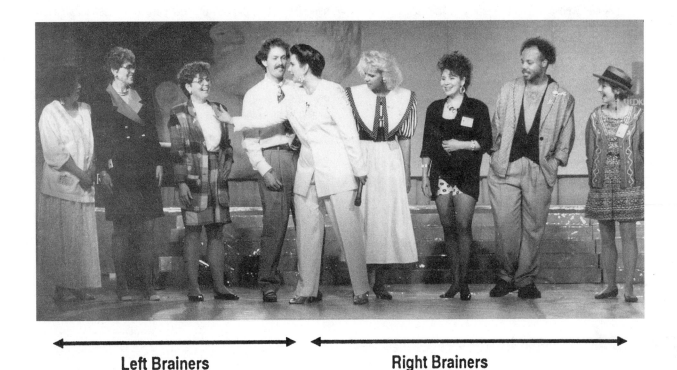

Left Brainers   **Right Brainers**

Fig. 10.5 Notice the difference between the left and right brain groups. (Special thanks to Redken Regional Program, Corpus Christi, Texas. Photo by George Orsatti.)

audience, "Why should I come in and have a facial in your salon?" Going around the room he received the following: "You are going to love how your skin feels." "It will help you relax." "I have luxurious products for your skin." "We have private treatment areas with soft comfortable chairs." "I give a wonderful massage." "You'll feel better."

Finally, a brave esthetician, after hearing all the others trying to "woo" my colleague, stood up and said, "I've noticed that you have some shaving irritation. My salon offers effective, results-oriented products and services. In just one short hour you will see an improvement on your skin." Bingo! She was the only person to speak to him in his language. She was quick, to the point, and factual. Her approach was left brained. She didn't try to sell him flowery, feel-good words.

The key to selling is to speak in words and phrases that match your client. The group of estheticians tried to sell by using right brain buzz words. Don't try to swim upstream. Sell people in their comfort zone, not yours.

Left Brain Selling

Remember the following when selling to a left brain dominant: linear, analytical, language, reading/writing, math, reason, logic/facts, organized, strong, details, critical, serious, experience, thinks. Stress the benefits, ease of use, price per unit, tested results.

- "Well, it would seem **logical** that we start with the **basics**. Keep your home care **routine quick and efficient.**"

- "After analyzing your hair, I **strongly recommend for maximum results** we should. . . ."

- "**The fact of the matter** is you need to condition your hair every three weeks. Doing so helps to **maintain** your color for a longer period of time."

- "Your **past experience** has shown that you need to have your hair trimmed every two and a half weeks. This allows you the **clean** and **tidy look** you desire."

Right Brain Selling

Remember the following when selling to a right brain dominant: visual, images, color, depth, rhythm, imagination, creativity, cluttered, gentle, big picture, appreciative, humor, new, feels. Stress fun to use, colors, shades. Create pictures and stimulate the imagination.

- "The **hot, new** makeup colors for fall just arrived."

- "Here, **feel** this **exciting, new** material."

- "The new pumpkin **colored** shirt is a **gorgeous shade** for you."

- "Can you just **imagine** what **reactions** your **new look** will bring?"

- "This **soft, gentle** cleanser will **feel** fantastic on your skin."

Can you see the difference between the left and right brain statements? Each personality type has a different tone and meaning. Learn to sell to your customers in their language. Can you imagine what would happen if you tried selling a left based on fluff and fun? It just wouldn't work. The same thing is true with a right client. Don't try and bog them down with all the details. Keep it light and fun and easy to understand.

If you are extremely left or right, you will have to stretch yourself to speak in your opposite manner. After a period of practicing the information you will find it becomes second nature and natural. You will find yourself adapting without forethought.

NEUROLINGUISTIC PROGRAMMING

In the previous section you learned the difference between left and right brain dominance. This section adds another dimension to understanding your clients.

Richard Bandler and John Grinder, two psychotherapists, developed an analysis theory called neurolinguistic program-

ming (NLP) that focuses on how people process information. Their studies revealed that there are three major ways people experience and process the world—visual, auditory, and kinesthetic representational systems.

Keep in mind a person favors the left or right dominant characteristic, and then favors one of the NLP patterns. Once again clients or family members will come to mind as you read each of the profiles. Jot down their names in the margins.

NLP Self-Quiz

Before you go any further in this section let's take a fun, short quiz to determine your representation style—visual, auditory, or kinesthetic. Select the answer that rings truest for you.

1. Which group do you prefer?
   a) Drawing, painting, reading, movies, photography
   b) Symphony, wind chimes, music, nature sounds
   c) Arts & crafts, massage, woodworking, ceramics
2. When you think back on a former partner, the first thing you remember is
   a) The way he/she looked.
   b) The sound of his/her voice.
   c) The feelings that surface.
3. When you physically work out your greatest reward comes from
   a) Your reflection in the mirror.
   b) The compliments from others.
   c) Feeling fit and being stronger.
4. When problems get you down, you
   a) Write them out so you can see them on paper.
   b) Talk them over with a friend.
   c) take some quiet time and sort them out internally.
5. Think back to an occasion when you met someone for the first time. What attracted you to this person?
   a) His/her appearance.
   b) Something he/she said or you heard.
   c) Your gut feeling.
6. When you have a task to do, do you want
   a) The directions written out?
   b) Everything explained clearly?
   c) to get a feel for the task before beginning?

7. When you go clothes shopping, once you spot an article do you
   a) Try it on immediately to see what it looks like?
   b) Chat with the salesperson or talk to yourself about the garment?
   c) Touch and feel the garment?

8. When you wake up in the morning, do you enjoy experiencing
   a) The sun beaming through the window?
   b) The birds singing or music?
   c) Staying in bed and snuggling in the blankets?

9. When planning a special event, the first thing you plan is
   a) What you are going to wear or what the setting will be.
   b) The music or entertainment.
   c) The mood or feeling for the event.

10. When you have completed a successful task do you
    a) See yourself moving up in the company?
    b) Replay your success scenario in your head?
    c) Feel intensely proud and satisfied?

11. Think back on one of your favorite movies. Do you remember
    a) Certain scenes flashing on screen?
    b) The soundtrack?
    c) The emotions and feelings the movie triggered?

12. When you need to get motivated, the first thing you do is
    a) Visualize yourself with extra energy and enthusiasm.
    b) Give yourself a pep talk.
    c) Feel yourself getting psyched up.

13. When you go to a museum, you are most likely to
    a) Stroll through and observe the works of art.
    b) Listen to the tour guide or headset explaining the artistic endeavors.
    c) Wander about just soaking up the experience.

14. You know you are going to be successful because
    a) You see yourself growing and developing.
    b) ou hear your inner voice reaffirming your success.
    c) You feel it. You know it will happen.

15. When you need to learn a new task, you learn best by
    a) Reading the material and taking notes.
    b) Listening to the instructor or audio cassette.
    c) Getting your hands into it.

16. When you go to the beach, do you prefer
    a) The ocean view and white sandy beaches?
    b) The sound of the waves crashing against the shore?
    c) The warmth of the sun on your skin?

17. What do you enjoy most about autumn?
    a) The vivid colors of the changing leaves.
    b) The sound of the leaves crunching underfoot.
    c) The crisp fresh air.

Count each category a, b, c and give yourself ten points for every answer.

a _____ points Visual
b _____ points Auditory
c _____ points Kinesthetic

The following section will highlight cues to look for when dealing with each personality. Over the years I've used six categories for determining each clients' profile. There are physical tip-offs, body styles, breathing patterns, hand gestures, linguistics (words and phrases), and eye-accessing cues. These patterns are natural treasure maps leading directly to the pot of gold if you know how to read the map.

Visual People

Visual people must see things in order to learn and understand information. They learn best by reading the information. If they read it or see it, the material sticks with them. Show me, don't just tell me is their motto.

Physical Tip-offs
- Large eyes and/or big fashion eyeglass frames.
- Bold, vibrant clothing colors.
- Favorite color is red.
- Intense projection of personal body space.
- Erect body posture.

- Clothes will be fashionable and chic.
- Expressive visually, physically and mentally.

Body Style
Visuals tend to be trim and tall, or a least they think tall. Visuals are concerned with what they see in the mirror. This is the customer that has to be facing the mirror watching what you are doing or have access to a hand mirror.

Breathing Patterns
Breathing is high in the chest and shallow. Most of their body movement is above the waist. They have a tendency to hold their breath while thinking.

Hand Gestures
Hand gestures are high in the air or around the eyes. Picture a mamma flinging her hands high above her head, flicking her fingers up toward the sky?

Linguistics
They will use words and phrases such as appears, focus, image, watch, picture, glance, dream, vague, glitch, scope, looks like, perspective, plainly see, point of view, and sight for sore eyes.

Eye-Accessing Cues
Their eyes will look up and left when they are accessing re-membered images (replaying what has happened in the past) and up and right when they are visually constructing images (building pictures in the mind). (Fig. 10.6)

Auditory People

Auditory people process the world through hearing and through sound. This is the group most likely to have the television and the radio on simultaneously. The first piece of furniture this group invests in is a stereo.

Physical Tip-offs
- Unobtrusive personalities.
- Their head turns toward you when they speak.

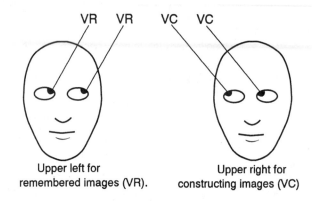

Upper left for remembered images (VR).

Upper right for constructing images (VC)

Fig. 10.6   Eye-accessing cues for visual people.

- They lean their ear toward you.
- Clothes style will tend to be conservative and understated, never loud.
- Notice the prominent size, shape, and placement of the ears on their head.
- Favorite color is navy blue.
- Easily disturbed by offensive noises.
- Incredible capacity to listen to others.
- Female auditories tend to wear lots of blush sweeping up toward the ears.

Breathing Patterns
Regular, even breathing utilizing the entire diaphragm.

Hand Gestures
Watch for hands flinging about shoulder height or waving by their eyes. Tune in to see if they are pulling, playing with tug-ging on, or pointing toward the ear.

Linguistics
Common words and phrases this group would use are ear shot, hush, speechless, loud, noise, screech, amplify, utterly, tuned in, tuned out, rings a bell, rap session, speak to me, hold your tongue, earful, manner of speaking, clearly expressed.

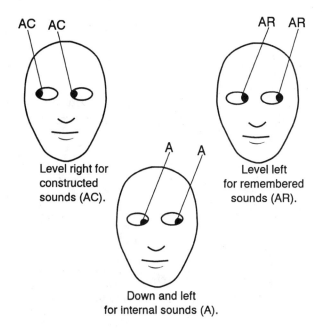

Level right for
constructed
sounds (AC).

Level left
for remembered
sounds (AR).

Down and left
for internal sounds (A).

Fig. 10.7 Eye-accessing cues for auditory people.

Eye-Accessing Cues
Auditories will look down and left when they are listening to internal auditory sounds (self-talk), level left for remembered sounds, and level right for constructed auditory sounds (How am I going to say . . . ?). (Fig. 10.7)

Kinesthetic People

Kinesthetic people process their world through their feelings or intuitive reactions. They may see the information presented or hear it, but until they "get a feel for it" or feel it inside, it really doesn't register.

Physical Tip-offs
- They're "touchy" people.
- They have a strong need to make physical contact.
- Look for texture in their clothing fabrics.
- Big, clunky, noisy jewelry.
- Comfortable, unrestricted clothing.

- Earthy or sporty look.
- Favorite color is purple.
- Hairstyle may have a fluffy soft look.
- Well-worn practical shoes.

Body style
Kinesthetic people tend to have fleshier or fuller bodies. This group can tip the scales toward the overweight side, especially since so many people use food as an emotional escape. Kinesthetics don't place much emphasis on what they see. You won't find this group lingering in front of the mirror, in contrast to the visual group.

Some researchers feel the athletic, sporty type is in the kinesthetic category. Over the past ten years I have been observing and teaching this information, and rarely does the true athletic type fall into this group. But keep your eyes open.

Breathing Patterns
Kinesthetics breathe low in the stomach and use the full diaphragm. Their respiration is altered by their feelings and by their mood. When this group is upset you will feel the difference in their respiration rhythm. Listen for long, drawn out sighs, or if excited they will fight to catch their breath.

Hand Gestures
Kinesthetics tend to wave their hands low on the body, fanning down low around the waist. They are usually doing something with their hands—fidgeting, playing with pens or pencils, doodling. They feel more secure when they have something to hold on to. Also notice that these people are the first ones to start hugging everybody.

Linguistics
They'll use words and phrases like handle, rough, upset, support, feels like, pain in the neck, grasp, worn, tight, hand in hand, hothead, pull some strings, underhanded, chip off the old block, come to grips.

Eye-Accessing Cues
True kinesthetics only look down and right when processing feelings. (Fig. 10.8)

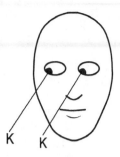

Fig. 10.8 Eye-accessing cues for kinesthetic people. They will look down and right.

TAP INTO EYE-ACCESSING CUES

How do you find out into which profile your client fits? First observe all of the physical tip-offs, breathing patterns, body styles, hand gestures, and linguistic patterns. Then ask a question that forces the client to retrieve information stored away in the brain. "What were you using before you switched brands?" "How long have you been thinking about changing your look?" Watch the eye movement. Did the eyes go up to the ceiling? Or did the eyes shift toward the left ear? Or did the eyes sweep down to the floor, swinging back and forth like a pendulum? (Fig. 10.9)

- Up and right—visual
- Level and left—auditory
- Down and right—kinesthetic

Eye Massage

Flash back to a time when you were having a bad day. Where did your eyes look? My guess is you looked down to the floor. "Poor me." "It's a bad day." "Things just aren't going right."

Do you know that it is psychologically impossible to send "Poor me" messages when your eyes are looking up in the visual pattern? So if you want to modify your negative mood, look up to the ceiling and roll your eyes from left to right several times. You should feel as if the movement is massaging the brain into a positive state. Great exercise during the day if you feel yourself slipping into a negative mood.

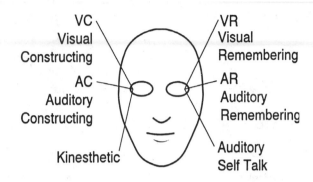

Fig. 10.9 Eye-accessing cues.

Speak Their Language

Once you have determined your client's profile, start to use words and phrases in his or her comfort zone.

Visual

How would you respond to a visual client? You would use descriptive words that paint pictures and stimulate the visual senses.

- "Well, Adam, it **appears** to me that you should switch your home care program. **Imagine** the results in a few weeks. From my **point of view,** you'll start to *see* some real changes."

- Alice, your appointment is scheduled for your new fall color update and fashion consultation. The **new** looks are **expressive** and **colorful."**

- "Toni, the new **hot pink,** off-the-shoulder cocktail dress you've been eager to own just arrived. It's so fun I can't wait to **see** this party dress on you. You'll be a **sight for sore eyes** in this little number."

Auditory

Choose your words very carefully. Definitely watch the tone and clarity of your speech. Be articulate and expressive without becoming wordy.

- "I hear what you are saying, Cameron. You have made it loud and clear. Let's start by modifying your new look. Let's tone down our original design."

- "The new fall fashions are clearly statement makers and will express your style."

- "Tell me what you had in mind. Speak to me."

Kinesthetic

Use words with flair, feeling, and emotion.

- "I can **handle** switching your skin care products. By using them together, **hand in hand**, you will **feel** the **softening** and **smoothing** results on your skin."

- "Do you have a **feel for** the color you'd like to alter your hair to be? Do you **support** going to the sunlit gold or could you **handle** the molten honey color?"

- "Kay, I have a **feeling** you'd love the new sand-washed silk suit that came in today. Wait until you **feel** the fabric. The suit is in your **smashing** signature style."

You may not normally use these words and phrases, but by incorporating them into your conversation you will be pushing the client's hot button, without being pushy. Watch the eyes light up, subconsciously, when you start using buzzwords in his/her comfort zone. (See Figure 10.10 for a list of words/phrases to listen for and use.)

Well, I hope so far in this chapter you have discovered a lot about yourself and your customers. Let's wrap up this section by putting the information to use. There are three final clues I want you to have for pulling all the personality selling together.

IMPLEMENTING PERSONALITY SELLING

Step Number One: Relax and Be Yourself

Don't feel you are being deceitful by implementing what you've learned about others' personalities. Keep focused on your objective to understand what makes your customers tick. They are all certainly different! Concentrate on the other person.

Your genuine openness and heartfelt understanding will start you on the right tRack.

Step Number Two: Observe Personality Cues

Access your mental computer scanning for personality traits. Listen for verbal cues. Are they sending signals of the left- or right-brain-dominant personality? Watch for eye-accessing cues. Do their phrases tip you off as being visual, auditory, or kinesthetic? Actively listen and observe. Keep going; the more you know about the person the greater your chances of uncovering treasures of information about their personalities.

Step Number Three: Mirror the Customer

Mirroring is subtly assuming some of the other person's personality cues in pace, breathing, linguistics, and body language.

Pace

Let your customers set the pace for the interaction. If they are fast talkers, you speed up your words. If their pace is slow then switch to slow play. The clients will dictate the pace of the dialogue by what's comfortable, but the stylist must control the evolution of the conversation from topic to topic.

Breathing patterns

You can speed up or slow down your breathing rhythm to synchronize with your customer. A private conversation or consultation is the best opportunity to mirror breathing patterns. Running around the store assisting two or three shoppers can be a little tricky. Think rhythm, harmony, and pacing. Inhale and exhale following the client's lead.

Linguistics

Talk in their language. Listen for clues into their favorite phrases. If the client is expressing visual, auditory, or kinesthetic patterns, follow suit.

Body Language

Practice mirroring body language but be cautious that your actions are not overt. After you've been building rapport start to

VISUAL	AUDITORY	KINESTHETIC
an eyeful	after-thought	all washed up
appear	articulate	bearable
appears to me	audible	boils down to
bird's eye view	blabber mouth	callous
clear cut	boisterous	charge
dim view	call on	chip off the old block
dream	clearly expressed	clear as a bell
eye to eye	converse	concrete
focus	discuss	cool, calm, collected
foresee	divulge	feel
glance	earful	firm foundation
glimpse of	express yourself	grab
hazy idea	gossip	grasp
illusion	give me your ear	grip
illustrate	hear you	hand in hand
image	hear you out	handle
imagine	hold your tongue	hang in there
inspect	inquire	heated argument
look	keynote	hold on
looks like	listen to me	hunch
mind's eye	loud and clear	impact
paint a picture	manner of speaking	lukewarm
perspective	oral	pain in the neck
picture	outspoken	pull some strings
pretty as a picture	proclaim	sharp as a tack
scope	rap session	slipped my mind
see to it	remark	smooth
shadow of a doubt	ring	soft
short sighted	roar	start from scratch
show	speak to me	stiff upper lip
sight for sore eyes	speechless	stuffed shirt
view	tongue tied	support
tunnel vision	unheard	tense
watch	voice an opinion	upset
witness	word for word	whipped

Fig. 10.10 Linguistic tip-offs. Color your conversation by using these words to match your client's language patterns.

subtly mirror the other person's body language or nonverbal cues. If her legs are crossed, cross yours. (If they are crossed at the ankles however, cross yours at the knees.) Do not "parrot" each gesture exactly. If he adjusts his tie, straighten your collar. If she tugs on her ear, play with your earring. If he clicks the counter with his finger, then fiddle with your pen on the counter. The key is to mirror the client, only after you feel you are harmonizing and in sync.

If you've been successfully mirroring the client and you want to check the progress, take the lead and subtly adjust your body language. Up until now you have been following the clients' lead. Now it's time to switch. For example, if your legs are crossed at the ankles, switch and cross them at the knees. If you are resting your hands on the chair arms, fold your hands on your lap. Wait and see if the client follows your lead. If she is "clicking" with you, the client will not even realize that she shifted her body to match yours. If the client's body language

follows your actions, she is "buying" what you are saying. You have successfully established rapport and tuned into each other. Getting the client to say yes to your offer will be a thousand times easier because she has subconsciously connected with you.

Now, the exceptional thing about mirroring is that if you are really tuned in to the other person, you will automatically, subconsciously mirror the other person, and vice versa. The actions happen naturally. You won't have to stage the action, it just falls into place, just like the perfect haircut.

The key to understanding personality traits and building rapport is to know yourself and to be flexible enough to shift into the other person's comfort zone. The chameleon can change his color to match his surroundings so that he blends in and harmonizes with his environment. Once you become tuned into the sections outlined in this chapter, notice how much smoother and easier your selling becomes.

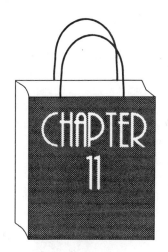

CHAPTER 11

RETAIL KILLERS AND SALES BUILDERS

Retail killers and sales builders are simple ways you can increase your revenues. Positive results are simple. Many of the following suggestions are as painless as changing your thoughts or phrases.

RETAIL KILLERS

We Close the Client's Wallet

Quite often clients' wallets are closed in your mind even before they utter a word. Don't shut off clients' potential to spend based on appearances. "They look like they can't afford it." "She doesn't look like she has $20 extra to spend, so I won't waste my time talking about the product." "Oh, I don't know if she has the money. If I sell her products then little Johnny may not get his new tennis shoes." Don't prejudge how little or how much money the client will turn loose.

One of my first retailing jobs was at a florist shop. The store provided all the beautiful blooming goodies one would expect, but they also had a thriving greenhouse business. One unusually hot, humid July day, a woman entered the store. She appeared to be out of place, not lost or confused, but unable to afford the store's prices. We were not the cheapest place in town. She approached the counter and stated that she would like fourteen flats of bedding plants. She looked as though she did not have that much money, and I surely didn't want to

waste my time hauling all those flats. Each flat was about the size of a school cafeteria tray and very cumbersome to carry. Earlier that day I had spent the entire morning shift in the greenhouse. The temperature was over one hundred degrees with 80 percent humidity. Not wanting to be rude, I told her the price, and she informed me with a shrug of her shoulders that it was "no problem."

She then bent forward, reached under the neckline of her dress, and pulled out a blue velvet Chivas Regal bag that had been securely nestled between her breasts. She loosened the bag from the chain to which it was attached and proceeded to unroll a wad of crisp $100 bills. Boy, did I feel stupid, and from that day forward I swore never to prejudge how much a client will or will not spend based on appearances.

The power of your mind can make or break a sale. I remember conducting a staff meeting and the topic of discussion was retail quotas. We were huddled around the conference table in my office when the power of mind became strikingly evident. At the time, three of the staff members were working toward a record-breaking month. The others were bemoaning and griping that their clients were out of town, the economy was bad, times were tough, and the customers didn't have any extra money. I found it puzzling that half the staff had great clients that were spending money like there was no tomorrow and the others had deadbeats. How could this be? The city of Wichita was not that big. I asked those three under the gun how their clients could be in such bad states, while the other three had managed to leap easily over their selling goals. Did they have the unfortunate luck of the draw to get the only clients struggling in bad times? It was absolutely shocking that half the staff had great sales and the other half were limping along. What could have caused the difference?

After a little prodding we finally uncovered that the three who were making it had the right success sales attitude, the right mind power. The other three were transferring their "poor me" attitude to their customers. If the employee didn't have any extra money then obviously the clients didn't either. They were closing the clients' wallets in their mind based on their own lean financial conditions.

After this episode, I went back over sales statistics and discovered a surprising piece of information. There was a direct link between the success of sales and the pay period cycles. The staff was paid twice a month. The three days preceding and the three days following the pay periods, sales went up. After discussing this phenomenon with the three who needed to bring up their sales, we discovered that if they felt wealthy, then that energy transferred itself to making the sale. If they felt a little lean in the wallet then sales went down. Either way, their minds were controlling the situation.

So the moral of the story is to guard your thoughts from closing the customer's wallet. Allow your client to give you the signals and go ahead for making the sale. Don't lose out by snapping their wallets shut before you have a chance to start.

Fear of the Word No

The fear or apprehension of hearing "No" can set up mental roadblocks that can keep you from closing the sale. "No" is the one word we all have heard thousands of times as little children. "No" is a tiny word that erects giant emotional blocks. You don't meet many people who enjoy being told no to something.

You've made the presentation, you've asked the client to buy, and she has said "no." What's the worst possible thing that can happen? The world will not open up and swallow you. The day doesn't come to an end. You won't die. The customer simply said no. Keep in mind she is not rejecting you personally, but your offering.

Don't allow a little word to hold you back from your success. Change the fear of no into go energy.

No Close

Three-fourths of selling situations will not end with a positive sale. Seventy-five percent of the world's daily selling transactions fail because someone did not close the sale. They simply didn't ask for the order. If you don't ask for the order, chances are it is not going to happen. I've only had one client rush into the salon and say, "Give me everything on this long list. I'm paying cash and I only have a few minutes." Retailing would be a cakewalk if every customer just volunteered to buy everything you have.

Selling has a beginning and an end, a start and finish point. Retailing is a skill like perming, cutting, color, facials, pedicures. There is a natural order to follow if you want to achieve fantastic results.

We Don't Listen

"Opportunity is often missed because we are broadcasting when we should be tuning in." Every day people hear, but the problem is they don't listen. They are too wrapped up in their own little corner of the world. They don't really listen to what is going on around them. It's much tougher to listen than to talk.

Tune in and really listen for selling opportunities. Ask your customers what problems they are having with their hair/skin/nails. Listen for the response. When they respond they are verbally handing you the sale on a silver platter. If you listen to the response, solve the problem, and make the sale.

Lack of Authority

You must radiate confidence and professional know-how. You cannot expect to be successful in sales if you are too meek and timid. Now I'm not suggesting you bulldoze your clients with aggressiveness, but you must display an aura of confidence and capability. "I strongly suggest" is an excellent way to reinforce your professional recommendation.

I was in a salon training its staff to sell. During the day I kept hearing one stylist ask her clients, "There isn't anything you need today, is there?" What a killer! I knew the stylist was in trouble when one client even answered back, "Well, now that you mention it, no." I was having heart failure, partly due to the poor sales question, but also because of the stylist's demeanor. She was looking at the floor, her hair covered 90 percent of her face, and she asked the question in a barely audible voice.

You have gone to school. You know your stuff. Let your questions and body language support your sales effort. Make the cash register ring by proudly and naturally displaying your professional know-how.

Lack of Communication

There are really two sales killers here—no talk and wrong talk.

Wrong talk—what do people in this industry tend to chat about with the customer seated in their chair? Yes, you guessed it. You will overhear conversations on such topics as travel, food, new businesses, hot spots, previous clients, your next client, who is doing what to whom, relationships, soap opera plots, news in the news, political activities, personal life dilemmas and tribulations, everything but beauty-related topics. The dialogue too often runs the gamut of every subject imaginable, except why the client is there in the first place. Center your conversations around the client's needs and wants.

No talk killers are when the technician performs the duties and there is little or no conversation. I remember having a facial in a very posh New York salon. During my two-hour visit I heard six words. "Follow me." "Lean back." "Thank you." There was no conversation regarding my skin's needs or special requests, no offer to reschedule, nothing. I couldn't believe the total lack of communication during the service. Not only did they miss the boat on product sales, but I would never return for their services. The lack of verbal contact gave me the impression that every treatment was exactly the same, with no regard for personal differences. Their standard treatments were straight off the factory line.

Avoid killing the sale with wrong talk and no talk. Remember that selling is talking and successful selling is channeling conversations directed toward the client's needs.

I'm a Stylist; I Don't Sell

Selling is a continuation of your artistic endeavor, not a separate duty. As a stylist you must convince your client that you are competent in your creative talent. Simply being skilled with your shears or hands is not enough. Have you ever worked on a customer and you knew that if she would only use Thus and Such you could solve her problem?

If you need to talk your customer into an updated version of her style you are really selling a new look. You are selling. Don't get caught up in the hype that true artists don't sell. Hogwash! You are giving clients the best possible service. Why send them home empty-handed? They need the products to recreate the look tomorrow morning. Don't cheat them. And don't cheat yourself. Proper home care, recommended by you, will give the client the home advantage.

I, I, I

Well I did such and such. I know all there is to know. I just went to Italy and I spent a fortune on new clothes. I went to a private party last night on Mrs. Megabuck's yacht. Who cares?

Watch statements that begin with I. It is the smallest word in the English language, and it is an insignificant word to your client. Of course there will be times when relating personal stories is appropriate, but be cautious.

One of my customers owned a unique clothing store. I strive to do business with people that do business with me, so one day when the mood to shop hit I decided to check out my client's new store. A rack of silk blouses caught my eye when the owner proceeded to flip through the collection and tell me, "I have this one in blue, and I also have this one in yellow and black." The little voice inside my head was saying that's great for her, but big deal. A few moments later I ran across an absolutely gorgeous dress. "Oh Carol, you are going to love this dress. My husband took me on a trip to Hawaii. I packed this dress in three colors, and I loved the way it traveled for me." Who cares? The point was that if she had purchased everything in the store, I didn't want to be a fashion copycat. By the time I left the store she had used the word *I* more times than I could count. Needless to say my shopping money never left my wallet. Obviously, the owner was too concerned with herself to care about the shopper's interest and needs.

Keep in mind that your clients are tuned into one radio station, WIFM, What's In It for Me. Keep the focus directed toward the client and away from yourself.

May I Help You?

I have a few rules, and this one is in the top five. This frequently used phrase can put the kibosh on making the sale. Absolutely, positively refrain from asking this seemingly harmless question. Strike it from your vocabulary!

Have you ever been in a store and the salesperson approached you and asked, "May I help you?" My guess is that your response was "No, I'm just looking." Now if the question is asked very quickly it could sound liked"Nelpyou?" And the lightening quick response is "No Juslkin." Asking "May I help you?" can prevent the conversation from going any further. Your potential sale will come to a screeching halt. This seemingly harmless phrase throws a giant wrench in the questioning process because it is a yes or no question. If the shopper says no you are stuck up the sale without a paddle. Avoid setting yourself up for failure. Never ask a client, "May I help you?"

If would not be fair of me to take away the phrase without telling you what you can use. Try "How can I help you?" "What can I do for you today?" "Hello, how can I assist you?" It may take a little practice but after a while you will start to catch yourself when this road-to-nowhere question starts to pass over your lips.

SALES BUILDERS

System Selling

If you heed nothing but this one sales building tip, I'll guarantee you that you could double your retail sales. That's a pretty big promise. Want to know what it is?

System selling is to sell matching products two by two. Every product on your shelf has a companion product; recommend and sell them as a set. If I said shampoo you'd naturally think of conditioner. Certain products are naturally "married" to each other. In the application sequence you do one then the other. Here's a few more: top coat and base coat. Gel and finishing spray. Base makeup and powder. Loose powder and compact powder. Nail polish and quick dry. Body shampoo and body moisturizing lotion. Eye shadow and mascara. I think you get the picture.

The first shop in which I sold cosmetics had a store policy—if you only had one item on the ticket you did not receive commission on the sale. The owner felt that if only one item showed up on the receipt that the staff was just taking orders and not selling the products and services. Her store policy sure lit a fire under me. No two items, no sale, no commission, no money. You learn quickly to monitor your tickets for two item sales.

Sell What it Does, Not What it Is

When you present products to your clients always stress what the product will do for them, not what it is. For example, sell what a perm will do for the client. The perm will save time, make the hair fuller and able to hold the curl throughout the day. Don't just sell the perm based on what it is, such as a nonalkaline perm with fourteen different herbs and conditioners that will take twenty to thirty minutes to process.

Emphasize how the product will help the client, how it will look, how it will solve the beauty problem. Punch the ultimate reason why the client would want or need that product.

I'd Be Glad To

A national board meeting was being held at the Pier 66 Hotel in Ft. Lauderdale, Florida. As a representative I had the unique pleasure of experiencing this remarkable hotel. My trip had been one of those horrible traveler's nightmares. I had arrived three hours late, without one of my bags, and was missing the opening business meeting. As I made my way to the front desk a very pleasant desk clerk looked up and said, "Welcome to the Pier 66 Hotel. My name is Lisa. How can I help you?" I responded with my confirmation number, and she politely announced that she'd be glad to make the room arrangement. Did I need help with baggage? We would be glad to ring the bellhop. Three sincere declarations of service. I was amazed. "Ms. Phillips, would you like to go on up to the room and freshen up? I'll have your luggage sent up," she continued. That sounded great to me.

After the bags arrived, I realized that the first meeting was by then over and I might as well dress for the dinner party. When I opened by suitcase I was in for a shock to see how everything was wrinkled. Well, a quick call to housekeeping and they could send up an iron. "I'd be glad to send up an iron, Ms. Phillips. Would you like an ironing board as well?" My trip lasted five days and I heard this sincere statement expressed from everyone on the Pier 66 Hotel staff—desk clerk, bell captain, manager, waitresses, even the housekeeping staff. Now, that's service.

The experience left me with such a positive impression that the phrase "I'd be glad to" was incorporated into salon dialogues. I would highly recommend that you incorporate this phrase too. When a customer requests something (appointment, literature, samples) add "I'd be glad to" with your response and watch the positive feedback you receive from the customer.

Review and Repeat

Have you had clients walk up to the front desk after a particularly relaxing treatment and appear to be a little foggy? They have that glazed-over look in their eyes because they are so relaxed? When many of your salon treatments are designed to pamper customers, you will need to review and repeat the necessary information, just to make sure they heard your home care advice.

We all process information differently and at varying speeds. Remember that some people learn through sight, others through sound, and still others through feeling. Keep in mind that the person you are addressing does not think the way you do and may need clarification of your directions. Review and repeat home care instructions, appointment time and day, location, or monthly offers or special directions.

Seventy-eight Percent of What People Buy Is What They See

Seventy-eight percent of the population purchases what catches their eye. Get the products out and visible. Change displays. Keep shelves clean. Make products accessible. Have point of purchase material available. You will not sell the merchandise if it's stuffed in drawers, dispensaries, back rooms, and boxes.

Clothing stores used to have you sit in a reception area and the clothes were brought out to you, either carried out or on models. With the exception of a few exclusive clothing boutiques, how many of these stores are still in business? Not many. Picture today's harried, hassled career woman lounging around while someone parades clothes in front of her without consideration of style, color, shape, and price. Hard to imagine? You bet!

Do you walk into a store, size up the lay of the land and instantly know where you want to head? It's really quite simple: people like to see plenty of merchandise to pique their interest before they turn loose their hard-earned cash. Who wants to shop in a place that looks empty, that has minimal inventory, that's been picked over? I don't and I'll bet you and your clients don't want to either.

Sell the Senses

People purchase products emotionally and support the decision with logic. They have to be excited, enthusiastic, or at least stimulated enough to make a positive decision and take action on your offer.

Pull up a very pleasurable memory you have of a favorite dining experience. Relive the evening in your mind's eye. What images are conjured up? Do you remember the food, the smells, the setting, the lighting, the greeting, the music? Chances are every nuance of the evening added up to a memorable and pleasurable experience. All the elements were working in harmony, subconsciously and consciously, to create a special event. Selling the senses puts the client in the right frame of mind to respond positively to your offer. Don't overlook the power of selling the senses.

Sell Solutions

Find out what problems the client may be suffering from, then eliminate the problem. Direct your questioning toward her hair/skin/nails. Ask the client: "What can I do for you today?" "Are you having any problems that you would like addressed today?" "Do you have any questions that I can answer regarding your home care program?"

You hear hundreds of problems every day in the salon. Too flat. Too thin. No body. Hard to manage. Makeup flakes. Makeup fades during the day. Nails chip and crack. Skin peels. Skin dry and tight. Pores clogged. Stressed. If you take into account the multitude of possibilities and the equal number of solutions your sales volume is unlimited. Find a problem and solve it.

Part Treatment and Part Products

Have clients feel the area that is to be treated. Have them get a good impression of the texture and condition of the area. After completing the service, ask them to feel the area again. "Notice the difference?" Make sure you get a positive confirmation. "The results are part treatment and part products." Now, how could they possibly go home empty-handed when they just confirmed the results?

If you simply said the result was due to the service, would they buy the products? No. If you said the results were due to the products, would they need you to administer the service? No again. Part treatment and part products covers your bases by truthfully declaring the results were obtained by the service and the products. The object is to plant the need for both your services and your products in the client's mind.

Expect to Make the Sale

You must go into the service expecting to make the sale. As many great positive thinkers have said, if you think you can, you can. If you think you can't, you can't. Either way you are right. You will not sell every single client that walks through your doors, but if you follow the steps, believe in what you offer, and expect to make the sale chances are you will succeed.

THE STEP-BY-STEP SELLING SEQUENCE

Well, this is it! The chapter all the previous chapters have been leading up to. In this chapter, you will discover the format, the game plan, the proven sequence for successful selling.

You already follow a logical sequence of procedures for assuring a successful service. Well, this is the logical, fun pattern for making the sale.

FORTY-THREE EXCUSES WHY PEOPLE DIDN'T MAKE THE SALE

1. Just yesterday the client bought $300 worth of stuff.
2. Retailing is too tough.
3. I just don't know what to say.
4. I get tongue-tied.
5. I was running behind and was trying to catch up.
6. My client had to leave.
7. Our products are lousy.
8. They can get shampoo in the grocery store.
9. But they are selling products at the flea market.
10. I needed some assistance.
11. I lost my voice.
12. I lost my nerve.
13. Why sell products? I'm not going to make any money.
14. The salon is too slow.
15. The salon is too busy.
16. I don't have any clients.
17. She said she didn't have any money.
18. I was having a bad day.
19. The client was in a cranky mood.
20. I can't take rejection.
21. We had a hard time "connecting."
22. He said he'd think about it.
23. I forgot the prices.
24. The phone was ringing.
25. I couldn't find the price sheet.
26. They were just looking.
27. The color she wanted was discontinued.
28. Our products are too expensive.
29. Our products are too cheap.
30. I need more product knowledge training.
31. She said she had tried one of our products before and didn't like it.
32. He only uses brand names.
33. She said she had sensitive skin.
34. When the service was complete the client was too sleepy and relaxed.
35. I didn't want to bother them.
36. They had spent so much money on other services, I guessed that they had spent their limit.
37. I was afraid to ask.
38. His sister sells products.
39. I don't sell products because I am an artist.
40. I assumed that they wouldn't want to buy anything.

41. We didn't talk about products; we talked about her dead-beat boyfriend.
42. We're such good friends, I couldn't possibly sell something to her.
43. I just didn't ask.

It's easy to talk yourself out of trying to make the sale. Excuses are a dime a dozen. People who make excuses are usually interrupted by people making things happen. Don't allow even one of these excuses to hold you back. You owe it to yourself and your clients to give them the opportunity to say yes to your professional services and products. After this chapter you will have the skills necessary to make the communication connection with each client.

Confidence comes with practice. Don't be afraid. Your temporary nervousness stems from a lack of knowledge. Once you finish this chapter you will be amazed at how natural and easy selling more products and services can be.

The four-point plan for making the sale is to garner the client's awareness, pique curiosity, build passion, then ask the client to take action on your product or service.

AWARENESS

The selling transaction begins with the initial client contact. You already know that you don't get a second chance at making a first impression, so your action here is instrumental in setting the stage for the remaining selling sequence.

It is critical to acknowledge the customer within the first five seconds she is in the salon. If you are not familiar with the client take the initiative and introduce yourself first.

"Good morning, I'm Juan. Welcome to the salon. Who are you here to see?"

Sales Dance

The beginning part of the selling sequence is a little like dancing—someone has to lead. You will be leading the client or she will lead at first. Simply use your common sense and follow the visual and verbal clues the client is displaying. If the client is looking at eye shadow, you don't want to talk about pedicures.

I was in a salon and literally saw an employee march up front to the retail area, pull the product out of the client's hand, slap it back on the shelf, and announce, "I am ready for you now. Follow me." I was in shock and so was the client. The stylist's militaristic approach made me want to click my heels and fall into rank. To this day I can't imagine why she didn't just carry the bottle back down the hall explaining the benefits of the product as the client was getting situated.

You must learn to respond to the situation at hand. Maybe the client has already been in the shop for awhile and is looking at a display of products. If the client has her hand on a product for oily hair and you can tell by looking at her that her hair is dry and chemically treated, you can respond to her by asking a question. "Do you feel your hair is oily? I see that you are holding XYZ Shampoo for oily hair." Then wait for her response.

Bye Bye, May I Help You

In the last chapter on Killers and Builders there was one phrase mentioned that should never pass your lips. Do you remember? This overworked phrase should be put to rest once and for all. The question "May I help you?"

You unfortunately have exercised your options and you have nowhere to lead the customer through the sale if you ask the Help You question and the client says No. The selling formula will come to a screeching halt before it has had the chance to flourish.

You may use:

- "How can I help you?"
- "What can I do for you today?"
- "Hi! My name is Larry, and you are?"

Anything but "May I help you?"

Perilous Pitfalls

The selling sequence begins as soon as the customer walks through the front door. The actions that happen during the first few minutes will set the tone for the client's entire experience. The client's initial reaction and visual observation can and will affect your sales. Some pitfalls that are unfortunately seen in salons are:

- Talking to other staff members and ignoring the client. Pull the client into the conversation. Turn to her and ask for input. "Gee, Toni what do you think about . . . ?" Or, "Mrs. Schnieder, we were discussing the new fashion colors for fall. Have you seen the new shades?" Pay close attention to the client sitting in the reception area. Not only is it rude to ignore the client, you may be alienating him or her when you try to make a sale later in the service. Even if the waiting client isn't your personal customer, make some kind of connection. Smile, greet him or her, hand him a salon brochure, ask if she needs coffee or tea. That client just may end up in your chair, and it will be tough to bridge the ill will.

- Chatting it up on the phone on a personal call while a client waits. If a client enters the salon or area you are working in, and you are taking a personal phone call, excuse yourself from the call and immediately hang up. Never take a phone call when you have the opportunity to give your attention and service to a client. Don't miss sales by talking on the phone, personal or business, while you have a live, breathing client standing in front of you.

- General indifference to staff and clients. Watch your body language and conversation. There are so many mirrors in the salon, you may not even be aware of all the eyes that are on you. If you want to increase your sales, it will be necessary to direct your focus and positive energy toward the people in the salon at all times.

Remember this section. Awareness building determines the direction the sales process will take. Watch the client's actions carefully at this stage. The goal is to make her feel comfortable and to start the selling sequence.

CURIOSITY

I have a little surprise for you. After you finish this chapter, you and I are going to Italy. What flashes through your mind? When are we going? How are we going to get there? Who is paying for the trip? How long are we going to be gone? What are we going to do once we get there? Can my family go along? Will we do any shopping? What kinds of restaurants will we dine in?

If you don't ask me questions, you don't have a clue as to what may happen. Selling is the same way. Your skill at asking questions is tantamount to successfully completing the sale. Asking questions is the only way to identify your customer's needs. Consult the client regarding lifestyle, likes, dislikes, and desires. Probe to find out beauty problems. By consulting the client you will then be able to determine the direction to take the sale.

Asking questions reveals to the client that you are interested in her, that you care. You are curious about her needs and wants. You want to uncover beauty problems and are willing to help solve them.

A client was sitting in the reception area of a salon. At the time she was minding her own business reading a magazine. One of the salon's stylists marched up to her, ran his fingers through her hair, then asked if she wanted it colored. No hello, no introduction, no questions, just straight to the "Do you want your hair colored?" You can guess what her shocked response was. "No!" In fact she was terribly offended and justifiably so. This is not the shortcut way to make a sale. The stylist jumped from Point A straight to Z. No questions, no sale.

There is only one way to find out what excites clients and that is to ask. Clients will describe in their own words exactly how to sell them. People like to talk about themselves. You just have to ask. The trick is to get out of the habit of telling the client everything. Ask me and I'll share my desires with you. Tell me or dictate to me and I'll shut you out.

If you tell people things they tend to doubt you. But if they tell you, they believe. Clients will respond a thousand times better if you ask them rather than tell them. If you impart your care and concern instead of dictating your opinion to the client, she will be more receptive to your advice and offering. It pays to ask questions.

Fact-Finding Mission

There is a journalistic formula for covering a story. A good journalist always covers the basics, the who, what, when, where, why, and hows. Your new selling skills will follow suit. You will be on a fact-finding mission to find out how you can help the client. To assist you on your discovery process here are different questions to aid you in piquing the client's curiosity.

As you are establishing a rapport with clients, ask permission first before you launch into your questioning process. "Before we begin may I ask you a few questions? I want your input and direction." Then direct your questions toward discovering the client's desires. Your customers buy solutions to their beauty problems. You will need to find out just what areas they feel need help. My first question to any client is, "What can I do for you today? What problems are you having with your hair/skin/nails?"

Now of course you will not ask all these questions, but study the possibilities. The goal is to have an arsenal of questions ready for taking aim at the sale.

What

What can I do for you today?

What products are you using now?

What would you change if you could alter one thing about your product?

What do you think about (name of product)?

What kind of product are you looking for?

What happens to your hair after a perm?

What results do you want to achieve?

What kind of look do you have in mind?

What are your favorite colors in makeup? In clothing?

What consistency do you prefer in a moisturizer?

What shade do you like?

What texture of styling aid works best in your hair?

What type of skin do you feel you have?

What problems are you having with your hair/skin/nails?

In what kind of lighting do you apply your makeup?

What inspired you to modify your look? Update your style?

What made you select our salon?

What problems are you having with application?

What can I do right now to get you to say yes?

What do you like best about this so far?

What products do you need to restock today?

What do you have and what do you want?

What results do you expect to see after your perm/facial/haircolor?

What areas do you want to treat?

What do you prefer?

When

When was the last time that your hair looked its absolute best?

When did you last change your look?

When would you like to change your hairstyle?

When would you like to see results?

When do you condition your hair?

When do you normally perm?

When do you mask?

When was your last appointment?

When do you apply eye cream/body lotion/nail polish?

When would it be convenient for you?

When would you like to start your makeover?

When would you like to have your first appointment?

When was the last time you had a pedicure?

When was your last fill for your sculptured nails?

When do you think you will run out of your old products?

When do you want to begin?

When is your birthday?

When is your special event? Party? Anniversary?

When would you like to have your massage/manicure/facial?

When would you be able to come back?

When did you first contemplate having a pedicure/leg waxing/makeover?

Where

Where are you applying?

Where are you going for your special date?

Where have you had a manicure/perm/color analysis before (locally or out of state)?

Where are you having troubles?

Where are you applying the eye creme?

Where have you been? I've missed you.

Where do you want your hair shorter? Straight? Cut? Curled?

Where did you find such a great scarf/pin/briefcase?

Where in the world did you find such a hot outfit?

Where did you learn that piece of beauty news?

Where do you store your cosmetics?

Where would you like to begin?

Where do you frequently travel?

How

How much of product A do you have left?

How do you apply your cosmetics?

How often do you condition? Mask? Perm? Schedule your trims?

How would you like to be one of the first to try this?

How can I help you today?

How may I help you?

How many do you want?

How about a change?

How about a new lipstick color?

How does your skin feel after cleansing?

How long after cleansing does oil show up in your skin?

Confidentially, how old are you?

How do you clean your skin?

How do you use your blower? Curling iron?

How do you hold your brush?

How would you like your skin to feel?

Why

Why are you waiting?

Why are you hesitating to change your look?

Why do you want a change?

Why do you believe that the product isn't working?

Why are you waiting to schedule your complete makeover?

Why are you apprehensive?

Why don't you give it a try?

Why is that important?

Why don't we sign you up for one while they last?

Who

Who referred you to the salon?

Who is your favorite designer?

Whose product are you using?

Who's getting married?

Who told you about product A?

Which

Which would be more convenient for you, morning or afternoon?

Which time of day is best for you?

Which product do you prefer?

Which color strikes your fancy?

Which strength of hair spray do you prefer?

Which family of colors do you like best?

Do you prefer . . .

Warm or cool colors?

Frost or nonfrosted colors?

Light or dark tones?

Matte or shiny textures?

Lipstick or gloss?

Clear or colored nail polish?

Black or brown?

Cream or powder?

Cake eyeliner or liquid?

Cream or lotion products?

Oil-based or water-based products?

Your foundation to be opaque or sheer?

Toner or astringent?

Working with one or two eye shadows?

Day cream or night cream?

A firming mask or gel?

Loose or compact powder?

Mascara or false lashes?

Bright or light colors?

Day or evening look?

Cleansing cream or lotion?

Soap or cleanser?

Straight or curly looks?

Soft or firm curls?

Long or short looks?

Spray or gel?

Perfume or cologne?

One or two colors?

Cash or credit card?

Are you

Are you sure you won't wait/change/reschedule?

Are you wanting a dramatic change or a gradual one?

Are you hoping to reduce stress/look younger/change your color?

Are you willing to modify your look slightly?

Are you willing to invest three minutes in the morning and at night to obtain results?

Are you holding on to that old product for a reason?

Are you ready?

Are you satisfied with the new look?

Are you happy with what we have created?

Are you sure you can repeat the look tomorrow?

Are there any questions?

Are you serious about this?

Have You

Have you ever tried a body massage?

Have you ever considered switching to another brand?

Have you ever scheduled a facial?

Have you ever treated yourself to a pedicure?

Have you noticed any change in your hair? Skin? Nails? Body?

Have you seen much improvement?

Have you tried our skin products?

Have you experienced any body waxing?

Have you been here before?

Have you used our recommended home care?

Have you filled out our confidential questionnaire?

Have you ever had your eyebrows professionally shaped?

Have you ever been color charted?

Have you had a makeup lesson before?

Have you seen our new brochure?

Have you imagined what the new you will look like?

Would You

Would you do this for me? Let's you and I work together for maximum results.

Would you like to flip through our catalogue?

Would you please have a seat?

Would you please feel your hair/skin before we begin the treatment?

Would you consider a new look/a darker shade/a shorter cut?

Will You

Will you consider this?

Will this program of products fit into your routine?

Will you agree with me on that?

Will you invest five minutes a day for a lifetime of better hair/skin/nails?

Will you do this for yourself and me?

Will you consider starting with the basic collection of products?

Will you be paying with cash or credit card?

Will you be bringing a friend with you? Will they want to have their hair done as well?

Miscellaneous Questions

Do you feel your skin is oily or dry? Normal or troubled? Smooth or rough? Large or small pores?

Does your skin get tight after washing? If so, when?

Do you like it?

If I could show you how, would you be interested?

PASSION

You have established the rapport with the client and you have invested time for the discovery process. Now, it's time to add a little spice to the process. Your client is buying plain old shampoo. What would make her invest in your super-rich, ultra-lather hair cleansing lotion? Soap is soap, or is it? How about adding a little sizzle to the sale? During this stage it is necessary to build some exictement and sizzle in the selling sequence.

As I've said before, people purchase products emotionally then justify their decision with logic. It is necessary for the client to become emotionally and physically involved in the presentation. Active involvement in the consultation and the presentation helps to stimulate the buying mechanism in the brain. Once clients' emotions are stroked, they are then ready to turn loose their hard-earned cash.

Stroking the Senses

The easiest way to stroke the emotions is to sell the senses. Incorporate many of the senses while working with the customer. Some ways to sell the senses are:

1. Sight: Start with a pleasant smile; show a video; have client follow along with a mirror or read a brochure or pamphlet; have displays at station.
2. Sound: Modulate your voice for appropriate selling scenario; monitor music choice and volume in salon; listen for annoying environmental noises.
3. Taste: Offer your client something to drink before or after your service. Have your drink selection be a little out of the ordinary, such as exotic teas, sodas, and coffees.
4. Smell: Hand the product to the customer and have them smell the aromatic quality of the product. Sniff out unpleasant odors in the salon and neutralize with air fresheners or diffusers.
5. Touch: The sense of touch is one powerful tool when trying to sell to your client. Touch your client on the shoulder or upper arm to make contact. Hand them a brochure or fashion magazine to hold onto during the treatment. Make sure your service area is kinesthetically appealing.

Client Participation

A key anchor appealing to touch is to get the client involved in the selling process. One way to get the client excited about your product is to build the client into the presentation.

Have you ever watched clients as they leave the salon and get into their cars? What is the first thing they do? They twist the rear-view mirror around and proceed to run their fingers through their hair. Right? It seems to be instinctive to put their own little touch to your finished work. Why not let them do that in the safety and comfort of your salon. Before you apply the finishing product, ask them to comb or brush their hair. Ask them if the cut feels right. Then, finish the look.

When I was in beauty school you absolutely, positively did not let clients comb or brush their own hair. And believe me, many tried to grab the brush out of my hand. I was missing the sales' boat back then. Don't you miss it today.

Touchy Sales

Have clients feel their hair before you even touch them. Ask them to get an impression of how their hair/skin/nails feel before you do anything to them, before you pick up a brush, cleansing sponge, or nail file. Many of your services will alter the condition. After you have completed the service, ask them to touch and feel again. Then have them recall the memory of the pretreatment condition. Will there be a difference? You bet! Now the client has a before and after comparison.

As you go through the service get the clients involved by handing them the product to apply. If it's mousse, hand the can to the client and tell her to turn the can upside down and press the trigger until a quarter-size dollop is in her hand. Then, have your client actually work the mousse through the hair. This eliminates the objection, "I couldn't possibly use the product. I don't know how."

Cries for Help

Have you ever had a client plead with you, "Could you be in my bathroom every morning?" If you are hearing this cry for help, you can bet your bottom dollar the client hasn't a clue on how to duplicate the look you have created. The goal here is to teach the client how to duplicate the look at home in the morning.

One of my favorite phrases is, "Words alone will often fail so demonstrate to make the sale." So much of our interaction with a customer is verbal. That is fine if the client has an auditory communication style, but many people have difficulty comprehending new information if they just hear the words.

Build the client into the presentation by:

- Giving the client the product to apply with your supervision.
- Handing her the blow-dryer and talking her through the proper way to dry her hair.
- Handing her a nail buffer and showing her the proper technique for buffing the nails at home.
- Applying makeup to the brush and handing the brush to the client to apply.

The trick is to incorporate as many of the senses as possible. As you involve your client in the treatment process and incorporate home care product use, you are solidifying the sale.

Remember, if clients hear it they will forget, see it they may remember. But if they see it, hear it, and do it they will understand and be more inclined to take action.

How Much People Remember:

- 10 percent of what they read
- 20 percent of what they hear
- 30 percent of what they see
- 50 percent of what they see and hear
- 50 percent of what they see and say
- 90 percent of what they say as they do a task

Product and Service Descriptions

When you describe to your client the benefits of a product or service keep the selling conversation simple. Remember to sell what it does, not what it is. Your clients are not buying hard, cold facts, but warmhearted benefits. Consumers today are better informed. But that doesn't mean you have to get technical and jargon-loaded when you describe a product. Keep uppermost in your mind how the product will ultimately benefit the client.

Little Yeses Add Up

Structure your presentation so you may receive minor agreements. Minor agreements are positive qualifiers. They are little questions that confirm the client is accepting your information. Once the customer has been honestly answering yes, it becomes increasingly difficult for her to say no at the end of the sale. Positive minor agreements lead the client to making the final commitment toward the sale.

Some trial closes are:

- Does that make sense?
- Is that all right?
- Is that fair enough?
- In your opinion . . . ?
- What would you prefer?
- Are you comfortable with what we have done thus far?
- Do you like the look?
- Does the product feel good?
- You can tell a difference now can't you?

These are minor agreements, little yeses that tell you if you are on track with the customer. But you will not stop here. You are now ready for the client to take action on your recommendation or offer.

ACTION

Well, so far you have established the rapport successfully, completed the discovery process, and fanned the flames of passion by building the client into your presentation. Now is the time to close the sale.

In a recent survey, salon clients were asked if they purchased their beauty products in the salon. An astounding 78 percent said, "No, I do not. My stylist never talked to me about them." That's seven out of ten missed sales opportunities. To close the sale, you merely give your client the opportunity to invest in your product/service. You set up an occasion where your client can take action on your professional recommendation.

No Overloading

Let me state right now, I don't want you selling clients anything they really don't need or desire. I don't want you to push unnecessary products. Don't load them down with bags of merchandise. The goal is to match the client needs with the right product.

Personally I don't like to sell too much on a visit, especially if it is a new client. I prefer to have the client invest $50 today, $50 next week, and $25 the next versus $175 on a one-stop shopping excursion. If, by chance, you have loaded a client up on products, that's okay. You just follow your client's lead. The idea is to get the client in the habit of shopping in your salon. And repeat visits help to establish the buying pattern.

Timing Is Everything

When do you close the sale? When the customer is ready to buy. You may be fortunate enough to have a client announce that she will take everything. For other customers it will be necessary to follow the lead of the client. Don't get caught in the trap of feeling that you have to tell the client everything you know about the service or product. Don't talk yourself out of the sale. Knowing when to close is similar to dancing—follow your customer's rhythm.

Physical Buying Clues

You are successfully following the sequence. As you lead your client through the process, you should be noticing certain physical body changes occurring in your customer. Customers can lie with their mouths, but not with their bodies. The mouth responds to conscious actions and influences. The body responds to the subconscious stimulus. The subconscious mind will be a truer monitor of the client's willingness to buy. She may be saying one thing, but observe the physical reactions for positive or negative confirmation of your presentation.

When the client has connected with you, you'll notice some or all of these tip-offs.

- The eyes will widen and even become brighter. The customer will look more alert. The pupils may even dilate.

- The client's breathing patterns will change. You'll notice a quicker, higher breathing pattern in visual clients. The kinesthetic types will be breathing deep, slow, thoughtful breaths.

- You may even notice hives flushing on the client's skin, especially if she has a thinner, more transparent skin type. If the client has on an open neckline pay attention to the neck and chest.

- Notice if the customer smiles and nods in agreement with what you are saying. You can physically get the client to agree with you by gently nodding your head. At first, when you try this you may feel like the little dog in the back of the car window. But do try it. You are merely getting the client in an agreeing stage. My staff had nicknamed this selling tip the N2 F2 sales tip for nod-nod and flutter-flutter. The flutter is when you nod and slowly let your eyes sweep the floor and then look back into the client's eyes.

- You may see your customer relax and slump slightly back into the chair. Notice if she leans back and tries to touch you if you are standing behind her. If she does, her body language indicates she has connected with you. Close the sale. You may see her lean forward or toward you if you are standing in front of her or are behind a counter. She will lean into your personal space when she has bought into what you are selling.

- Notice if the customer picks up a product or brochure and examines it. Look to see if she is calculating the product/service in her mind. You should be able to see her thinking.

- If your customer reaches for her purse or wallet, you are on the home stretch. She has closed herself. Say no more and put the products in the bag.

Verbal Buying Cues

Clients will voice their I'm-ready-to-buy cues:

- Listen for the point where they ask for more information. They are verbalizing their interest by asking for additional information. "Do you have this in bright red?" "How often should I condition my hair?" If clients are interested, they'll ask questions. If they don't give a hoot, they will not waste their breath.

- Listen for agreements. When they agree with your suggestions, they are selling themselves. "Yes, I agree that I need to treat myself better." "Yes, I know I should be conditioning my hair." "You know, what you are saying makes sense." Agreement equals acceptance. Acceptance equals sales. Sales equal more money for you.

- Tune in when your customer requests repeat information. "Now, tell me again, how do I use this product?" If they are taking the time to have you review the steps, you can be sure the client has purchased the item in the mind already.

- Listen to hear if the customer is referring to possession of the product. "I will like using my new lipstick tonight." "I'll have to remember to add this to my home care routine."

    As you interact with your customer, tune up your sales-honing mechanism. Pay close attention to your client and look for the visual and verbal signs. The greater the number of agreements, the easier the close of the sale.

Nailing Down the Sale

You close the selling sequence by asking for the order. Closing the sale is giving the customer the opportunity to say yes to you, your product, and/or your services. You are suggesting, recommending, and prescribing proper products or services. Your goal is to get the client to say yes, so you can put the products in the bag.

Yes/No Taboos

When you close a sale avoid questions that are yes/no driven. Asking such closed-ended questions can cut your selling process off because you'll have only a fifty-fifty shot of the customer saying yes to your sales question. So the first thing we'll eliminate is asking the client a yes- or no-based question. Instead, ask open-ended questions that force the client to respond with more than one word.

- Avoid "Do you need any product?" Use "What do you need to restock today?"

- Avoid "Do you want to buy any products?" Use "What products do you want to take home?"

- Avoid "Do you want to take any products home?" Use "What collection of products would you like to start with?"

- Avoid "Do you want to reschedule?" Use "What day in the week would be most convenient for you?"

    It's tough for the client to say no to one of these questions. They have to come up with some answer that will then lead you into the close.

COLOSSAL CLOSES

This close gives the client the opportunity to select options and state preferences. This close is easy and comfortable to use.

- "Would you prefer a lotion or cream moisturizer?"
- "Would you like to use your Visa or American Express?"
- "Do you like your lipstick to be cream or frosted?"
- "Would you prefer two bottles or one?"
- "Would you like the travel or the economy size?"

    I remember trying on a very expensive coat one day. As soon as I tried it on, I knew I had to have it. The only close the salesperson used on me was, "You have your choice of monograms. We offer your name in script or block letters. Which would you prefer?" Needless to say I purchased the coat. She had me hook, line, and sinker. Just think how you can use it for beauty products?

Assumptive Close

Assume the client is going to buy what you are suggesting. I feel I must caution you on this technique. It will work great if it is not overused. Definitely assume in your mind the client will accept your recommendations and that she will buy the product. When you are demonstrating the product and working with the client you may refer to situations as if she already has the product at home.

"Tomorrow when you are applying your new lightweight moisturizer, make sure to pat the cream on gently around the eyes and throat."

Related Close

Use this when the customer has selected an item and you recommend the companion product.

- "Since you have selected the Ravishing Red Nail Polish today, make sure you apply the Long-Lasting Super Top Coat over the color to help keep the color fresh."

- "You will need a skin freshener to follow the cleansing step. The toner completes the cleansing process and helps to keep your makeup in place."

- "I'm delighted you have selected the Sunless Tanning Lotion. Your skin will appreciate the care. For maximum results before you apply the Sunless Tan, take a minute and slough off the dead cells first with Super Smoother Body Scrub."

Every product in your salon has a companion product. Practice matching up products until it becomes a natural reflex to suggest the related product close.

Instruction Close

Put on your teaching hat here and show the customer how to use the product, how to open the container, amount to use, sequence of application. Share with your customer tips and secrets you personally have discovered about the product.

- "Before you open the lid of the cleanser, turn the bottle upside down and gently tap the lid on the back of your hand. I have found that this step helps to get the product out of the bottle easier."

- "Here's the mirror. Now, follow along with me and we'll use the prescription pad to go over your home care steps."

- "In the morning, before you apply any product, make sure you cleanse the eye area first. Take a cotton pad and saturate it with the eye makeup remover. Gently lay the pad on the eye and whisk away any residue."

- "You'll be using a quarter-size mound of texturizer. Work it through your hair, but concentrate on applying the full body texturizer at the base of the hair especially at the scalp. Here, you try it."

Standing Room Only Close

It's similar to trying to get tickets to a hot theater production. You know you've got to get those tickets because if they are that hard to get the play must be really good. Remember the Cabbage Patch Doll frenzy when all the kids wanted them and a limited edition was sent out before Christmas?

- "We are bringing in a guest makeup artist and there are only twenty appointments available. I'm sure you'll want to be one of the lucky ones. Let me see when the first available appointment is."

- "This is a limited supply. We could only get a small quantity from our distributor and this is it. If you want to get in on the bargain you'd better take it with you today."

- "Alex is only taking five new clients this month. Do you want to be on the list?"

Impending Close

If you have ever watched the Home Shopping Network you have seen this close at its best. This is when there is limited time to buy and limited quantity. Stress the fact that it is a limited time offer.

- "Christmas is three days away. What would you like to include on the gift certificate?"

- "There are only two days left on the after-summer beauty special. When could you get in for the reconditioning treatment?"

- "Time is running out. If you want your hair to look its best we'd better start right away."

- One of my personal favorites is "The sooner you start, the sooner you'll see and feel results."

You Owe it to Yourself Close

Some customers feel they shouldn't spend money on themselves. Others take spending to a new artform. Either way, you're covered with this close. Just emphasize the pleasure and need of being good to yourself.

- "If you don't take care of you who will? You work hard. You deserve a little treat."

- "As the commercial says, you owe it to yourself. After all you're worth it."

- "A full day of beauty is just what the beauty doctor orders. You deserve to come in and let someone take care of you for a change."

Service Close

You will close the sale by the added bonus of your service.

- "I want you to be happy with your new products. If you have any questions please give me a call."

- "Here's my card. If you have any concerns or questions about your new home care routine just give me a ring here at the salon. I'd be glad to help."

- "Before we select any products, it's my pleasure to administer a complimentary consultation."

- "Let's select the perfect shade of color to match your outfit."

- "I want your input in formulating the bath gel. Together we can make the perfect softening bath gel. Do you want it to be soothing or invigorating?"

Pro and Con Close

Weigh the advantages and disadvantages of a product or service.

- "Yes, this is a small jar, but you'll use such a little amount it will last you a long time."

- "The home care program that we have put together is a little bit more expensive, but the results are definitely worth it."

- "The Vanishing Wrinkle Cream is an investment. But I know you wouldn't want to skimp on quality."

Summary Close

Group products into collections. Summarize the benefits and uses for each collection. Get an agreement and then move onto the next group of products.

"Here are the three basic products for you to use at home. Start with the cleansing lotion, follow with the rinsing agent, and sparingly apply the day moisturizer. These three will start your personal home care cleansing basics. Do you have any questions? Great, then we'll move onto the intermediate collection." You will present each set, receive an agreement to purchase, then move onto the next collection.

MORE TIPS

Silence Is Golden

The hardest part of retailing after simply starting is to know when to quit talking. I have seen stylists talk themselves right out of a sale. Once you have asked your closing question for the client to take action, don't say another word. Keep your lips zipped. Most people can't stand silence. Your customer will be quick to respond to your close if you keep quiet. A successful negotiation technique to remember is that the first one who talks loses. Now you are not out to pull one over on your client, but on the other hand don't sell yourself short by talking too soon.

Ahead of the Game

If you have been following the selling format, your chances of closing the sale are 75 percent higher right now. You are seven and a half times ahead of other stylists. Hopefully you will be hearing clients saying yes to your recommendations, especially if you have based the product and treatment suggestions upon solving the customers' beauty problems.

If the customer does respond negatively, take heart. You may hear four to five nos before you get a yes. That's okay. You will not close 100 percent of your clients. No one can do that.

But what happens if the client says no?

HANDLING OBJECTIONS

You've gotten this far in the selling sequence and the client says that dreaded little "No." What do you do? I've seen stylists become mad, discouraged, offended, or confused and a few who have wished the ground would open and swallow them up.

Many people quickly respond with a no because they are afraid of making the wrong decisions. Seven out of ten people do not like making decisions so, when asked to make a commitment to a purchase they are likely to say "No" even if they want to say yes. It is physically and emotionally easier to say "No" than to say "Yes." This apprehension is called anticipated agony. Customers have made mistakes before when selecting beauty items.

If you do get a no from your client that's great. Now before you think I have lost my mind, let me assure you that I haven't. When a client tells you no, she is voicing an objection to your offer. Her no is not a personal rejection. Don't take it personally. She is not rejecting you as a person. Objections are red flags that more information is needed to make a decision. A no can mean the client is not convinced yet. It can mean she simply needs more of your professional knowledge to make a logical decision or that she is confused by your description, offer, or price. It can also mean that the client just doesn't understand how your suggestion will help her.

Remember you live and breathe beauty products and services. Your client may not have the foggiest idea what you are talking about. In your mind you can see that the client truly needs the product. It is obvious to you, but not so obvious to your client.

Objections are not sales killers, they are sales makers. I get concerned when a client doesn't object to something. Use an objection as a confirmation that the client is seriously involved with your presentation. If she really didn't give two hoots about what you were saying, she wouldn't care enough to object. When a client is rejecting your offer she is indirectly asking for more proof. She is questioning her own need for your offering.

Defensive Back

When you hear an objection, do not get defensive or argumentative. At first your natural defensive mechanism will want to kick into overdrive, but keep your hostility down. Objections are red flags for more information. Objections should not have the same effect as waving the red flag in front of the bull. Your positive mental outlook will help you overcome the instinctive defense mechanism until you are comfortable. Eventually, when you hear an objection, you will get excited knowing that your client is contemplating your advice. Keep your loving optimistic attitude and you will see your way through the objection process. Remember tough customers are better than no customers.

Six Steps to Overcoming a No

Hear Them Out

When a client starts to object to your offer, give the client your full attention. Block out all other activity and tune into what the client is saying and not saying. Remember to keep your defenses in check. Let the client state her case in its entirety. Under no circumstances should you interrupt your customer midsentence.

Objections can come from outdated information. Customers may object because of some magazine article they read years ago. The red flag is being waved to get your attention. What additional information does your client need to make a commitment? You will need to find out.

Neutralize the Objection

Pleasantly surprise your client. After she voices an objection, sincerely neutralize her defenses by accepting her current feelings. You are verbally pulling the two of you together to help solve the problem.

In a positive and professional tone, state one of the following: "I can understand why you feel that way." "Yes, I agree with what you are saying." "I'm glad you brought that up." "Yes, I can relate to what you are saying."

Question the Objection

"I'm glad you brought that up. Now your hesitation is because . . . ?" State the objection back to the client word for word.

Some objection examples are: "I'll never get a permanent wave again. When I was ten, my mother gave me a home perm in the kitchen and fried my hair." "I don't like mineral oil in products." "I had a fungus infection and had to quit wearing artificial nails." Do you have a technical response for these objections?

Answer the Objection

Once you are clear on the client's objection, your mission is to update her information. The examples above are due to the client's lack of updated information on services and products. This is the time to share your technical expertise with your client.

Confirm the Answer

Now that you have brought her into this decade with your information, the next step is to make absolutely sure she understands the information. Be sure that she comprehends your information. If you skim over the confirmation step you will be back to square one when you try to close. Get a confirmation. "Now does that clear up any confusion about home perms?"

Roll Back In To Close the Sale

Once you have received positive feedback on clearing up any misinformation you are safe to ask for the close again. "Well, that eliminates your hesitation. Would you prefer to try the four-ounce or eight-ounce bottle?"

I remember a new client who objected to using loose powder. Her objection was that loose powder made her skin dry. As it turned out the powder she had been using months before had oil-absorbing ingredients, which would have been fine if she was in her teens, but this client was pushing a beautiful fifty. Once she understood that loose powder would help keep her makeup on all day and that she needed a moisturizer on under her base makeup she gave up her reluctance to loose powder. Loose powder wasn't the culprit. The lack of a

moisturizer surely would cause more dryness than a loose powder.

Common Objections

Here are a few common objections you may be hearing in the salon. Study the responses and you will have ready-made answers. Do you hear?

"I have products at home already."

"I'll never use it."

"I tried it once and I didn't like it."

"I can't afford all those products."

"I ONLY use product XYZ."

"I don't have time for all of that."

"I want to think about it."

"I don't know."

"I'll need to ask my husband."

"Salon products cost too much."

"I have products at home already."

GOAL: Find out how much stuff is sitting in the bathroom. I'm sure your client will have some things at home, but are they the right product to suit the beauty need? How old are they?

Many products lose their effectiveness and some can be unsafe if kept too long. Target those with short shelf lives. "How long have you had your current tube of mascara?" "How much is left in your jar of moisturizer?" Watch their eyes scan the contents of the bathroom. You will be able to watch the client "read" the contents of the bottles and jars.

Many of your clients have bottles and jars stashed in drawers and cabients. The memory of buying errors can nudge clients when they are thinking of buying a new product. They start hearing that little voice screaming in their ear reminding of all the money wasted over the years. And here you are again getting ready to buy more stuff. Gently ease the client's buying anxiety.

- "I understand that. I personally have thrown out boxes full of cosmetics. That's one major benefit of purchasing your products here in the salon. You have access to professional advice and recommendations from trained stylists. Together, we can avoid any further buying errors."

- "When will you be finished with Product A?"
- "Is there someone in your family that could use product A?"

Try suggesting alternative uses. Face tonic used as after-bath splash. Face cream used as body lotion. Hair shampoo used for the family pooch.

Once you have inquired, don't be surprised if the client announces, "Well, I am about out of such and such." Your response is, "Great, let's start there. I'll send a sample for you to use as a companion product. I want you to see and feel the difference the proper products make."

"I'll never use it."

GOAL: Find out why she would never use it. There has to be an underlying factor in the objection. Maybe she doesn't know how to use the product. Maybe it's a time issue. Maybe it looks confusing. So instead of accepting your advice, she throws up this objection as a smoke screen. Hang in there and ferret out the real objection. "Tell me why."

"I tried it once, and I didn't like it."

GOAL: Find out what happened during her last experience. Don't lead the client by giving her a multiple choice answer. Ask your question then wait for the response. "Boy, that's too bad. Tell me what happened when you tried the product." Look for misuse of product, wrong sequence of application, wrong product for the beauty solution. Not all beauty products are created equal. Maybe she did have an unpleasant experience with another brand of products.

Don't lead the client with a verbal checklist of excuses. Say, "Tell me what you specifically didn't like about the product," then wait for her response.

"I can't afford all those products."

GOAL: Find her spending comfort zone. People buy what they want when they want it. Don't prejudge the client's ability to afford your offering. Remember she is buying products somewhere.

Have you every found an item while out shopping and then proceeded to talk yourself out of buying it by telling your-

self you couldn't afford it only to walk into the next store and find a new item you just can't live without? Did you think twice about plunking down the money? Clients do the very same thing.

Before she skips out of the salon, ask your client, "How much did you budget for today?" Don't panic and think I'm asking you to be rude. But how many of your clients actually walk into the salon with a predetermined budget in mind? Very few, I bet. This question helps them grab a dollar amount in their comfort spending zone. If the response is $20, that's great. Select the best products from your collection that fit the budget and beauty needs. If it's $50, same story.

- "I'll be glad to work your beauty program within your budget. You can always add to your professional home care collection."
- "Let's just start with the bare necessities. Which ones do you feel are most important?"

Another way to work out of the objection is to reemphasize the customer's beauty problem. "You mentioned at the beginning of our session that you have a problem with dry skin. The only way to eliminate that problem is to use moisturizer."

Good things are seldom cheap, and cheap things are seldom good.

- "Wouldn't you agree that it is better to pay a little more than you expected, than a little less than you deserve?"
- "I understand budgets. When do you feel you would be able to add these products?"
- "If it helps, we offer Visa, MasterCard, and American Express charging privileges here. Some of our clients prefer to charge some and write a check for the balance. Would that help make it easier for you to start working with these exceptional products?"

"I only use Product XYZ."

GOAL: Find out the client bond with the product. "I'm delighted you have found a product to use. Would you share with me what you like about the product?" The bond could be any number of things, but more than likely she is just afraid of changing. Listen to the reasons for the bond, then ask, "If you could change one thing about the product you are currently using what would that be?" Of course, you just happen to have a product that features the brand she'd like to make her current product.

"I don't want to switch because I've used this product for years."

GOAL: Find out how long the customer has been attached to the product. Evaluate whether the product is working. Is it up to date or are there new and improved products that would better benefit the customer?

A sales possibility is to use the build-up angle. You have seen the gradual reduced results a product offers over extended periods of use. If you can see signs of the product not working up to its potential try overcoming the objection with this, "How long have you been using this product?" Wait for the response and if it has been years, inform the customer that "the product selected years ago is a very good one. However, it is not providing you with the best possible results. If you were to eat the very same foods day in and day out you would get pretty bored at mealtime. The body is the same way. Seasons change, styles change, and quite often it is necessary to switch product to receive the best possible results. I want you to look your best and I know you do too. That's why I strongly recommend . . ."

"I don't have time for all of that."

GOAL: Find out how much time the client will invest. First of all, don't show the client twenty things she needs to use at once. You'll terrify your customer.

Start by finding out her current beauty program. "How much time do you spend in the morning getting ready?" Listen for time-wasting efforts. A lot of women make looking good harder than necessary.

"What are you currently doing? Well, this new home care routine will save you over fifteen minutes a day!"

For nonproduct users try, "The total process will not take longer than ten minutes. If I promise a quick and easy routine that guarantees results, would you invest ten minutes or less a day for a lifetime of better hair/skin/nails?" Make her hair care routine as easy as possible. Only show the client two or three products. Gradually build up the customer home care routine.

"I want to think about it."

GOAL: At least get a yes or no. It is sales suicide to prolong the decision. Out of sight, out of mind couldn't be truer than with sales. The client needs to act one way or the other. Some of your customers may feel that the word no is too final, so to soften the blow, they cushion bringing the sale to an end by stretching out the inevitable. They want to think about it.

"That's fine Lynn, obviously you wouldn't take your time thinking about it unless you were seriously interested. I want to be of assistance. Please tell me what it is you want to think over; maybe I can help. Is it the potential results? How to use the product? The company's integrity? Or maybe, I haven't clearly explained how it will benefit you?" Stop. Wait for her to grab onto one of the reasons. Then go on from there, clear up any confusion that is preventing the customer from making a decision.

If push comes to shove and she can't make a decision go ahead and send a sample home with her to use. By the time she returns for her next visit, she will have had time to decide. You will just need to remind her. Refer to your client chart.

"I don't know."

GOAL: Help the customer clarify her needs and the benefits of acting now. Give your customer reasons for taking action today. People are afraid of making decisions. Bring to light the necessary reasons for wanting or needing your product.

"You mentioned earlier that you were having a problem with oily hair. Let's recap the benefits of Product XYZ. Now you know that the product doesn't work in the bottle. So, if you start today with Product XYZ you will start to see the results you want."

My personal favorite when I have a tough time getting a client to budge is this one: "I strongly suggest Product A." Now make sure you back this up with an authoritative voice. Let the depth of your conviction come up and out of your throat.

- "Shirley, I can sense that you are a little hesitant about the beauty program we have discussed today. Let's keep it simple. I professionally recommend that you at least start with the eye cream."

- "We have spent the last hour together working on your beauty program. Judy, would you go to your doctor, have a treatment, take the doctor's recommendation and prescription, and then go home and ignore his advice? Of course, you wouldn't. The quicker you start with the program, the quicker you will benefit from the results."

- "At the beginning of your service you mentioned you were about out of Product A. Your next appointment is not for three weeks. Will you have enough to last or can I save you a trip back?"

"Salon products cost too much."

GOAL: Educate the customer on professional products. Most clients assume all products are created equal. But you and I know that is not the case.

- "There are different qualities of products. Take cars for an example. Is there a difference between a Honda and a Mercedes? Of course. Yet both have tires, an engine, steering wheel, a couple of doors. Just as there are differences between autos, there are differences in beauty products. Which one would you rather have, the Honda or the Mercedes of hair care?"

- "There are thousands of ingredients that can be used in products. And in most cases each ingredient has many levels of quality and grade. Some product companies reach for the bottom of the barrel and dump in inadequate ingredients. Then there are other professional salon manufacturers that insist on top ingredients. The professional salon-only manufacturer and I are both concerned with the quality of your hair/skin/nails. I'm concerned with the long-term results a product can give. I won't risk my reputation recommending an inferior product for you to use. My integrity as your beauty professional is too important to skimp on a few cents. I know you're worth it. Even if that means the product may be a dollar or two more."

- "You know when we started the salon our company made a basic decision. We decided that it was easier to explain price one time than to apologize for quality forever."

- "It amazes me that consumers would be taken in by advertising. Many mass-produced products are being touted as salon comparisons. If salon products weren't superior to begin with, why would advertisers keep trying to bond their mass-distributed product to salon-recommended and -tested products?"

REMEMBER THE FORMULA

You have just discovered the formula for making the sale. First you have to garner the client's awareness, and you do that by your greetings, avoiding the perilous pitfalls, responding to the client's actions. The second stage is to pique her curiosity, and do you remember how to do that? You ask questions and listen carefully to the responses. The third section is to build the passion during the interaction. You do that by involving the customer in the process. Hand her a product, and show her how to use it. The final stage in this formula is to ask the client to take action. The one rule here is to avoid questions that can be answered by a simple yes or no. Use one of the colossal closes for helping the client take action on your offer.

Don't mix up the sequence and you'll do great. You follow a sequence for your treatments; you now have a formula for sales.

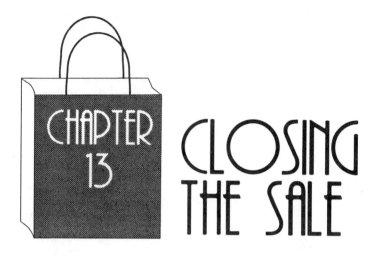

CHAPTER 13

CLOSING THE SALE

In this chapter, we will go over the different closing zones within the salon. You will find yourself in many varied positions when you want the client to make her purchase decisions. Knowing when and where to position the product will improve your ease of selling and increase your closing rate.

POSITIONING THE PRODUCT

Tantalizing Trio Collections

One way to capture sales is to simply give the client a choice. The best way is to cluster the recommended home care items into three collections—the basic collection, the intermediate collection, and the everything-you-ever-thought-you-needed collection.

The Basics

This set contains the bare essentials the client needs to start her home care program. For the basic collection, select the two or three items that make up the essential foundation for your client, i.e., cleanser, toner, and cream.

The Intermediate

In this collection, you can round out the basics with one or two additional key products. This collection features the basics plus the next two items the client would need for her specific look or problem.

The Everything-You-Ever-Thought-You-Needed Collection

Yes, that's exactly what I call it. In this collection, you can include the basics, the intermediates, and any specialty items your client will need to effectively duplicate the look the next day. These products are unique or fashion items, the unusual tools you reach for as a professional to help you create the latest and greatest looks.

The hair basic collection includes shampoo and conditioner. The hair intermediate collection includes shampoo and conditioner, plus styling product and conditioner. The hair everything collection includes shampoo and conditioner; two styling products; conditioner plus intensive conditioner; and fashion agents such as a gloss, brush, or wet comb.

The skin basic collection includes cleanser, toner, and day cream. The skin intermediate collection includes cleanser, toner, and day cream plus eye makeup remover, night cream, and mask. The skin everything collection includes cleanser, toner, and day cream; eye makeup remover, night cream, and mask; and day eye treatment, body lotion, and sloughing mask.

The nail basic collection includes top coat, nail enamel, and body lotion. The nail intermediate collection includes top coat, nail enamel, and body lotion plus polish remover and base coat. The nail everything collection includes top coat, nail enamel, and body lotion; polish remover and base coat; and strengthener, cuticle cream, nail file, and glue.

Tell the client the price for the entire collection. "The basic collection is $18.75" rather than "The shampoo is $4.95, the conditioner is $8.50, and the finishing spray is

$5.30." Keep in mind that many people, those right brainers in particular, have difficulty with mathematical equations. Help them out and simply give them the price per kit. If they feel they need to know the individual prices, then by all means tell them.

Go over the three collections of products. Then ask your client, "Which collection of products would you like to start with today?" You are letting the client close for the sale herself. You just present the information and the client will select the best collection for her. You don't have to sell anything. The client will confidently choose the one that best fits the beauty needs that day.

Which collection do you think clients are most likely to select? If you guessed the intermediate collection you are absolutely correct. More clients will select the middle kit because they don't want to be too cheap, and they don't want to break the bank; middle kit is the safest choice for the majority.

Fill In the Blank

In the passion-building section of the selling sequence we talked about the importance of building the client into the presentation and service. To get the client involved is to get her interested in your professional recommendation.

The best way to get the client involved in the learning process is to have her fill in her own home care recommendation sheets. (Fig. 13.1) This gives you the opportunity to recap the necessary steps and the client can make any notes she chooses to help her retain your suggestions.

Have the client fill in the blanks because this process helps to reinforce the tips and techniques you have shared. Some clients learn visually, some learn by hearing, and others learn by feel or touch. Having the client fill in the blanks allows you to cover your bases with all three learning styles.

Another great reason is that when the client writes her own notes, the chart and information becomes hers. It's not a carbon copy sheet you have handed to every client. This personalizing step brings the information back to the client sitting in your chair and helps to bring you one step closer to the sale.

If you are using preprinted forms or computer analysis printouts, personalize the sheets by highlighting the products needed and ask the client to take the marker and star the items she knows she wants to take home with her. If you feel

you don't want the client to have to work, you can do all the highlighting, but at some point ask her to write down a special secret styling tip. My goal is to have her make at least some personal notations. This warms up the preprinted, one-for-everybody style of paperwork.

One additional reason for clients filling in their own charts is pretty practical. Clients may not be able to read your handwriting if you fill out the chart.

Keep plenty of writing tools close at hand. Brightly colored markers and highlighting pens draw more attention to the notes on the prescription pad. I shy away from pencils because they don't have the same visual impact.

Hot Hair Sales

There are two key places to close the sale with a hair customer. The first place is when you are administering a wonderful shampoo. The client is comfortably relaxing in the chair, warm water is caressing her scalp, and your wondrous fingers are releasing tension and stress from the neck and scalp.

This is the perfect time to talk about proper cleansing and conditioning steps. Evaluate the client's scalp and overall hair condition. Don't skimp on the shampoo time.

Make sure you have reviewed her product purchase history before you begin her session. Scan the information for products the client has not previously purchased from you. See what shampoo, conditioner, and intensive conditioner the client is or isn't using and how long she has had certain products. Use the client record card as a map for leading the sales and analysis.

The second place to close the sale is when you are starting the finish work. Remember to get the client involved in the procedure. If you are going to suggest a new product or styling tool, hand the item to the client and have her apply it for the first time. Once she gets her hands involved, you won't get, "I could never do that." She did it during the appointment. Once you have had the client use the product at your station, put it back and set a new retail product on the station in the client's view but out of your way. Do this for the products you want her to use at home.

When you have finished or are close to finishing, start to recap the steps you "professionally recommend" or "strongly suggest" that the client use at home tomorrow morning. It's

Chapter Thirteen: Closing the Sale   165

HAIR HOME CARE RECOMMENDATIONS

CLIENT:_____

DATE:_____LOOK:_____

These are the following products and steps I professionally recommend for you today, for achieving the maximum results with your hair. These steps will help you to duplicate the same look we created today in the salon.

Make every day a perfect hair day!

_____

Your Stylist

THE BEST PRODUCT FOR YOU

SHAMPOO   _____   _____Daily

Deep Cleanse   _____   _____x week

Color Balance   _____   _____x week

CONDITION   _____   _____x Daily

                  _____   _____x Weekly

                  _____   _____x Monthly

STYLING   _____   Creates_____

                  _____   Creates_____

                  _____   Creates_____

FINISH   _____   Light Hold_____

                  _____   Medium Hold_____

                  _____   Firm Hold_____

SPECIAL NOTES _____

_____

_____

YOUR HAIR MAINTENANCE SCHEDULE:

    Haircut   _____

    Color   _____

    Perm   _____

Fig. 13.1 Hair home care recommendations.

best to be face-to-face with the client. Walk around and face the client directly. Don't talk to the client through the mirror to emphasize your point. Briefly walking around from behind the chair stresses your commitment to the client.

Facial Sales

During the initial consultation, listen for cues for product needs. You can close the sale at a couple of spots during the actual treatment. If this is the client's first visit, go over the home care program during the last mask. Tell the client that on the first session you have a lot of information to go over so you'll take a few minutes now while she is masking and then you'll let her rest. When you start to go over the home care items, tip the facial chair up slightly and swing your stool over to the side of the chair so you are facing the client. Go over your recommendations and close the sale. Say, "I have selected the products that would work best for you. Once you've made your selection I'll tip your chair back and let you have some rest while I organize your home care products and information."

Now if you feel dead set on letting the client sleep during the masking stage, you can wait and close the sale at the end, provided you've allowed time. You'll realistically need ten to fifteen minutes at the end for a new client home care instruction.

NOTE: Charge more for a first-time client. If you normally take one hour for a treatment, add fifteen minutes to properly instruct the client on home care and charge more for the first appointment. Some salons charge $5 to $15 dollars more for the first time. Then clients go on a maintenance price schedule if they maintain their treatment schedule every four to five weeks.

Nailing Down Sales

It can be tough for weekly or bimonthly nail clients to be your main retailing source. They can only use so many new polish colors. But there is a way to capture sales when the client is in the chair for a manicure or pedicure.

Use the nail analysis sheet to set up the selling sequence.

Once you have brought a nail problem to the client's attention, she will need the corresponding product to solve the problem.

Select universal products the majority of your clients can use, for example mascara, body lotion, shampoo. Select a product of the week. Feature the item on the stations, reception area, and cash-out desk. Make a minidisplay with a product benefit card to post on your station. Talk up the product of the week to your weekly clients. If the majority of your clients are on two-week cycles, rotate the products every two weeks instead of weekly. As a professional nail artist you can easily recommend products in addition to your regular selection of nail care products.

Maximizing Makeup Sales

Lesson Sales

The makeup lesson is designed to teach the client how to do her makeup. The session is structured so the client can learn by doing. As you take the customer through the steps, have her mark the home care form. (Fig. 13.2, on pages 167–168) Give her the product, tell her how to put it on, watch the client's technique, then have her fill in the color name and any special application tips. Proceed to the next step in the client's application.

Once the entire makeup is applied, recap the techniques by taking the client over the form again, this time filling in the chart with actual makeup products. Ask the client to star the items she already knows she wants to take home. You are allowing the client to make her own choice; you don't even have to feel like you are selling.

If you have the space to schedule two clients together, make sure you keep their respective colors separated on the counter. The same techniques apply here as in a single lesson.

Pull the retail items out of the cases and place them in two separate areas to make checking out easier. After you show the client the makeup technique, pull out the colors or product you have selected and start a pile per client. Using two different colored mats works great. If you have the space, block the pile from the client's direct line of sight. Place the products, say, behind you or on another counter. As you get ready to mark the chart, you can pull one item at a time and present the retail product as the client marks the chart. No testers are in sight when you go to close the sale.

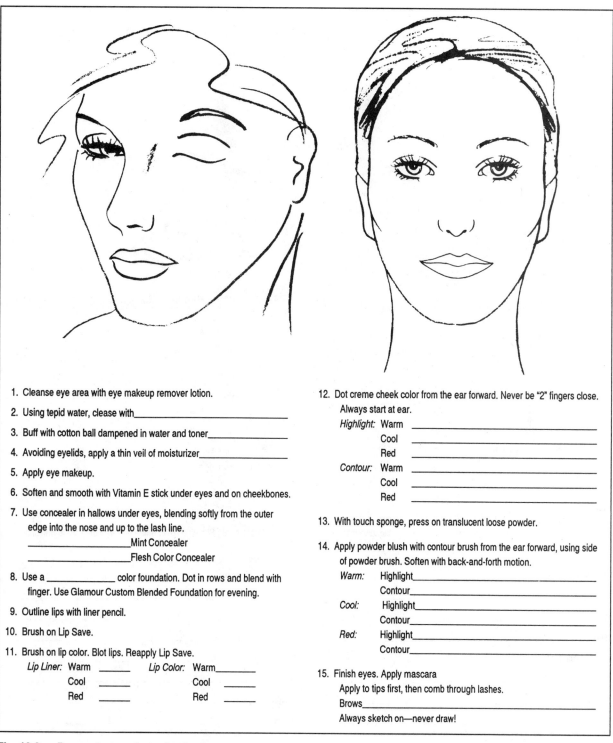

1. Cleanse eye area with eye makeup remover lotion.

2. Using tepid water, cleanse with_____

3. Buff with cotton ball dampened in water and toner_____

4. Avoiding eyelids, apply a thin veil of moisturizer_____

5. Apply eye makeup.

6. Soften and smooth with Vitamin E stick under eyes and on cheekbones.

7. Use concealer in hallows under eyes, blending softly from the outer edge into the nose and up to the lash line.

   _____Mint Concealer

   _____Flesh Color Concealer

8. Use a _____ color foundation. Dot in rows and blend with finger. Use Glamour Custom Blended Foundation for evening.

9. Outline lips with liner pencil.

10. Brush on Lip Save.

11. Brush on lip color. Blot lips. Reapply Lip Save.

Lip Liner:		*Lip Color:*	
Warm	_____	Warm	_____
Cool	_____	Cool	_____
Red	_____	Red	_____

12. Dot creme cheek color from the ear forward. Never be "2" fingers close. Always start at ear.

    | *Highlight:* | Warm | _____ |
    | | Cool | _____ |
    | | Red | _____ |
    | *Contour:* | Warm | _____ |
    | | Cool | _____ |
    | | Red | _____ |

13. With touch sponge, press on translucent loose powder.

14. Apply powder blush with contour brush from the ear forward, using side of powder brush. Soften with back-and-forth motion.

    | *Warm:* | Highlight | _____ |
    | | Contour | _____ |
    | *Cool:* | Highlight | _____ |
    | | Contour | _____ |
    | *Red:* | Highlight | _____ |
    | | Contour | _____ |

15. Finish eyes. Apply mascara
    Apply to tips first, then comb through lashes.
    Brows_____
    Always sketch on—never draw!

Fig. 13.2a   Personal cosmetic application form.

Client Name:_____   Advisor:_____

Date:_____   Look:_____

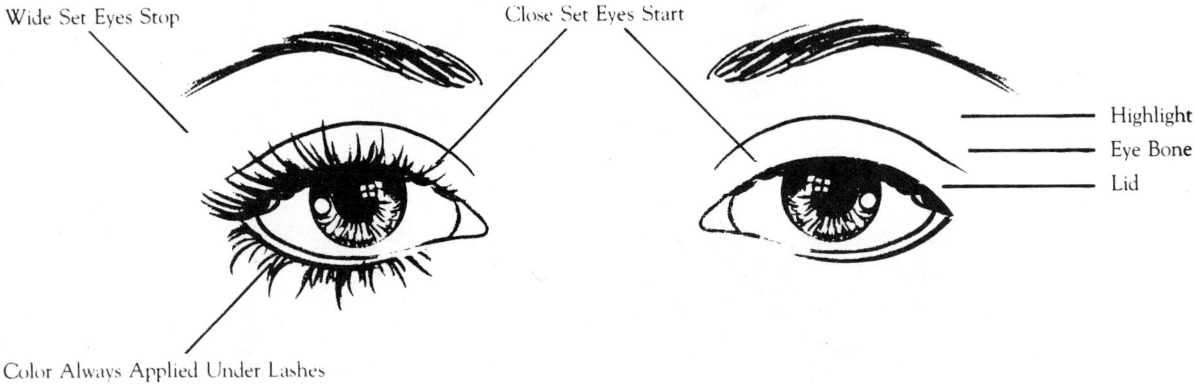

Wide Set Eyes Stop   Close Set Eyes Start

                                                                    _____ Highlight
                                                                    _____ Eye Bone
                                                                    _____ Lid

Color Always Applied Under Lashes

Eye Makeup Tips   **Under Eye Area**

1. Apply before base and concealer.   1. Vitamin E stick on bone.

2. For upper lids: Look into mirror with chin up and eyes down.   2. Mint concealer if needed.

3. For under eye: Look into mirror with chin down and eyes up.   3. Flesh concealer_____

Eye makeup remover lotion leaves no oily residue. Use morning and evening.

WARM

Crease Proof Pencil - Sketch on over entire eye area then blend with finger.

Base_____

Translucent Powder_____

Highlight_____

Lid_____

Bone_____

Crease (center of lid)_____

Liner_____

Mascara_____

Brows_____

COOL

Crease Proof Pencil - Sketch on over entire eye area then blend with finger.

Base_____

Translucent Powder_____

Highlight_____

Lid_____

Bone_____

Crease (center of hall)_____

Liner_____

Mascara_____

Brows_____

Fig. 13.2b   Eye cosmetic application form.

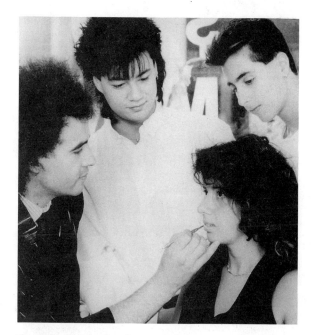

Fig. 13.3   Application demonstration.

Makeup Applications

Makeup applications can be fun services to perform, but can fall short of retail sales. (Fig. 13.3) The main tip to remember is to present the client with a touch-up kit. This kit includes travel size hair spray, compact powder, lip pencil, lipstick, and blush. Present the touch-up kit in a cosmetic bag for a special price. This technique helps to capture retail sales.

If the client keeps asking technique questions, sell her on the benefits of the makeup lesson. Answer a couple of her questions, but if you have perfected the lesson skills, the client will benefit a hundred times more if she goes through the lesson series. "I appreciate your interest in learning how to improve your makeup. Today your appointment is for professional application for your party tonight. Why don't you sit back and enjoy being pampered. Then when you are done, we'll schedule a makeup lesson series where I can spend more time going over the step-by-step look and teach you some fun makeup secrets. What day in the week would work best for you?" Sell her on your lessons, and you can dramatically increase your retail sales.

WHERE TO POSITION THE PRODUCT FOR CLOSING

Is there a more successful spot for placing products? The answer is yes. Depending on your location, there are a couple of powerful positions for placing product.

The main rule of thumb is to remember to visually show only new retail product to the client. You will use your station product, but when you go to close the sale have only brand new products in sight.

If you don't have shelving and display for retail merchandising by your station, take the customer through the home care fill-in sheet. Get the client to agree to a product collection. Walk the client to the reception desk, hand the prescription form to the receptionist, and turn the filling process over to the front desk. "Ashley, Mrs. McKowen has selected the intermediate collection for today. Please pull those items we have marked for her to take home. Mrs. McKowen, do you have any last questions on your new home care routine? I'll look forward to seeing you in four weeks. Thank you."

Behind the Counter

If you are assisting a client and working from behind the counter present the product in collections. Keep extra items out of sight. Show her collections or products that are sold through the system-selling technique. (Fig. 13.4)

Avoid lining up tons of product in front of the client, even if she needs all your suggestions. If the client sees a battalion of products lined up like soldiers, her first reaction may be to run and take cover. What would you feel if you saw ten products lined up?

What you want to do is present them as the client would use them at home the next day. Show cleanser and toner together, then set them aside. Next show day cream and base makeup, and set them aside. Show products for the night home care routine together. Watch for buying signals and close when the client is ready to buy. Get an agreement for the collection you are discussing, then go on to the next collection of products.

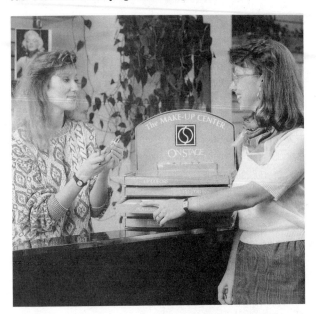

Fig. 13.4   Cosmetic counter selling. (Photo by Michael A. Gallitelli on location at Rielms Hair Salon, Latham, NY.)

Styling Classes

Group styling classes are an excellent way to increase your retail sales. These can be scheduled one on one or in a group.

The individual styling class is a predetermined appointment where the client is coming into the salon to learn to style her hair. She may need help achieving different looks, blow-drying options, subtle switches for after work. The goal is to teach the client the steps for achieving the right look. By the way, this should be a paid appointment time, or a bonus service for a good chemical service client. (Fig. 13.5)

Talk your way through the styling class. This may very well be the toughest part for you. Your goal as a teacher is to be able to thoroughly explain the techniques, without touching the client's hair. The customer must learn the tips and techniques herself. You already know how to do the looks; the best way for the client to learn is to get her hands in the middle of it.

For group classes, schedule as many clients as stations or work areas. Team up staff to students. The stylist is there to support and encourage the clients and to lend a helping hand. The stylist will not dictate the entire look. The program leader will take the students through the paces and control the class format.

Have plenty of product and tools at each work area for the students. If they get their hands on the proper products and tools, it is easier for them to buy. For selling in a group, have a styling class worksheet available for notes or sketches. Leave room for suggested styling products for each look you show the client.

To close the sale, the client can highlight or star the products she knows she wants to take home. If your product line provides a collection of fashion styling aids, offer the students a bag deal or class bonus.

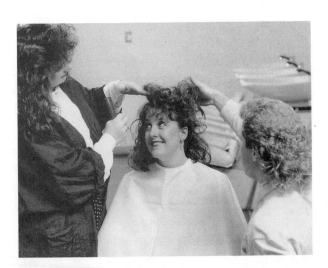

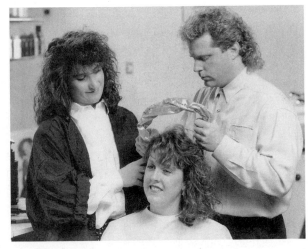

Fig. 13.5a and b   Styling lessons. (Photos by Michael A. Gallitelli on location at Rielms Hair Salon, Latham, NY.)

Selling in Groups

If one of your marketing efforts is to go out of the store and do group programs there are a couple of things you can do to maximize sales. When you structure your program, make sure you feature two or three unique services and products. You will give the audience nuggets of information, but remember to feature a few key products.

Take a small inventory of the key products you mention in the program. These universal selling products can be made available after the class for those who want to try the new look the next day. Strike while the iron is hot. You won't need to take the entire store; a handful of items will be enough. Take a tester of each product that you plan on suggesting to pass through the audience. You want to tempt them by allowing the audience to feel, see, and smell the product.

And remember to bring along your appointment book to schedule post-program appointments.

PUTTING IT ALL TOGETHER

In the last chapter you discovered all the right things to say to the client to get her to say yes to your products and services. In this chapter you have learned how to add placement and positioning to your growing repertoire of information. Keep up the good work. I promise it will get easier the more you use the techniques.

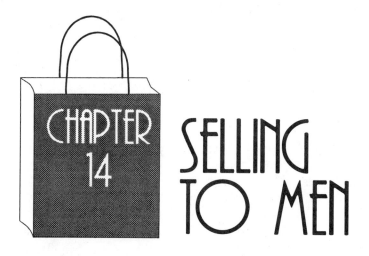

CHAPTER 14

SELLING TO MEN

Selling to men can require a different strategy. In this chapter, we will take a look at several ways to set up the selling environment to make your male clients comfortable having services and buying retail products. The principles outlined in other sections will definitely work for your male clientele, but I want to share additional tips with you for easing into retailing grooming products.

A PROFILE OF THE MALE CLIENT

Men that come into salons today want suggestions. They are looking for professionals who are not afraid to strongly suggest a new look, service, and especially product. Men are used to gathering professional advice. It is common for men to gather information and then harvest the results by making their minds up quite quickly. These men make great retail clients. If you believe that the product or service you are recommending is beneficial to the client, and state your case accordingly, men will follow your lead. How often do you hear, "Well, you're the professional, what do you recommend?" It's your area of expertise.

Salon male clients are looking for professionals who are not afraid to make suggestions and professional recommendations. When you are selling a product to your clients, make sure you stress how the product or service will benefit their looks or life. Stress the ultimate reason they would want or need your offering. Keep it short and sweet. Learn to use words that trigger the male ear.

Men are working out like crazy. They may be pumping iron, running, surfing, roller blading. But whatever the form of exercise they choose, they do it because they want to look good. If they have healthy bodies, they should also have healthy hair and skin.

My best retail clients were men. Not only were they punctual with their maintenance appointments, but they purchased products in twos and threes. My favorite male client would schedule his appointment before the salon opened. He would stroll in, hand me his huge cigar, grab a specialty coffee I stocked for him, and then was ready for his treatment. During the session, he would give me his list of products, and every one was in threes. He was a big guy and I couldn't image how he would need so much product but even if he was bathing in it, I didn't mind. After all, he was simply requesting the goodies.

DESCRIBING PRODUCT AND SERVICE TO MEN

"I'd lost my way in Bloomingdale's and stumbled on something called the Aramis Lab Center, where I was set upon by strange, yet friendly people dressed in white lab coats (scientists? doctors?), speaking of skin hydration and mechanical exfoliation of microscopic cellular debris. I didn't speak the language." This was taken from an article in *Vogue* that was obviously written from the male perspective.

Can the salon industry scare off the male checkbook-toting species? I think so. One surefire way to capture the heart and credit card of the male shopper is to learn to talk in his language.

Selling Snafus

During one part in a program I was giving on marketing your salon, I asked the group why a gentleman would go into a skin salon for a facial. The answers were: to feel good, to look better, the massage is so soothing, the room is relaxing and comfortable, my training. No one in the group thought of the male need for a facial. When men in the audience were asked why they would schedule a facial, their responses were shocking to the females in the group. They would go in for skin advice, to reduce shaving irritation, to seek professional guidance for skin fitness, to make the skin look better. The big mistake the women in the audience made was to assume the men would respond to the same buzzwords and benefits as the women do. The women were using "feely" words rather than factual result-benefit dialogue.

Men's Words

Learn to use words that simulate the buying center. Men want words that are crisp, short, and to the point. Keep the fluffy, kinesthetic words to a minimum. Here's a few for you to try out.

cleaner	potent
commanding	powerful
condition	precision
control	primitive
dynamite	reduce irritation
electric	results
face fitness	rugged
healthy	straightforward
intense	strong
knockout	tough
manageable	vigor
peak performance	vital

The Female Voice

Have you been around couples who debate the fact that she talks too much, and he never listens? Research seems to indicate that women do talk more than men, five times as much in some cases. The communication problem surfaces when she supposedly talks too much and he tunes her out—the old selective-hearing technique.

When women are selling to men, they should guard their sound level and voice quality. Go back to chapter 9 and review the verbal skills section. Your voice can support your success, or it can pull the plug. Record yourself and listen for clarity, sound level (too soft or too loud), nasal tones, whininess, breathiness, and rate of speech. If you are falling victim to any of these voice saboteurs you are reducing your success potential, especially if you are dealing with male clientele. Pay attention to your voice and your male clients will be paying you.

SELLING SERVICES

Here are a few tips on selling services to your male clients.

- Haircuts: Today's grooming is more than a shave and haircut. One question I like to ask the men when they return after their haircuts is, "How did the cut work for you? Did you notice when it started to lose its neatness?" Quite frequently you will hear that the cut lost its shape in three weeks, yet they come in every five weeks. This will give you the opportunity to move up their cut cycle. "So you can look your best every day, let's schedule your next appointment for three weeks." (Fig. 14.1)

- Commanding color: Men will want to wash away gray just like women. Keep a few leftover clippings from a haircut and experiment with color options. When your client comes in for his next appointment show him your color findings to introduce haircolor options. Look at recommending color-enhancing shampoos for subtle changes. Don't forget that beard and mustache areas may need a touch of color too. (Fig. 14.2)

- Powerful perms: Men will like perms, especially if they can make getting ready in the morning faster and easier. Give him hair control and manageability with your perms.

- Super Bowl of skin care: Men are entering the previously female-dominated facial rooms. Skin care treatments are excellent ways to tackle skin problems as well as being relaxing outlets. I have found that there are two main groups of men who seem to take to skin treatments. The younger men turn to estheticians as they face skin problems and

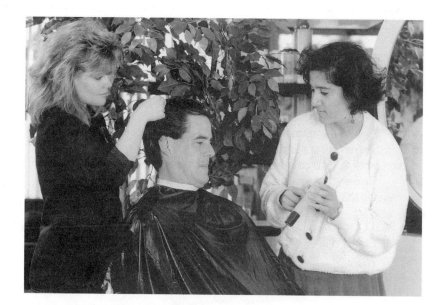

Fig. 14.1   Men have become more knowledgeable about the cut, style, and condition of their hair. (Photo by Michael A. Gallitelli on location at Rielms Hair Salon, Latham, NY.)

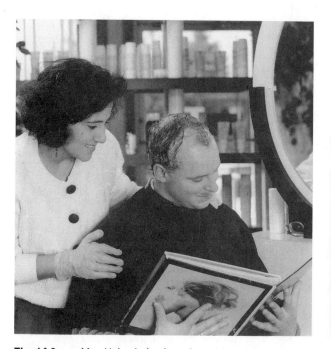

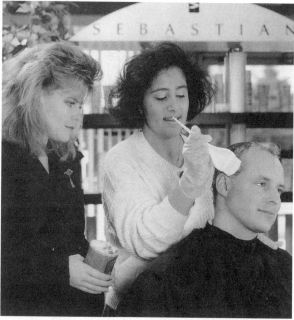

Fig. 14.2a and b   Haircoloring is an important service for the male clientele. (Photos by Michael A. Gallitelli on location at Rielms Hair Salon, Latham, NY.)

Men's Skin Fitness

In three simple steps you can control breakouts, reduce shaving irritation and get a closer, smoother shave. The staff at our salon has discovered that by changing a few of the basics of your morning routine you can achieve a smoother, closer shave.

Call the salon today at _____ to schedule your private 20-minute consultation. Our professional staff will share some down-to-basic facts about skin protection and design a shaving routine especially for your beard type.

Before you drag a razor across your face give us a call and see how you can stop shaving irritation.

Salon Logo
Address
Phone number
hours

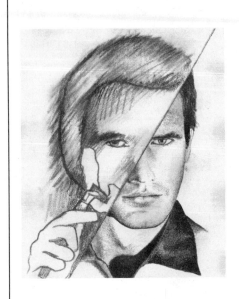

Fig. 14.3   Men's shaving system.

breakouts. The mature male clients have been exposed to barber-shaving services and hook up with estheticians for in-depth skin treatments. Target your treatments to attract these clients into your facial rooms. By the way, avoid using the word "facial." Use skin treatments or skin therapy.

- Shaving consultation: One of my favorite services to offer men is the shaving consultation. Many men learned to shave by watching dad and emulating his actions. A twenty-minute consultation covers the best way to shave and take care of the skin and ways to reduce shaving irritation. (Fig. 14.3)

1. Dampen the skin with tepid water. Work a small amount of shaving cream onto the skin. Using a single-edged razor, very gently remove the beard in the direction of the hair growth. Start where the hair is the thinnest leaving the coarser areas to continue softening. Suggested starting places would be the sides of the cheeks or neck. Leave the lip and chin areas for last.
2. Splash with tepid water to assure all traces of cream have been removed.

3. Splash or spray on skin freshener to complete the cleansing process.
4. Apply lotion very sparingly from the cheekbones down and the eyebrows up. This lotion will act as a barrier to fight the environmental effects that can cause damage on the skin.
5. In the evening only, add a few dots of eye and throat cream around the eye, on the cheekbone under the eye, and directly beneath the brows.

Shaving Suggestions

1. Avoid using very hot water on the skin. Splashing with scalding water will strip the skin of the natural protective oils that cushion it from the razor.
2. Shower before shaving to help presoften the beard. Use the steam from the shower to start softening the stiff hairs.
3. Try using a water-soluble cleanser rather than soap on the skin. Soap can have a tendency to be drying.
4. It is healthier for the skin to go through two shavings a day rather than one ultraclose shave.

- Hair-razing tale: When you are going through your consultation with the client, make sure you check the brows, neck line, and ears where unruly hair tends to grow. Look into waxing services and possible electrolysis for permanent hair removal.

- Face sculpting: If men don't want to part with the facial hair, look into offering beard-sculpting sessions for designer beards and special sessions for conditioning the skin under the beard.

- Nailing down nail care: Men today don't necessarily want the dandy look of highly polished nails, but healthy hands and nails are definitely in. After well-cared-for shoes, people notice the hands and nails.

A Male-Friendly Environment

When you are designing your salon or remodeling, keep in mind the mix between male and female clients. You will have a difficult time trying to attract male clients if the salon is decorated in pink lace and latticework. Now, I wouldn't go to the extreme and hang elk heads over the stations, but keep a balance between fluff and tough.

Designing Decor

Take a look and see if your chemical area is out in the open. Even enlightened men are a uncomfortable if they are plunked down in the middle of all the hubbub and made to sit there with gray and pink rods dangling off their heads. Have a separate area in the salon for private sessions. If you have a high traffic of male customers, you might consider a private men's room. Set up a station and work area that is decorated in unisex or male directions. This allows you to decorate the area and not have it visually conflict with the rest of the salon.

Captivating Color

If your salon is of the upscale, old-money mind-set, then look toward rich, hunting club-type colors—hunter green, burgundy, navy—and luxurious woods such as cherry wood and mahogany. If your male clientele is up and coming, starker black, chrome, and glass looks great. If your male clients are "good old boys," use blue and woods in pine and oak.

Testy Temperature

Men tend to run a few degrees warmer than your female clients. Keep the temperature down a few degrees to keep them from becoming overheated.

Odd-Time Appointments

If you want to attract a larger percentage of men to the salon be prepared to take odd-time appointments. Extend your appointments beyond the normal working hours. Busy executives will want to schedule early-bird or night-owl appointments. The client I introduced you to earlier insisted upon coming in before the rest of the staff and clients, because he was so tall his feet would stick out the facial room door and he was uncomfortable with others strolling by. For an average $300 ticket, if he wanted to show up at dawn it was okay by me.

Cutting Capes and Robes

When you are shopping for robes and capes make sure they are unisex or male directed. If you have the man change into robes make sure you have small, medium, and large sizes. Offer a separate place for men to change into the robes. Add a wooden valet stand for their clothing or specialty hangers for their suits. Have a chair in the area so they can sit and put on their shoes or boots.

Visual Stimulants

Show men in photos having a range of services. Hang up posters showing men using grooming products. When setting up displays don't forget to use masculine props such as weights, shaving kits, razors, cowboy hat and paraphernalia, aviator glasses and Red Baron scarf, model cars, footballs, baseballs, tennis balls.

Make the men more comfortable by utilizing props from their everyday lives.

Staff Support

Salon Specialists

If your salon is large enough, have people on staff who specialize in men's grooming treatments. Maybe you have a cutter or two who are exceptional with men's hair. Promote the specialists. Men trust professionals and will seek out those they feel are more knowledgeable than the rest of the pack. Have specialists in cutting, chemicals, manicures, beard trimming and sculpting; skin consultants with a hook for shaving programs; and a massage therapist that specializes in sports massage and stress reduction.

Appropriate Attire

This should go without saying but pay close attention to the attire you select if you are working on male clients. I have seen some stylists look more like cocktail waitresses than beauty professionals. Clothing says a lot. Be careful of the message.

Salon Safety

When I first opened the salon, we would get undercover calls from the vice squad of the police department. Do you do full-body massage? Who does the massage? I'm sure if you have been around this business for any length of time you have heard all kinds of wise or not-so-wise cracks. If your services

are to be performed in private, have another staff person with you in the salon at all times. If your setup allows, leave the door slightly ajar to dissuade uncomfortable comments. I never promote body massage in print or ads to reduce the number of crackpots that mistake a salon for a parlor. I promote those services in the salon and through referrals. Play it safe.

MALE PRODUCT MIX

The products that you are carrying in the salon more than likely can be recommended to men as well as women. But here are a few tips for maximizing your sales. (Fig. 14.4)

- Product mix: Look for products that are easy to use, are not sticky, and require minimal steps. Don't overlook scalp-to-toe-care for men. Men do buy basics in skin-care cleansers, toners, skin-protecting lotions, and exfoliants.

- Product names: Before you reach to the shelf to suggest a

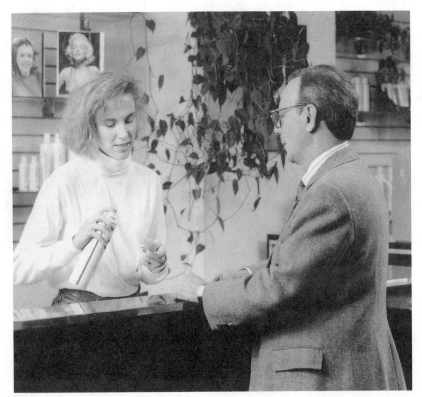

Fig. 14.4   Maximize your sales with a complete male product mix. (Photo by Michael A. Gallitelli on location at Rielms Hair Salon, Latham, NY.)

product, remember the name of the item you're recommending. If you're grabbing La Fleur Fragrance Luxurious Hydrating Cream, hold your horses. Male shoppers will buy and use grooming products if the product is effective and the name is straightforward.

- Products that work in the shower: Most men hit the floor running in the morning, and they are in and out of the shower and out of the house in record time. Recommend products that can be applied and work while they are in the shower. To save time and hassle combine grooming steps while showering.

- Shaving kit: Prepackage the essentials for a shaving kit. Face wash, skin smoother, protecting lotion and razor. Market the items in a shaving duffel bag.

- Shower kit: Prepackage the simple steps a guy would need to perform the necessary showering procedure. Pull together the four steps necessary: shampoo, conditioner, styling product, and finishing product. Add a comb and brush so the men have everything at arm's length.

- Travel kit and gym bags: Keep it as simple as possible for men to administer the grooming routine. If they have to shuffle products between shower and gym and travel bags the routine is likely to become flushed down the drain. Show them the travel sizes of your products. Offer them the larger sizes for home use and the tiny travel companions for gym and travel use.

MARKETING TO MEN

If you are going to go big game hunting you have to go into the jungle. If you are desiring to increase the number of men walking through the front door, you'll need to focus on where they are.

- Health clubs: Post flyers, host men's grooming consultations, promote spa and fitness products, see if you can sell/give professional products for use in the dressing rooms.

- Tennis clubs: Feature fun-in-the-sun products and body massage; donate gift certificates for auctions and club fund raisers.

- Local sports courts: Distribute flyers at the local courts highlighting your services that cater to men. See if you can post flyers.

- Father's Day: Pull out all the stops before Father's Day. Feature gift certificates that your current female clients can purchase as presents.

- Radio personalities: Tune into your local DJs and invite them into the salon for a complimentary service. Select your DJ carefully and search for ones that are positive and chat up their personal activities. Once they come into the salon, you will stage a positive salon experience and tune in the next day. Chances are you'll be hearing them tell the tale of the Salon Adventure.

- Men's magazines: Check out your area for men's sports and fitness magazines. Target paid ads, press releases, publicity articles, and even photos of your work.

- Men's organizations: Scout out clubs and organizations that attract high-profile executives. Offer to do a presentation at a club meeting or do a direct mail campaign to the members encouraging them to visit your salon.

- Talk it up. I have found over the years that men are open minded and fun to talk to when it comes to grooming services and products. Use your powers of persuasion when you are simply talking to men. Find out if they are having any grooming problems or difficulties, then offer suggestions for solving their problem.

CHAPTER 15
SELLING SERVICES

This chapter is divided into two main areas. The first section covers the personal beauty needs that will drive clients into your salon. The second section covers the main service areas in salons with direction on how to sell the service. I have included some unique tips for increasing your service sales. Try them and see what happens to your sales.

FINDING YOUR CUSTOMERS' INDIVIDUAL BEAUTY NEEDS

There are ten common areas that surface for a client to take action for your product and services. These ten areas need to be addressed as you listen to your client's answers during the consultation and service time. Keep focused on the client's needs. What is playing in her head? Your clients are the lifeline in your business. What will make them turn loose their hard-earned cash, write a check, or whip out the charge card? Match your services to the key personal beauty need.

The ten key individual beauty needs are:

1. **Dominance.** This is the client attracted to power and authority. **Sales:** Market products with super strength, extra hold, fortified. Wardrobe planning and dress for success seminars, personal shopping services that feature power dressing, VIP client cards.
2. **Understanding.** This client has the need to learn and comprehend techniques and styling tips. **Sales:** Makeup lessons. Home styling classes. Consumer seminars. Image consulting. Body analysis workshops. Makeover packages.
3. **Consistency.** This is the need for order and cleanliness. She has the need to predict the outcome of the look, to know that this service will be just like the last appointment. **Sales:** All cleansing products, soaps, shampoos, astringents. Computer imaging so she can see the end result and know what to expect before any work is done. Well-documented client cards support sales.
4. **Independence.** This is the need for making one's own choice, having options and alternatives. Daring to be different. **Sales:** Custom-blended products. Create the look that sets off your unique features and ways to modify the look. "Seven Ways to Style Your Hair."
5. **Stimulation.** The need to charge up one's senses. To electrify some or all of the five senses. **Sales:** Aromatherapy facials and body treatments. Smells from the product. Paraffin hand and foot treatments. Body, face, foot, scalp massages. Color analysis session. Simultaneous services.
6. **Nurturing.** The need to receive help, support, comfort, to feel taken care of. **Sales:** All salon services touching the client especially facials, body massage, manicures, pedicure. "Pampering" packaging. Full- or half-day beauty days are great.
7. **Sexuality.** The need to establish sexual identity and attractiveness. **Sales:** Products that are decidedly masculine or feminine in use and packaging. No unisex products. Colognes and perfumes. Hair accessories, long wigs, hair pieces.
8. **Exhibition.** The definite need to be noticed and visible. Willing to be on display and walk away from the ordinary

and common. **Sales:** Distinctive jewelry. Bright colors in clothes, hair, makeup. Flashy accessories. Progressive looks and styles.

9. **Diversion.** The need for a break from routine, a play day. The need to be entertained. **Sales:** Service with a friend. Mother/daughter makeovers. Half-day packages. Fashion shows. Party looks.

10. **Novelty.** The need for a change and diversity. **Sales:** Costume party preparation. "New Do for a Day." "Holiday Hair." "Big Bash Night." Temporary haircolors. Wig and hairpiece sales.

The successful stylist and cosmetologist will match the selling strategy with the client's personal beauty needs.

SERVICE BENEFITS

In this section you will get some new ideas for selling services. For each category you'll receive a basic statement, benefits of the service, and my personal selling hints. Let's take a look at the key service areas in salons.

The hair salon service menu focuses primarily on four key areas: cuts, color, condition, and curl. Here are some ways to boost your service sales in the four "C" areas.

Haircuts

Today's cosmetologist is widely versed. In designing an ideal look for a client, the stylist must take into account the face shape, bone structure, wave pattern, and hair density. Once those areas are evaluated, a suitable look is then cut.

Selling Hints

The major fear clients have when facing a stylist is that the stylist is scissor-happy, that he or she will cut off too much. Try easing the anxiety by telling them, "Before I pick up a comb or pair of scissors, you and I will talk to determine the look you desire."

Schedule regular appointments every four to five weeks to keep hair looking its best. If the client waits too long, he or she can go from smashing to shabby. A regular trim allows the hair to look its best every day of the month.

Evaluate the entire staff. See if there are different looks on everyone on the beauty team. The staff should be a walking, breathing catalogue of new looks. Regularly offer makeovers for the staff. If everyone is sporting the same style, then you can't expect your clients to be adventurous with their looks.

Get in the habit of talking about new looks with each season. As the client starts shopping for that new fall or spring wardrobe, emphasize the need for updating the hairstyle. It may not have to be a dramatic change, but a few new twists and curls can add sparkle and sizzle to the new clothes. You'll set the stage for seasonal changes. Once you start working with the client on seasonal hot looks, it will become a habit—a good habit, I might add—especially if the client has been hanging onto the same old style for years.

Styling Options

When you are discussing new looks with the client also stress the fun of creating different finished looks with the same design cut. One cut, four different looks—one for day, one for the office, one for night, and one for romantic looks. Showing clients options will also increase your home care styling product sales. To create the different looks, they will need the proper tools. Schedule a separate appointment where you show the client the options. Make it a paid service appointment.

Make sure you and your client are singing the same song before you release your creativity and techniques. The majority of unhappy-client problems start with miscommunication. Remember that a phrase can have drastically different meaning to your client and to you. (Fig. 15.1)

Haircolor

It's no secret that baby boomers are graying. Haircolor services will dramatically increase in this decade. There are so many different techniques for coloring hair today that I will concentrate on converting that resistant client to a color client.

Proper haircolor can make clients feel better about themselves. The advances in haircolor give clients options for adding color without that just-dyed look. In years past, when a woman colored her hair everyone knew. The breakthroughs in products' formulations and techniques have opened up a rainbow of coloring possibilities.

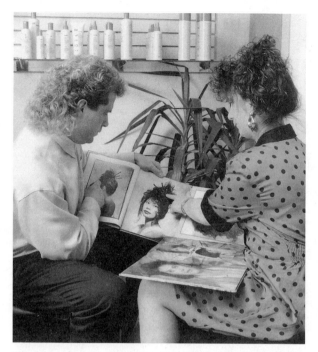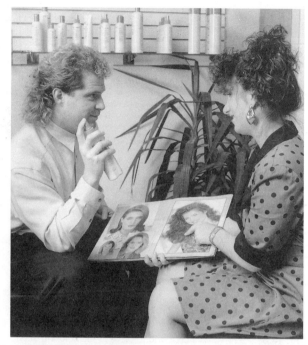

Fig. 15.1 a and b   Discussing hair cutting and styling services with a client. (Photos by Michael A. Gallitelli on location at Rielms Hair Salon, Latham, NY.)

Selling Hints

Start a resistant client off gradually with haircolor services. The consumers don't have your eye for imagination and color, and it may be very difficult for them to "see" the finished look you are describing. Ease them into color with temporary or color washes that will go down the drain with shampoo. No risk. No stress.

The next time you cut a client's hair, collect a handful of the cuttings. When you have some down time, take the hair and divide it into four or five bundles and color the client's samples with looks you feel would be good for her. When they are finished attach them to a card with the client's name. At the next appointment, say "After we cut your hair the last time I got to thinking about haircolor options for you. I designed several looks that would be great on you. What do you think?" This is a great lead into the color sale.

Keep several wigs in basic cuts but different colors on hand. If clients can see a range of looks, and some look great and some look good, their resistance to haircolor will soften.

Keep a swatch book in the reception area. Let clients shop through the book at their leisure. If you have a color swatch ring, hang it by a high-traffic mirror to encourage playing and testing. (Fig. 15.2)

Hair Curls—Perms

Chemically restructuring the hair can give clients the curl they have dreamed of. Perms bring about dramatic change in the look of the hair and the internal structure, from volume-producing curls, to tiny ringlets framing the face. Clients are apprehensive because they are afraid the curl won't take, it will be too tight, or it will be frizzy.

To provide the client with the perfect perm results begin by determining the hair's texture, condition, and length, and the desired result. Your expertise will reassure the client of the importance of in-salon perming.

Some consumers still refuse to perm their hair because years ago they received a home permanent. Unfortunately, the bad results seem to last permanently in the memory.

Perming the hair will give the client curl, texture, shape, fullness, waves, bounce, ease of style, and it will save time.

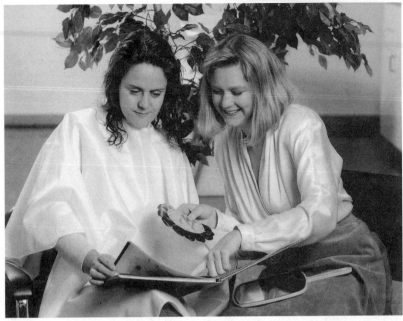

Fig. 15.2   Have visuals on hand to discuss haircoloring services with clients. (Photo by Michael A. Gallitelli on location at Rielms Hair Salon, Latham, NY.)

Perms can provide a variety of looks. The proper perm can support a cut and design by restructuring the hair's natural wave pattern. (Fig. 15.3)

Selling Hints

Prepare a visual display of curl options. Have a board or poster that will show the client the different intensities of curl. To your client, a firm, tight curl may mean deep, waving ridges. To the stylist, that may mean breaking out the yellow rods. If you have a chart the client can look over, you will be assured that you are both talking the same language. Have the client pore over hair magazines and note any looks she is interested in.

Reassure the client that "permanent" doesn't mean forever Chemically altering the curl will last for three to four months. Some clients refuse to perm because they feel they will have to live with the outcome forever, or until the hair grows out. That is not true. Use the words perm or chemically restructuring rather than permanent to soften the resistance.

Conditioning

Beautiful hair is healthy hair. In-salon conditioning treatments should be a foundation in your hair care menu. If the hair is in poor shape, it is difficult to sell chemical services.

Long hair, in particular, takes a beating. A monthly deep conditioning treatment is a must. The hair needs both protein and moisture. Conditioning treatments can replace and restructure the condition of the hair. Chemically treated hair is fragile. Conditioning treatments help to protect and strengthen the hair shaft.

Selling Hints

For starters, make sure the in-salon conditioning treatment is different from the one the client can do at home. It would be tough to sell a service that the client can do herself. Add unique salon conditioning packs and masks that are different in application and appearance from the do-it-yourself type.

If a client is reluctant to spring for a conditioning treatment, ask if you can do one side of the head and let her feel

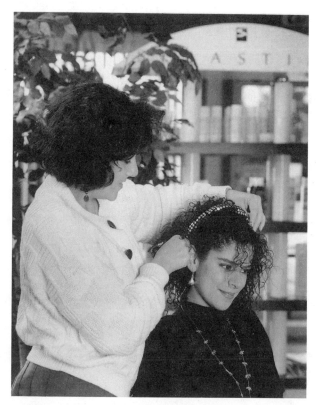

Fig. 15.3 Perm services can provide a variety of looks for the client. (Photo by Michael A. Gallitelli on location at Rielms Hair Salon, Latham, NY.)

the results. When the client runs her fingers through the hair, she will feel an immediate improvement.

Hair Extensions

"Short today and long tomorrow" could be your new motto in the salon if you offer hair extensions. There are clients that just can't wait months or years for their hair to grow out. Hair extensions could be the new instant gratification service of the decade. Extensions can instantly add fullness and length. No wait. No fuss.

Selling Hints
Suggest extensions or pieces for your male clients who want flexibility with their look. Maybe he'd die to have a ponytail but

corporate policy forbids it. Poof, instant ponytail for the weekend.

SELLING COSMETICS SERVICES

Cosmetics should be the fifth C in the dynamic selling services category. They are a natural extension of hair services. Once the hair style or color has been altered, the very next step is to update the makeup look. A modern hairstyle and outdated makeup will clash.

Makeup Lessons

Consumers look to salons for professional advice and guidance. One way to lock them into your salon is to offer makeup lessons. There are several ways of doing the lessons, but I am only going to concentrate on the most effective way for increasing client loyalty and retail sales.

Break up the lesson into two or three sessions—one lesson on eye makeup, one lesson on base, blush, and lips. During the third lesson, the instructor will help select another color family and review the previous lessons.

Shorter lessons work with the shortness of the client's natural attention span. If you tend to keep the client for one or two hours a session, she will only retain a very small percentage of the information. There is so much to grasp with shadow placement, blending techniques, highlights and shadow, and color selection that it is necessary to separate the techniques and have the client return for each session. This technique also sets you apart from the department stores. Have you ever had your makeup done? For the entire lesson your eyes are closed and they paint your face and you're supposed to learn how to do your new look. I don't think so.

Clients can stop guessing what products and colors work for them. A trained makeup instructor will help ease the confusion.

Clients actually save money by building a relationship with the makeup technician. Together they can create new looks and mix and match colors that fit the wardrobe or season. No guessing, no purchasing errors.

Selling Hints

Clients will learn by doing. They will actually be putting on their own makeup while the technician helps them with color selection and blending. The goal is for the client to be able to duplicate the look the very next morning because she did the original application.

I used to do one-half of the face then ask the client to match it on the other side. Every reaction was the same. "My side doesn't look as good as yours." And they were right. I had years of experience on them. When it came to increasing the sale I had to swallow my artistic persona and realize it was more important for the client to be able to do the look. Learn to talk your way through an entire makeup lesson. The only time to touch the client is to help her blend.

In-Salon Makeup Application

Party looks are fun to do. Stress selling makeup applications for parties, special events, photography sessions, yearbook pictures, and bridal parties. (Fig. 15.4)

A professional makeup artist can enhance any complexion. When a woman is going to be in a new environment or at a special occasion a makeup artist can make her look her best. New scenarios can leave some women quaking in their pumps. Knowing that you look your best will help shore up any weakening self-confidence.

Selling Hints

If the client wants to learn how to do her makeup then switch her over to a makeup lesson appointment. Reserve your applications for artistic expression and creativity.

Show "before and after" special occasion looks. Have a bridal photo on hand where the bride did her own makeup and

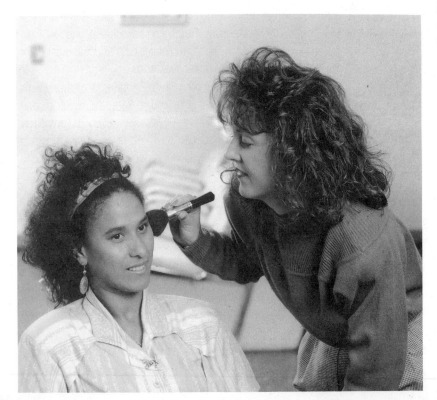

Fig. 15.4 In-salon makeup application. (Photo by Michael A. Gallitelli on location at Rielms Hair Salon, Latham, NY.)

a comparison photo where the makeup was professionally done in your salon. They will be able to see the difference in the clarity and appearance of the face.

Drop a press release to the local high school paper close to prom and homecoming time featuring your makeup services. If you offer acne or troubled skin treatments, send a before and after photo for makeup services when class photos are being taken.

New Year's Eve, Valentine's Day, Mother's Day, company party, if the occasion calls for a new dress, then the appropriate makeup look is needed to finish the picture.

SELLING BODY AND NAIL CARE SERVICES

Skin Treatments

Minor skin problems are frequently caused by improper cleansing and misinformation about skin care. A thoroughly trained professional can increase sales in the salon both in retail dollars and consistent services. Using the four Cs to skin care—cleaning consistently to correct the complexion—your clients will have the glow of health and softness that is unbelievable.

Skin cleansing treatments are extremely important for preserving healthy skin and controlling problem complexions. A facial can be designed to accomplish several objectives depending on the client's needs the day of the treatment.

Facial treatments help to keep the skin healthy by deeply cleansing the surface, increasing the elimination of toxins within the skin, maintaining muscle tone, and improving the skin's texture, plus the esthetician can work with the client individually to coach her on the proper home care program.

Selling Hints

Look at your facial room door. Clients see people entering and leaving the room, but they may not have a clue as to what goes on behind the closed door. Make a sign for the facial room door that describes the services and benefits that take place in the room. Allow the signage to start the sale especially if the esthetician is behind the closed door all day and can't make personal contact with the clients.

Catch a client while she is still under the dryer and offer to treat her skin to a masking session. The hot dryer can cause

dehydration and a soothing and hydrating mask can ward off the potential damage.

Take one of your skin-sloughing creams and treat one hand of a client who has never had a facial. "The results you are feeling now are only minor compared to how the skin will feel after a skin treatment. What day in the week would be convenient for you to try your first facial?"

I like to have the client schedule two treatments back to back, one week apart. This gives the technician the opportunity to reevaluate the skin and its progress from the first session. After the two, then set the client up on a maintenance program, usually every twenty-one to twenty-eight days after that for maximum results. The client will have three sessions within five to six weeks on this program. Once she starts to see and feel the results, she will be more inclined to stick to the recommended skin routine. It is harder to see marked results in one treatment every three to six weeks off the bat.

Some clients will laugh and tell you they are too old for such things. Stress that the skin renews itself every twenty-eight to thirty days. Remind them that it's never too early or too late to start a skin care system.

Body Waxing

Waxing can be one of the most profitable areas in the salon next to retailing. Your set-up cost is minimal and the speed of service is remarkable. If you don't have a private room in the salon, you may still be able to offer face and neck waxing services.

Most consumers shy away from body waxing due to misinformation. They fear that hair in waxed areas will grow back thicker and darker. That is not true. Waxing on a regular basis, every three to four weeks, will actually slow down the hair growth rate. The fact is that during waxing the entire hair shaft is removed and the growth center is stunned. It will take the follicle at least three weeks to produce an entire new hair.

When you wax, a thin film of product is applied to the skin. The technician will then efficiently and quickly remove the wax and the unwanted hair at the same time. The pull will feel a little like removing a bandage, but the results are three weeks of smooth, satiny soft skin.

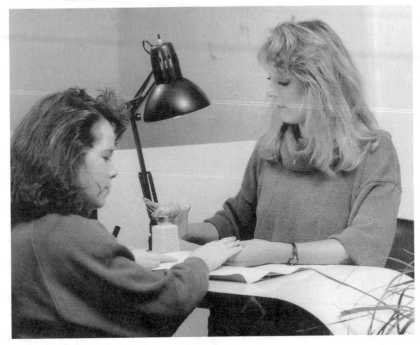

Fig. 15.5   The foundation for nail care services is the manicure. (Photo by Michael A. Gallitelli on location at Rielms Hair Salon, Latham, NY.)

Areas to wax are brows, upper lip, cheeks, jawline, men's necklines, under arms, full arms, full legs, bikini lines, and men's backs.

Selling Hints

Start stressing waxing services in March for summer-smooth skin. This allows clients to have three to four months of treatments before they hit the beach.

Suggest a body scrub and body lotion as home care products. The body scrub helps to prevent ingrown hairs by keeping the dead cells from sticking on the surface, making the finer, thinner hair recoil and turn back into the follicle.

Nail Care

Nail Care sales can be a hands-down winner in your salon. The astronomic increase in nail salons and nail services have been staggering. Whether you have one station or several, selling add-on services is easy.

Manicures

The foundation for nail care services is the manicure. Clients can cover their bodies with clothes, their hair with hats, their faces with cosmetics, but unless they are willing to don gloves all day, the hands are always exposed. (Fig. 15.5)

Manicures condition the nail itself, smooth and soften the skin, and clean up the cuticles for picture-perfect digits. The treatment smooths and polishes the nail surface and surrounding cuticles. The increased circulation from the massage helps to reduce any fluid increases and helps the blood flow to the nail growth center.

Take a few minutes and thoroughly evaluate the nail condition. Putting more emphasis on the treatment and technique sets you apart for the basic paint and polish service.

- Does the nail bend easily?
- Are there visible splits or breaks?
- Does the nail appear yellow?

- Is the tissues under the nail pink and healthy?
- Are the cuticles rough and dry?
- Are the cuticles overgrown?
- Do the cuticles appear thick and lumpy?
- Are the tips of the nails peeling?
- Has the client filed the sides of the nails?
- Are the nails filed squarely?
- Do the nails curl?
- Are the nails all the same length?

Selling Hints

One way to emphasize the importance of proper nail care is to take the client through an analysis of the hands and nails.

Take before and after shots of hands that you have treated, especially if you put a nail biter on a regular nail treatment program. Frame the results and put a set on each station to show the customer what you can do for stubby nails.

Sell add-on nail services—nail charms, freelance designs, glitter dusting, striping, and custom airbrush polish designs. Introduce nail accessories for special occasions. For Christmas the salon that does my nails lets clients select a nail striping or rhinestones. They give this service for the holidays as a gift to their good clients. (It is a nice way to introduce new services to clients.) Once a client has experienced a novelty nail, she will be inclined to request the service in the future.

Make a "flower arrangement" using decorated plastic nail tips on a tall dowel. Feature seasonal looks, charms, new colors, or new techniques.

Paint nail tips in every color of polish you have in stock. Label the back of each with the color name or number. Punch a small hold in the narrow end of the tip, and hook each tip onto a key ring. Place a nail enamel color selector at each station. The client can sit and flip through your assortment without leaving the chair or rummaging through bottles.

Pedicures

The feet take a beating. They walk an average of 115,000 miles in a lifetime. Pedicures smooth and condition the often neglected areas of the feet and toes. The feet are soaked, buffed, smoothed, massaged, and polished to perfection. The nails are trimmed and filed down to prevent any irritation in shoes. The more than seven thousand nerve cells in each foot respond wonderfully to the massaging and buffing treatment. The client will notice reduced swelling, and the skin texture will take on a healthy glow.

Selling Hints

Incorporate a warm wax paraffin to your pedicure. The warmth from the paraffin seals in the moisture and intensifies the softening of the tissue. The paraffin wax envelops the entire foot for ten to fifteen minutes. The heat and wax work wonders on the rough, dry areas.

When it gets close to sandal season, start to stress the importance of pedicures. I would suggest you start selling pedicures as soon as the snow melts. The toes need extra care before they exposed in spring footwear.

Body Massage

The mere mention of a body massage makes most people purr. A professional salon body massage does wonders for reducing stress. It helps you deeply relax, relieves mental and physical fatigue and tension, improves circulation and elimination, reduces swelling and fluid retention. And on top of all that it feels great!

Selling Hints

All you have to do is start massaging a client's shoulders and as she starts to melt talk to her about the benefits of scheduling a full massage.

When the massage therapist has time, have her walk through the salon and introduce herself and offer to do a mini hand and arm massage. Let the client know the massage hours and the benefits.

Stress the privateness of the treatment. Assure the client the only area of the body that is exposed is the area the masseuse is treating. Remember, some people aren't comfortable with their bodies and a suggestion of a massage may be too much, unless they understand the privacy efforts taken.

Use the selling hints to support your sales. You are proficient in your craft. The general consumer doesn't have your level of artistic eye. Support your explanations and descriptions with the selling tools.

I am confident that you are probably more comfortable selling services. The next chapter will help make selling products as easy as suggesting that new cut, new polish, or leg waxing.

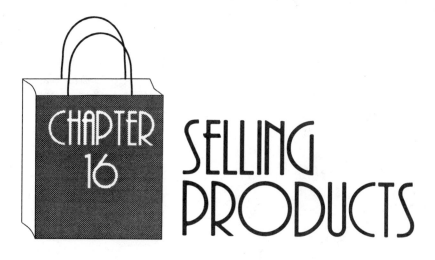

SELLING PRODUCTS

CHAPTER 16

In this chapter you are given examples of how to sell products for every category in the salon business. You'll find a brief description of the product, a general application procedure and recommended sequence of application. There is also a system selling section that gives you three products that are naturally grouped together to help trigger sales.

HAIR CARE

Most beauty salon retail sales are hair care items. With the plethora of product possibilities the consumer has to choose from, you'll need to have some off-the-cuff responses.

One great way to retail additional hair products is to offer hair checkups. If you should service your car every three thousand miles or three months, whichever comes first, why not offer your clients and even potential clients the opportunity to have their hair evaluated? The change of seasons and styling modifications require a different set of home care products. Hair care checkups put clients in your chair. They are in the perfect spot to hear your product recommendations and suggestions. Education makes the sale.

Hair products are generally broken down into four main categories: cleansing, conditioning, styling, and finishing.

Cleansing Products

Shampoo

Statement: This shampoo is designed to thoroughly clean your hair, without damaging the natural condition. Use it to gently wash away pollution, dust, debris, and product residue. The result is shiny, healthier, manageable hair.

Application: Soak the scalp and hair with tepid water. Take a quarter size amount of the shampoo and work it through the hair. Lather well and rinse. If the scalp is oily you may need to lather a second time for maximum results. Rinse the hair completely.

Sequence of Application: Wet hair, shampoo, lather, rinse, shampoo again if necessary, condition, and follow with selected styling products.

System Selling:
1. Shampoo 2. Conditioner 3. Spray
1. Shampoo 2. Conditioner 3. Weekly conditioner
1. Shampoo 2. Mousse 3. Spray

Selling Hints: As a practicing professional, you are aware of the differences between brands of shampoo and other hair products. Your client doesn't have the hands-on exposure to products that you do. Make it your mission to educate the client about the differences. (Fig. 16.1)

Color-Enhancing Shampoo

Statement: Color-enhancing shampoo is used to maintain hair that has been previously color treated. This specialty product should be used after a fresh color treatment to keep the hair looking its best.

Application: Use as you would any shampoo, but leave the lather on the hair for one or two minutes. Rinse well and condition.

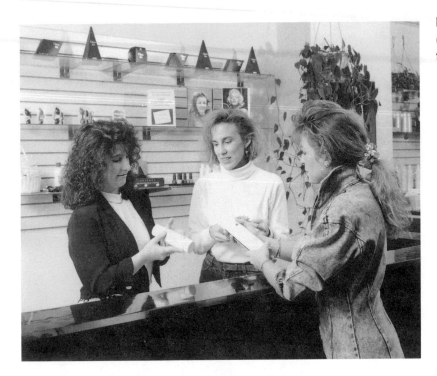

Fig. 16.1 Selling shampoo products. (Photo by Michael A. Gallitelli on location at Rielms Hair Salon, Latham, NY.)

Sequence of Application: Thoroughly wet hair and work shampoo through hair from scalp to ends. Rinse and follow with recommended conditioner.

System Selling:
1. Color-enhancing shampoo 2. Daily shampoo 3. Conditioner
1. Color-enhancing shampoo 2. Conditioner 3. Intensive conditioner
1. Color-enhancing shampoo 2. Mousse 3. Spray

Selling Hints: This particular product is perfect for clients who have color-treated hair, especially in the red color family, which tends to fade quickly. Suggest clients use the enhancing shampoo the next time they cleanse the hair after the color process. Depending on your recommendation, they may need to use the product daily or alternate with another shampoo.

Use this product as an introduction to color services. Show them how to spice up their natural color without committing to a permanent color.

An option is to sell a "colorless" color-enhancing shampoo. The sole purpose is to brighten up the natural color without changing it. Brighter and shinier, without the color risk!

Swimmer's Shampoo

Statement: Chlorine and mineral salts in swimming pools can play havoc with the hair. Swimmer's Shampoo has been formulated to remove all trace minerals from the hair after swimming. Have fun in the sun without damaging your hair's condition.

Application: Use after each dip in the pool or Jacuzzi.

Sequence of Application: Make sure the hair is thoroughly saturated with water before you get into the pool. Just like a dry sponge can soak up more than a wet sponge, you'll want to make sure the hair is soaked with plain water first. Don't allow the hair to dry out before you have a chance to shampoo. Once you're ready to use swimmer's shampoo, wet the hair and lather as normal. Rinse well and repeat.

System Selling:
1. Swimmer's shampoo 2. Plain shampoo 3. Conditioner
1. Swimmer's shampoo 2. Conditioner 3. Intensive conditioner
1. Swimmer's shampoo 2. Sunscreen 3. Lip and eye balm

Selling Hints: Swimmer's shampoo is not just a fun-in-the sun product. You may be able to retail this item year round. Look for clients who swim at the gym or use Jacuzzis. Even clients in rural areas have indoor-outdoor pools.

Your client's water source at home may have additional minerals and deposits that need to be removed from the hair. This is especially true for the clients with well water. If they do, recommend swimmer's shampoo, or deep cleansing shampoo. This client should use the product one to two times a week to remove the mineral traces from the hair.

Conditioning Treatments

Healthy hair is easy to spot. You see it flowing and glistening in the sun. It's hair you want to touch. It's hair with gorgeous color and natural wave, and the sunlight dances off each silky strand. Every client who walks over the threshold of your salon can have the perfect perm or captivating color, but it all starts with healthy hair.

Beautiful hair is hair in good condition. Make that a priority for every client. When you are prescribing home care programs, make sure you add a daily conditioner and an intensive one for repairing and restructuring the hair. Pollutants, water, sun, poor hair products can aggravate the condition. If you want to sell additional perms and colors, the success of those services is in direct proportion to the health of the hair. (Fig. 16.2)

Leave-in Conditioners

Statement: Hair takes a beating, and it is necessary for healthy hair to be conditioned between salon visits. Leave-in conditioners are easy to use and effective.

Application: Shampoo the hair, rinse well, blot off excess water, and massage in about a nickel size drop of product. Comb and style hair as desired.

Sequence of Application: Shampoo, massage in conditioner but do not rinse, then select next styling product.

System Selling:
1. Leave-in conditioner 2. Intensive conditioner 3. Shampoo

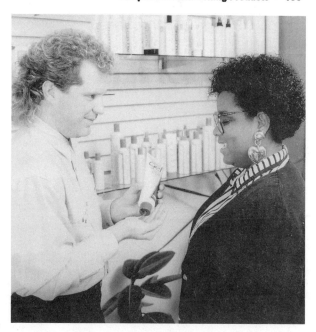

Fig. 16.2   Selling conditioning products. (Photo by Michael A. Gallitelli on location at Rielms Hair Salon, Latham, NY.)

1. Leave-in conditioner 2. Shampoo 3. Color-enhancing shampoo
1. Leave-in conditioner 2. Shampoo 3. Body shampoo

Selling Hints: With pollution and sun damage taking their toll on hair, it is critical to get your clients in the habit of conditioning their hair. A lightweight leave-in conditioner adds moisture and protein to the hair.

Leave-in conditioner makes a great detangler for adults as well as children.

Look for ones that don't leave a buildup in the hair to attract dirt and oils.

Intensive Conditioner

Statement: Once a week, treat your hair to a deep conditioning beauty session.

Application: Apply the intensive conditioner. A nickel size for short hair and a quarter size for longer hair should do the trick. Massage the conditioner through the hair. Wrap the hair with a plastic bag and warm towel. If you have access to a hooded dryer, sit for ten minutes under medium to hot temperature for deep penetration. Use once a week for maximum shine.

Sequence of Application: Cleanse with shampoo, rinse, blot out excess water, apply intensive conditioner, wait ten minutes, rinse well.

System Selling:
1. Intensive conditioner   2. Leave-in conditioner   3. Shampoo
1. Intensive conditioner 2. Gel 3. Spray
1. Intensive conditioner 2. Facial mask 3. Body lotion (My connection here is that when the client is doing her primping session, she can be masking and hydrating the body at the same time.)

Selling Hints: Pollution, smog, dirt, sun, stress, water conditions, tugging, pulling, and poor nutrition will have a negative effect on the hair. Intensive at-home treatments need to be a regular part of every client's home maintenance program. It is easy to spot those people who don't take the time and pay attention to the conditioning of their hair.

Styling Aid Selections

Styling aids are essential to great-looking hair to protect it from styling damage, heat, and even air drying. When left to dry on its own, hair rubs and scrapes against the cuticle and roughs up the outer cuticle. This unfortunately leaves the hair looking like it has been overprocessed. Styling aids encourage the hair cuticle to be flatter and therefore to look shinier and healthier.

Mousse

Statement: The new curly style we have designed today will need a mousse to give you lift and volume in the hair. This will dry quickly, not weigh your hair down, and it will close down the cuticle layer of the hair, giving you a shiny, glossy finish. (Fig. 16.3)

Application: Turn the can upside down and squirt out a small mound of product into your hand. Work the mousse through the hair, concentrating on the base of the scalp for extra lift. Comb the mousse through the entire length of the hair.

Sequence of Application: Shampoo, condition, mousse, style, spray.

System Selling:
1. Mousse 2. Shampoo 3. Conditioner
1. Mousse 2. Gel 3. Spray
1. Mousse 2. Styling brush 3. Blow dryer

Selling Hints: Great for your clients with curly hair who want that soft, tousled, and tumbled look.

Show your client styling options—a day look, office look, evening look. They will need the proper products to recreate the styling options.

Caution your clients on mousses that are alcohol based. Using the wrong product can lead to dry and damaged hair.

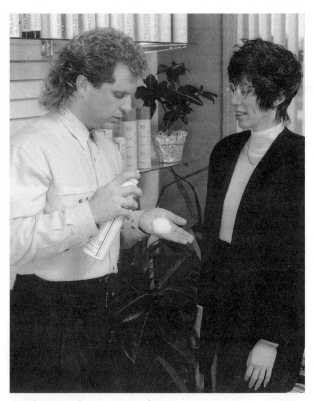

Fig. 16.3 Selling mousse. (Photo by Michael A. Gallitelli on location at Rielms Hair Salon, Latham, NY.)

Gel

Statement: For your smooth, sleek look this styling gel will give you extra body and hold. Since you want to create that forties' sleek style, use the gel and comb waves into place.

Application: Work the gel through the hair, paying close attention to the scalp. Comb and style hair.

Sequence of Application: Shampoo, condition, gel, style, finish spray.

System Selling:
1. Gel 2. Mousse 3. Spray
1. Gel 2. Shampoo 3. Conditioner
1. Gel 2. Intensive conditioner 3. Color-enhancing shampoo

Selling Hints: A sculpting Gel is super for those looks requiring a more dramatic and exaggerated shape.

Gels are a favorite of men. Sculpt and go with a gel. It is easy and quick. Two pluses for your male clients.

It is great for wet looks too!

Gloss

Statement: Add brilliance and sheen to the hair with gloss. Glosses are ideal for the client who has permed hair. The chemical process leaves the hair looking dull and flat. Adding a whisk or two of the gloss will bring the shine back to the hair.

Application: Apply a tiny amount of gloss to your hands and rub the product through the hair. This is the last step in the styling session.

Sequence of Application: Apply after shampooing and conditioning. Rub a small amount of gloss into the hair and comb in place. You can also apply the gloss to hair that has been dried and styled.

System Selling:
1. Gloss 2. Shampoo 3. Gel
1. Gloss 2. Gel 3. Spray
1. Gloss 2. Color-enhancing shampoo 3. Conditioner

Selling Hints: Add a gloss to the home care routine when the desired finished look is for super shiny hair.

Great for enhancing hair if being photographed.

Finishing Products

To top off your crowning glory, selecting the right spray is key. The primary activity for a spray is to lock the curl or style set into the hair. Women don't have time to touch up throughout the day, so the perfect spray is the answer for saving time.

When I was starting out in beauty school, we reached for the spray gun in hopes of anchoring the curl into place before it fell out. Our school motto was "spray and pray."

Sprays come in varying strengths:

- Light hold for those clients not used to hair spray or for those who don't want a set look.

- Medium hold for those who need a little extra power in their finished look and for those clients who don't have time to fuss with their hair throughout the day. Medium hold spray will give you the hold without being stiff.

- Superhold. For the client who can get caught in a hurricane in a convertible and still look like she just stepped out of a salon.

Sprays

Statement: Finish off your look with a super hair spray. Keep your style looking fresh throughout the day.

Application: Hold the container eight to twelve inches away from the head and spray. Allow a fine mist to cover and settle over the hair.

Sequence of Application: Shampoo, condition, styling product, then set style in place with hair spray.

System Selling:
1. Spray 2. Gel 3. Shampoo
1. Soft spray or superhold spray 2. Gloss 3. Color-enhancing shampoo
1. Spray 2. Shampoo 3. Leave-in conditioner

Selling Hints:
One selling hint is to make sure the sprays you sell to teens are water soluble. They tend to get heavy handed with the spray and will need it to wash down the drain.

Check to see if your sprays have sunscreen in them to help shield the hair from the ravages of the sun.

Many clients still prefer the aerosol spray but are environmentally conscious. Ask your product supplier or manufacturer if the CFCs (chlorofluorocarbons) have been removed from the spray. Many manufacturers have addressed this concern and are already producing and environmentally friendly products. If your products are safe, don't hesitate to sell an aerosol spray. There are thousands of women who want a spray that sprays, not pumps.

SKIN CARE

Selling skin care should be an integral part of your retailing mix. If your client is suffering from a flaking scalp, chances are she is also having problems with her skin. Selling skin care can be a natural as selling a shampoo or spray.

Cleansing Systems

Skin care sales today require deeper analysis and explanation than in years past. If you have been out of the beauty business for awhile you may need to go back to the books and refresh yourself on anatomy and physiology.

Cleansers

Statement: Cleansers are designed to remove all traces of surface debris. Cleansers whisk away pollution, makeup, dust, and dirt. Cleansers are recommended for all skin types, both male and female. Today I'll select the appropriate cleanser to match your beauty needs.

Application: Cleansers are used both morning and night. In the morning cleansers prepare the face for makeup application. At night they cleanse the dirt and makeup away before you apply a night moisturizing treatment.

Sequence of Application: Using lots of small dots, apply the cleanser directly to the skin. Work the cleanser in little circles, being careful not to move the skin. Wet a natural sponge or cloth and rinse the cleanser off with tepid water. Splash to remove any traces of cleanser left on the skin. Try to avoid the eye area as cleansers, especially ones for oily skin, tend to dry out that delicate area. Cleansers should be used from the eyebrows up and the cheekbones down.

System Selling

1. Cleanser 2. Toner 3. Day moisturizer
1. Cleanser 2. Eye makeup remover 3. Toner
1. Cleanser 2. Body shampoo 3. Shampoo

Selling Hints : Always suggest a companion product such as a toner with a cleanser. The cleanser and toner are "married" together. You use your cleanser, then you use your toner.

Allow your client to feel the product, even if only on the back of her hand. This helps to incorporate her senses.

Remind your client of the importance of softening the dead cells to prevent a cloudy or dull look to the skin.

Eye Makeup Remover

Statement: Eye makeup remover is used to gently dissolve all eye makeup. This specially designed cleanser will melt away eye shadows, eyeliner, and even stubborn mascara.

Application: Saturate a 100 percent cotton pad with the remover. Place the pad on the eyelid and lashes. Wait a few seconds and gently whisk away the mascara and shadows. Always use a clean cotton pad for each eye. Never reuse a soiled cotton pad.

Sequence of Application: Use the eye makeup remover at night to dissolve all eye makeup. Also use eye makeup remover in the morning to remove any trace of eye treatment cream.

System Selling:

1. Eye makeup remover 2. Face cleanser 3. Toner
1. Eye makeup remover 2. Eye cream 3. Eye mask
1. Eye makeup remover 2. Eye shadow 3. Mascara

Selling Tips: Present the eye makeup remover during the cleansing sequence. Start all face cleaning with eye makeup remover.

Eye makeup removers are lighter in consistency than most facial cleansers. This lightweight formula has fewer oils that when left on the lid can cause the eye shadows to run and smear.

Try using eye makeup remover as a precleanser for lipstick.

Toners

Statement: Toners and skin fresheners remove all traces of cleanser and film left on the surface of the skin. These products are used as rinsing agents to complete the cleansing cycle. Anyone who uses a cleanser on the skin should follow with the appropriate toner.

Application: Thoroughly saturate a cotton pad with toner and completely rinse the skin until the skin drips with toner.

Some toners can be sprayed onto the skin. If they are sprayed, the client should take a clean cloth and gently buff the skin clean to pick up any remaining traces of dirt or cleanser.

Sequence of Application: Use after every time the cleanser is used, both morning and at night.

System Selling:
1. Toner 2. Cleanser 3. Day cream
1. Toner 2. Day cream 3. Night cream
1. Toner 2. Mask 3. Sloughing mask

Selling Hints: Difference in toners usually refers to the strength of the product.

Tonics or herbal waters feel good on the skin and contain no alcohol. They are great in spray form for use after toning the skin and before before applying moisturizer.

Fresheners are the mildest form of toner. They have a lower percentage of alcohol and are used basically on sensitive and dry skins.

Astringents have additional kick to them . They are the strongest form of toner and are used on very oily or troubled skin.

Protectors and Treatments

Day Moisturizers

Statement: These products provide a film that seals in the skin's natural moisture. This film helps to slow down the skin's water evaporation. Moisturizers protect the skin much in the same way that clothes protect the body from the environment.

Some form of moisturizer should be used all the time by all skin types and by both men and women. Even people with oily skin should have some form of protection. Select one that protects the skin without causing irritations or overdrying.

Application: Day moisturizers can be used with or without makeup. Moisturizers should be applied from the cheekbones

down and the eyebrows up. Never apply day cream directly around the eye unless the manufacturer recommends it. The regular face creams can be too heavy for the eyes. Treat the eye area separately.

Sequence of Application: Day moisturizers are best used during daylight hours. Have the client cleanse the skin, follow with toner to complete cleansing, then apply cream or lotion to face and neck area.

System Selling:
1. Day cream 2. Night cream 3. Eye cream
1. Day cream 2. Cleansers 3. Toner
1. Day cream 2. Body lotion 3. Eye cream

Selling Tips: Check to see if your client prefers to dip into or pour the product. Some clients just don't like to dip into pots or jars of creams. Give them the option to choose.

Evaluate the skin's needs for moisturizer, especially as the seasons change. The protection and moisture levels may need to be switched. Seasonal checkups are a must. The moisturizer that works well in the freezing winter months may be too heavy and greasy for lighter summer days.

Night Creams

Statement: These products can be slightly heavier than day moisturizers. The skin needs a layer of protection from the elements, even during the night. Night creams often have intensive ingredients that work best without makeup.

Everyone should have some formula as night protection. The general condition of the skin and age will determine the best formula for results.

Application: Although day creams can be used at night, it is recommended that night creams only be used at night. Some may include certain ingredients that, when exposed to sunlight, can cause photosensitivity.

Sequence of Application: Gently pat a small amount of the selected night cream to the complexion, after completing the cleansing and toning steps of the home care routine. Make sure you apply the lotion from the cheekbones down and the eyebrows up.

System Selling:
1. Night cream 2. Day cream 3. Eye cream
1. Night cream 2. Body lotion 3. Eye cream
1. Night cream 2. Hydrating mask 3. Sloughing mask

Selling Tips: Introduce night treatment products with the day cream selection.

Depending on the skin condition, you can layer intensive treatment products at night. Adding too many layers during the morning routine may cause the makeup to run and smear.

Seasonally check the home care prescription. The skin changes with the seasons. Monitor clients' formulations. Make sure they are rotating their products with each season.

Masks

Statement: Masks are used to refine, firm, and clarify the skin, depending on the formulations. Any skin type and age can benefit from an at-home mask.

For maximum results, masks should be used at least two times a week. Depending on the skin condition and desired results masking could be administered one to three times a week.

Application: Cleanse and tone the skin. Apply a thin film of mask to the complexion. Wait approximately 10 minutes, then splash off with tepid water. Finish your process by applying the face moisturizer, day or night depending on the time.

Sequence of Application: Masks are always applied from the eyebrows up and the cheekbones down. Masks should never be applied directly to the eye area, unless you are using a specially formulated eye mask. You should cleanse the skin, tone, apply a thin film of mask, wait desired time, rinse, and follow with appropriate moisturizer.

System Selling:
1. Hydrating mask 2. Sloughing mask 3. Eye cream
1. Mask 2. Cleanser 3. Toner
1. Mask 2. Eye treatment 3. Body lotion

Selling Tips: Consistently working with a home care mask helps to smooth and soften the skin surface.

Many women have the misconception that masks have to get hard, that they have to lay down with their feet propped up and chilled cucumbers on the eyelids for a mask to be effective. Who has time for all that? I'm sure you don't and neither do your clients. If your client has some time to pamper herself those treatments are wonderful. They are not, however, necessary for mask results.

Complete at-home cleansing should include cleanser, toner, mask two to three times a week, and moisturizer.

To magnify the benefits of masking, have the client apply mask to one-half of the face. Wait five to ten minutes and splash off. She can then see the immediate benefits of incorporating a mask into her home care routine. I've tried this selling tip with many customers and some skins look a quarter to a half-inch higher and firmer on the masked side. It is easy to sell when the client is looking in the mirror and seeing one side of her face firmer and younger looking. (Fig. 16.4)

Sloughing Treatment

Statement: Sloughing treatments give the skin a fresh, light look. Dead cells can make the skin appear lifeless and dull. Masking or scrubbing lifts off the accumulation giving the skin a healthy, smooth finish.

Most skins will benefit from using a sloughing treatment cream or mask. For normal to dry skins a treatment once a week will keep the skin looking its best. Oily skin will benefit from whisking away the thick layer of accumulated cells.

Application: Normal to dry skin once every seven days. Delicate or sensitive skin once every seven to fourteen days. Oily or thick skin, once or twice a week.

Sequence of Application: If the product is in a cleanser form, have the client remove all traces of makeup then gently wash the skin. Use the sloughing lotion just like a cleanser. Work a little water into the palm of your hand and add a nickel size amount of product. Work the product over the skin, being careful to avoid the eyes.

If the formula is in a mask base, cleanse and tone the skin. Apply a thin film of sloughing mask and allow the product to dry for five to ten minutes. Once the product feels flaky and dry, begin to buff the mask off with your fingers. You will see the mask flake off. Rinse the skin after most of the product has

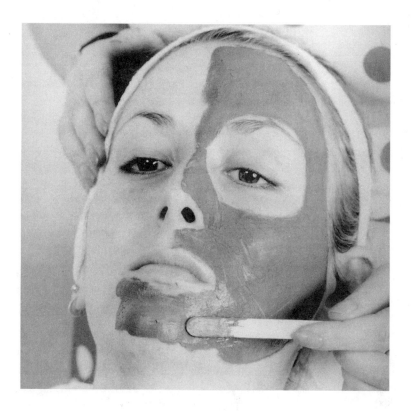

Fig. 16.4 Demonstrating the benefits of masking.

been removed to complete the cleansing process. Follow with appropriate moisturizer.

System Selling:
1. Sloughing mask 2. Hydrating mask 3. Night cream
1. Sloughing mask 2. Base makeup 3. Loose powder
1. Sloughing mask 2. Body scrub 3. Moisturizer

Selling Tips: If you want the skin to look its best, say for a photograph, use your sloughing mask or lotion prior to applying your makeup. You will notice how smoothly the makeup goes on.

An easy way to sell this product is to apply a small amount of the product on the back of your customer's hand. Let it sit as directed. Then have the customer buff or rinse off the product. Ask her to feel the difference between the treated side and the untreated side. Big Difference. Big Sales.

I remember introducing a new sloughing mask product in the salon. Using this simple technique, we were able to close over 65 percent of the clients. Try it. You'll like the results, and your clients will like the way their skin feels.

Ampoules and Serums

Statement: Ampoules and serums are concentrated levels of active ingredients. The product is packaged in individual vials due to the delicate nature of the formulations.

Application: Thoroughly cleanse and tone the skin. Carefully break open the top of the vial, and pour the lotion into the palm of your hand. Gently work the product over the skin until it has penetrated.

Sequence of Application: Cleanse, tone, apply serum, follow with appropriate day or night cream. Use for seven consecutive days for maximum results.

System Selling:
1. Ampoule 2. Day cream 3. Night cream
1. Ampoule 2. Cleanser 3. Toner
1. Ampoule 2. Sloughing mask 3. Hydrating mask

Selling Hints: Ampoules have many different functions. Study the manufacturer's directions carefully.

Look to see if your serums have aromatherapy benefits. The essential extracts can be a selling plus if the fragrance is pleasing.

If the vial is glass, make sure you show your client how to break the seal. The last thing you want is for the client to get cut while she is performing her home care beauty routine.

Serums and vials can be expensive. Suggest a trial run during the facial. Price your service package to utilize one of the vials during the facial. After the treatment, the client takes the rest of the package home for intensive work for the next six days.

Eye Creams

Statement: The eye area is the most delicate region on the face. Aging will show here first. To slow down telltale lines gently apply this ultralight nourishing eye cream.

Application: Take a small amount of the product and gently tap on the hollow under the eye. Then tap along the crease in the eyelid. Your body heat will naturally blend the lotion into the skin. Do not rub or pull on the tissue.

Sequence of Application: Cleanse the eye and face. Rinse with toner and apply face moisturizer, being careful not to apply it to the eye. Take the selected eye cream and carefully apply to the upper and lower eye area.

System Selling:
1. Eye cream 2. Day moisturizer 3. Night cream
1. Eye cream 2. Eye makeup remover 3. Mascara
1. Eye cream 2. Cleanser 3. Toner

Selling Hints: Stress the importance of treating the eye area separately. Many lotions when used on the eye can make the tissue swell and puff up. If a product is too oily then the eye makeup won't stay on as well and will be prone to creasing throughout the day.

Sell jars of eye product in smaller quantities. When you retail a two- to three-ounce jar, the product will more than likely go rancid before the client can use it all.

MAKEUP

The salon is the perfect place to sell makeup items. The clients are exposed to new looks, new techniques, and the latest and greatest fashions. Makeup is the next step. (Fig. 16.5)

Makeup products are great impulse items. Color is fun and makeup can be an inexpensive morale booster. A few well-chosen selling phrases and product displays can help boost your daily sales average. Makeup can make up the difference in sluggish sales.

Colors and Concealers

Base Makeup

Statement: Base makeup is used to create a flawless finish on the skin. Foundation is worn to bring harmony and balance to the skin's surface.

Application: Lightly dot the base over the complexion. Add a little extra product over the T-zone. With a sponge start to connect the dots. Keep blending until the base is smooth and there are no telltale signs ringing the jaw.

Sequence of Application: Prepare the skin by thoroughly cleansing and toning. Apply the day moisturizer. Dot and blend base makeup.

System Selling:
1. Base makeup 2. Loose powder 3. Compact powder
1. Base makeup 2. Concealer 3. Loose powder
1. Base makeup 2. Blush 3. Lipstick

Selling Hints: Check the client's base color when you tip her back in the shampoo bowl. If you are seeing a ring around the jawline, bring up changing makeup colors for the season.

Bases come in many forms and consistencies—cream for those who like maximum coverage; souffle that is whipped; oil-free for oily skinned clients; water-based for those who prefer their base to have less oil than normal; oil bases for those who need an oil-rich product; liquid, which is a good old standby base that is sheer and smooth; camouflage for serious cover-ups; sport weights to wear while working out or for minimal coverage. Check with your client to see what weight or benefit she would like the base makeup to impart.

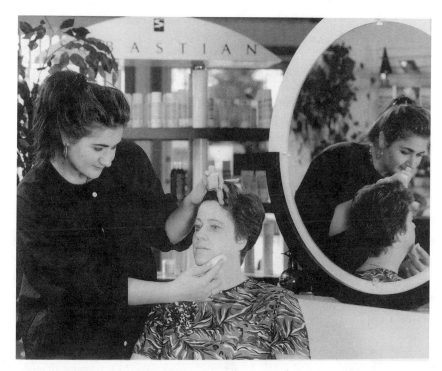

Fig. 16.5 The salon is the perfect place to sell makeup. (Photo by Michael A. Gallitelli on location at Rielms Hair Salon, Latham, NY.)

Test the color of base along the jawline and neck. Don't swipe the color along the hand and expect to get an exact color match. If the client has on a truly wrong color, leave it on the skin. Just clean a small test area. This gives you visual appeal when she looks in the mirror and sees her color glowing back at her while the color you've selected looks so natural. The base is practically in the bag.

If you have access to natural light in the salon, take the client over to the window and check the color match. Make sure the color you've selected looks great in the salon, but also when she gets outside in the sun.

Use the matching tools when you are instructing your client on base application. Show makeup brushes and sponges. You don't sell fingers. Show the client how to work efficiently with professional tools to obtain professional results.

Loose Powder

Statement: Loose powder is used to set makeup. Loose powder will absorb ten times its weight in oil and perspiration. Loose powder will help keep your makeup on all day.

Application: Take a cosmetic sponge and gently press the powder onto the base makeup. Continue tapping the powder into place. Dust off any excess. Run your hands over the base. If the skin still feels damp you may need additional powder. Double check the blush area. If the skin is still damp, applying powder blush over it may cause streaking.

Sequence of Application: Apply base makeup, cream cheek color, then loose powder or base makeup, loose powder, then powder blush. If you don't use base makeup you can apply loose powder, blush, then powder again to soften.

System Selling:
1. Loose powder 2. Compact powder 3. Base makeup
1. Loose powder 2. Compact powder 3. Cosmetic sponge
1. Loose powder 2. Blusher 3. Powder brush

Selling Hints: Notice the texture and consistency of the loose powder. Many are refined and silky to the touch. Loose powder will leave a soft, velvety feel to the skin.

Clients with oily skins should definitely use loose powder to absorb surface oil and combat shine.

New colored powders allow you the option to alter the finished look. If you need a hint of color try one with a touch of pink or peach. If the skin looks a little sallow, dust a touch of lavender powder over the finished look. Watch the skin perk up.

Travel Tip. If the powder is in a pot or jar take the plastic liner out. Insert a large piece of plastic wrap over the loose powder. Replace the hard plastic liner over the wrap. This travel tip helps prevent any powder from spilling out into your suitcase or gym bag.

Compact Powder

Statement: Compact powder is designed to keep makeup fresh throughout the day. Compacts are used for touch-ups to eliminate shine and perspiration.

Application: Gently rub the powder puff over the pat of powder. Press gently over the face concentrating on the T-Zone.

Sequence of Application: Compact powder is best used as a touch-up product. Compacts can be used any time throughout the day or night. Use your Loose Powder to set the makeup during the morning application and save your compact for touch-ups.

System Selling:
1. Compact powder 2. Loose powder 3. Blusher
1. Compact powder 2. Powder brush 3. Extra puffs
1. Compact powder 2. Concealer 3. Lipstick (Touch-Up Kit)

Selling Hints: Show loose and compact powder together.

Compact powder doesn't have properties for setting the makeup. Compacts are so compressed into the pat that they lose some of the adhering properties. For maximum staying power, use loose powder in the morning and carry the compact for quick touch-ups as needed.

Eye Shadow

Statement: Eye shadow is a colored powder used to accentuate the eyes and bring out the features of the face.

Application: Depending on the desired look, shadows can be applied with an eye shadow sponge or fluff brush. Gently tap the desired color onto the selected brush. Hit the side of the brush on the side of your hand to remove any excess shadow. This helps to eliminate the excess powder from flaking off onto the cheekbone.

Sequence of Application: This depends on the desired look. Coach your client on the easiest way to apply the color. Make sure you teach your client how to professionally blend the shadows for a polished, smooth look.

System Selling:
1. Eye shadow 2. Mascara 3. Eye pencil liner
1. Eye shadow 2. Cake eye liner 3. Pencil liner
1. Eye shadow 2. Concealer 3. Mascara
1. Eye shadow 2. Eye makeup remover 3. Makeup brushes

Selling Hints: Determine the client's preference of color family; don't show her forty colors at once. Preselect the best colors for the desired look. Ask what tone or intensity she prefers. Ask for input and listen.

Show eye shadow collections in threes. Select highlight color, medium tone, and contour color. As you work with each selection, make sure to match the appropriate makeup brush to complete the look. Show fashion or seasonal accent colors.

Learn to mix and match the client's colors if she has some product at home. Ask her to bag the products up and bring them to the salon for you to look over. If some are okay, select one or two colors the client can add to her existing collection.

Mascara

Statement: Mascara brings out the eyes. This luscious mascara will lengthen and darken your natural lashes, bringing out their natural shape.

Application: Take the tip of the mascara wand and lightly coat the tips of the lashes. Sweep through the tips then turn the wand so that it is parallel to the lash line. With long sweeping motions comb the mascara from the base of the lash up and out to the tips. Once the tips have been coated you won't need as much mascara through the lashes. This helps prevent lash clumping.

Sequence of Application: Apply mascara at the end of the makeup application. Allow time for the top lashes to dry before you apply the product to the lower lashes.

System Selling:
1. Mascara 2. Eye makeup remover 3. Eye cream
1. Mascara 2. Eye pencil 3. Cake liner
1. Mascara 2. False lashes 3. Lash curler

Selling Hints: The preservatives in mascara weaken after the tube has been open for ninety days. Date the bottom of the tube ninety days from the date of purchase. For eye safety the customer should replace the product at that time.

Never share mascara or any tube eye product. It is very easy to spread infections. Avoid cross contamination by keeping your products for yourself. Teach teens the importance of eye makeup safety.

If your client has a problem with dark circles under the eye, use black mascara on the upper lashes and suggest brown or brown/black mascara for the bottom. Softening up the color will help eliminate the dark shadows.

Stress the importance of removing the eye makeup every evening before retiring. Mascara buildup can cause the lashes to become dry and brittle. Notice if your customer has any gaps of lashes missing. Chances are she is skipping over this important cleansing step.

If your customer has a problem with eye makeup staying on and mascara smudging, check into the method of cleansing the eye. A heavy oil can leave a residue giving the eye product reason to slip and slide. Refer to eye makeup remover.

Eyeliner

Statement: Eyeliner is used to maximize the eye shape. Liner is great for making the lash line appear thicker and fuller. Cake liner is mixed with water to create a sharper, more defined line around the eyes. Pencil liner comes in a variety of colors. Use a sharp pencil to trace around the lash line. Sketch color on and soften with an eye shadow sponge or cotton swab.

Eye shadow can be substituted as liner. Take the angle brush and press the shadow up along the base of the lashes. This allows for a softer, more delicate liner look.

Automatic liner comes in a form similar to mascara. The brush with the tube helps to draw on a fine or wide dramatic line. This creates a stronger look with staying power.

Application: For top lashes, have the client tip the chin up and look down the nose. This position tips the lashes down away

from the lid. Lay the selected brush along the lash line and apply color. For lower lashes, tip the chin down and look up. Start at the outside of the eye and work the color along the lash line.

Stress eye safety importance. Some clients like to apply their liner to the inside ridge of the eye. Show your client how to get shape and definition, without rimming the ridge on the eye. There have been reported cases of permanent eye damage from pencils ripping the cornea of the eye. Why take chances? Keep the liner under the lashes.

Sequence of Application: Following the application of eye shadow, use eyeliner to define upper and/or lower lashes. Mascara is then applied to thicken lashes.

System Selling:
1. Eyeliner pencil 2. Angle brush 3. Eye shadow
1. Eyeliner cake 2. Fine eyeliner brush 3. Mascara
1. Eyeliner 2. Eye makeup remover 3. Loose powder

Selling Hints: Clients should always sharpen pencils before and after each use. This helps to prevent eye damage and creates a sharper more defined line.

Suggest a darker liner for top lashes and a lighter color for bottom, especially if client is plagued with dark bags under the eyes.

Try overlapping colors. Use liquid liner first, then gently lay eye shadow over line to smudge and blend.

Purple-based colors are more prone to eye sensitivity. If client is sensitive prone, avoid purple-based colors. Stay in the neutral family.

Lipstick

Statement: Lipstick adds drama or subtle color to the lips. There are many new forms of lipstick to test and try. You can choose from matte colors, high shine and frost, lip gloss, ultra-wear colors, conditioning lipstick, to name a few.

Application: For long-lasting lip power, apply a thin film of base to the lips. Lightly dust loose powder over the lip and trace the outside edges with a lip pencil for a defined lip edge. Take a lip brush and paint the color onto the lip. Take a tissue and press firmly over the color and blot. Repeat, but just a touch of color back over the lips.

Sequence of Application: Base, powder, lip pencil, lipstick.

System Selling:
1. Lipstick 2. Lip pencil 3. Lip gloss
1. Lipstick 2. Lip brush 3. Lip pencil
1. Lipstick 2. Lip moisturizer 3. Lip gloss

Selling Hints: First find out if the client prefers lipstick or gloss. What intensity of color is she comfortable wearing? What color of clothing would she like the color to match? Next select three choices from your inventory that you feel would be flattering to the client. Have the client look in the mirror. Now one at a time, hold the tube up to the cheek and notice how the color reacts to the skin. After you have tested the three colors, hold all three up to the cheek and ask the client, "Now that you have seen the selection, which color do you prefer?" Get the client's reaction.

Offer lip lesson makeovers. Blot out all color, apply base to lips, and show the customer a new and possibly daring way to accentuate the lips and face. (Fig. 16.6)

Lip Pencils

Statement: Lip pencils help frame the lips and bring added focus and dimension to the face. Lip pencils are great tools for keeping the lipstick from bleeding.

Application: For a stronger look, outline the lips and then fill them in completely with the lip pencil. If the desired look is softer and more natural, apply the lipstick with a brush, then lightly trace around the lip edges after you have applied the color.

Sequence of Application: You have three options—base makeup on lips, lip pencil, lipstick; lip pencil, loose powder on lips, lipstick; lipstick, lip pencil, loose powder over lips and pencil.

System Selling:
1. Lip pencil 2. Lipstick 3. Lip gloss
1. Lip pencil 2. Sharpener 3. Lip brush
1. Lip pencil 2. Lipstick 3. Nail polish

Selling Hints: Match a lip pencil to the selected lipstick.
Always sharpen the lip pencil before and after each use.
If the lead in the pencil feels a little hard, gently press

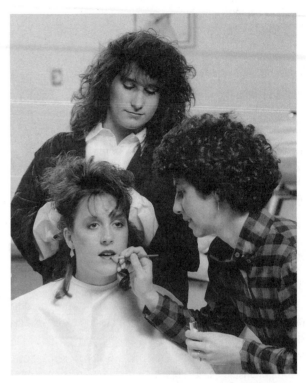

Fig. 16.6 Offer lip lesson makeovers to your clients. (Photo by Michael A. Gallitelli on location at Rielms Hair Salon, Latham, NY.)

it between the thumb and index finger. Hold for a few seconds while the heat of your hand warms and softens the lead.

Due to the color dyes in lip pencils, avoid using them in or around the eye area. Some color additives can cause severe eye irritation, so it is better to use lip pencil on the lips only.

Most women need three colors of lip pencils: a red, a warm or cool tone, and one in the neutral or nude family.

Concealers

Statement: Hide those pesky dark circles under the eye with concealer. Camouflage the darker area with this easy step.

Application: Take a small amount of concealer on your ring finger. Look into the mirror and tip the chin down. Starting at the outside corner of the eye, gently tap the concealer under the eye. Once the color has been applied take a small sponge and blend in the concealer. Make sure you don't rub too hard and whisk away the product.

Sequence of Application: Apply concealer, then delicately dot on the base makeup over the rest of the complexion and under eye area.

System Selling:
1. Concealer 2. Base makeup 3. Loose powder
1. Flesh-colored concealer 2. Mint concealer 3. Base makeup
1. Concealer 2. Eye shadow 3. Mascara

Selling Hints: Some makeup companies offer flesh-colored concealers and specialty colors for added coverage. Look into colors such as mint for added benefit of covering blue dark circles. Some have yellow tones for clients who suffer from whiteout under the eye.

Blush

Statement: Use a hint of color to kiss the cheek or create sculpted cheekbones with the proper use of blush-on cheek color.

Application: The application of blush may vary depending on the desired effect. Have your client look into the mirror and tip the chin down. She should see her natural cheekbones. Follow the ridge for contour placement and the top of the bone for highlighting color.

Sequence of Application: Base makeup, then cream cheek color, loose powder or base makeup, loose powder, powder blush.

System Selling:
1. Cream blush 2. Loose powder 3. Base makeup
1. Powder blush 2. Blush brush 3. Contour brush
1. Powder blush 2. Highlight blush 3. Brush for blending

Selling Hints: Start by showing a base contour color. Then select accent colors based on wardrobe, warm, cool, red, and neutral tones.

Blush does get old, frequently before the product is used up. Look to see the condition of the top of the blush. If it dis-

colored and streaked with cakes, suggest to your client that it is time to toss it out or trade it in.

Blush is one item that should be worn fresh each season. A color that is too dark, or too light will not balance with the season's clothing, a sure sign that the client is behind the times.

BODY CARE

With today's hurried and hassled pace, body care items provide a much needed escape from reality. Whether the products are for pampering and soaking or targeted specifically for smoothing and softening the skin, don't overlook the sales possibilities with body care items.

Body care sales in the salon are a piece of cake. These products are uniquely easy to sell because of their universal properties. Body care items are usually single-benefit products.

Scrubs and Loofahs

Body Scrubs

Statement: Body scrub is a great item for whisking away dead cells from the body. It leaves the skin silky smooth and fresh.

Application: After cleansing the body in the shower, gently massage body scrub over skin. Rinse thoroughly to remove all traces of product.

Sequence of Application: Body cleanser, body scrub, body lotion.

System Selling:
1. Body scrub 2. Body cleanser 3. Body lotion
1. Body scrub 2. Facial scrub. 3. Loofah
1. Body scrub 2. Body oil 3. Body lotion

Selling Hints: Give the client a small amount to try on the back of her hand. Let her work the product on the skin and rinse. After the client has finished ask if she feels a difference on the skin. Once you get a confirmation, the product is practically in the bag.

If you offer body waxing, a body scrub is an excellent product to suggest to your clients. Used daily in the bath or shower body scrub can help eliminate ingrown hairs. Body scrub keeps the cell buildup off allowing the hairs to break through the skin surface. Start scrubbing the day after waxing.

Loofahs

Statement: A unique body sponge for eliminating dead cell buildup.

Application: The loofah is used wet and liberally saturated with body cleanser.

Sequence of Application: Cleanse the skin, then buff over the body with the loofah. Rinse thoroughly and follow with body lotion after shower or bath.

System Selling:
1. Loofah 2. Body cleanser 3. Body lotion
1. Loofa 2. Body scrub 3. Body oil
1. Loofa 2. Bath sponges 3. Aromatherapy oil

Selling Hints: Loofahs need to be replaced every couple of months, before they become moldy.

Look for loofahs that are not too abrasive on the body. Some can feel like you are using industrial grade sandpaper. Natural body sponges will also exfoliate the skin, and may not be as hard on the delicate tissues.

Lotions and Oils

Body Lotions

Statement: Envelop the skin in this luxurious body lotion. Hydrate and condition the skin using the body moisturizer.

Application: After you have stepped out of the shower or bath, leave a tiny trace of water on the skin. Rub the body lotion into the skin to seal in the natural moisture as well as the hydrating properties of the lotion.

Sequence of Application: Body cleanser, body scrub or loofah, body lotion.

System Selling:
1. Body lotion 2. Body cleanser 3. Body scrub
1. Body lotion 2. Hand lotion 3. Cuticle cream
1. Body lotion 2. Face moisturizer 3. Eye cream

Selling Hints: Keep a tester of body lotion in the bathroom, at the front counter, and at each manicure station. A good body lotion is a great impulse purchase item. Keep it handy for the clients to try.

Aromatherapy Oils

Statement: People have been using aromatic oils for healing and beautifying for centuries. Aromatherapy oils are intense and active oils used for the face, body, and scalp.

Application: For body oils, after bath place a few drops of the designated oil on the soles of the feet and up the heel. It is not necessary to rub the oils into the skin like a lotion. The skin will absorb the properties.

For bath aromatherapy oils, add a few drops to a tub of warm water and soak away the cares of the day.

Sequence of Application: Bath, aromatherapy oil, body lotion.

System Selling:
1. Aromatherapy oil 2. Bath oil 3. Body lotion
1. Aromatherapy oil 2. Body scrub 3. Body lotion
1. Aromatherapy oil (body) 2. Aromatherapy oil (face)
   3. Soothing bath bubbles

Selling Hints: It is best to recommend aromatherapy oils after massage or body therapy work. Many companies offer target-specific products, for example for stress, to enhance deep breathing, etc. This is super because it helps to eliminate the guesswork between oils.

Listen for clues in your conversation. Many clients will casually mention physical problems that would benefit from aromatherapy oils, especially fluid retention, tension, and stress. A word of caution: follow manufacturer's guidelines in recommending oils. Do not try to treat medical problems.

Sun Products

Consumers are finally waking up to the fact that baking at the beach is going to cause skin damage. With the number of skin cancer cases on the incline, many people are reaching for sun block. Keep your clients out of the drug store aisles; offer a competitively priced sun care line.

Sun products are available in varying strengths. The products are coded according to their sun protection factor or SPF. A sun product will have a rating on the bottle that tells you how long you can stay in the sun without burning while wearing the sun product.

- Maximum Protection: SPF 15+ to 12
- Moderate Protection: SPF 10 to 6
- Minimal Protection: SPF 4 to 2

Sunscreen

Statement: Whether you are planning a play day at the beach of simply driving your car to and from, you'll need a sunscreen for protection.

Application: Sunscreen should be applied daily for nonbeach activity and reapplied every ninety minutes if you are basking at the beach.

Sequence of Application: Apply selected body and/or facial moisturizer, then massage on a liberal amount of sunscreen.

System Selling:
1. Sunscreen 2. After-sun hydrator 3. Lip balm
1. Sunscreen 2. Body scrub 3. Body lotion
1. Sunscreen 2. Sunless tan 3. Body lotion

Selling Hints: Quite often, clients forget the need to protect the skin if they work indoors. They will be exposed to the sun driving to work and to the fluorescent lights during the day. Even on a cloudy day the skin can still react to sun exposure. Make sun protection a basic part of any home maintenance program.

Your customer may need a wardrobe of products—a lower SPF for use under base makeup and in the office and a stronger formula for outdoor adventures.

Suntan Oils and Lotions

Statement: Suntan oils and lotion are great products to help you achieve the tan you desire while still protecting the skin.

Application: Once you are stretched out at the beach, generously massage on suntan lotion. Pay close attention to delicate tissue not normally exposed to the sun.

Sequence of Application: Still apply a sunscreen before exposure, and then apply oil or lotion every ninety minutes. Apply frequently if you are in the water, even if the product is waterproof.

System Selling:
1. Suntan oil 2. Sunscreen 3. Lip balm
1. Suntan oil 2. After-sun hydrator 3. Body lotion
1. Suntan oil 2. Sunless tan 3. Body scrub

Selling Hints: You can get color on the skin, even wearing a high SPF product. But if your client still wants that bronze goddess glow, a suntan oil or lotion is the ticket.

Avoid using baby oil as a suntan oil. Think of what happens to an egg when you put it on oil. The skin can get just as crispy with baby oil and the sun. You are asking to be fried if you slather on baby oil and bake. Baby oil may be cheaper, but in the long run your clients will be paying the price for the damage. Stress an SPF suntan oil or lotion.

Sunless Tanning

Statement: Grab a tan without breaking a sweat. Sunless tanning creams give you that back-from-the-islands look without baring your skin to the sun.

Application: Make sure you use a body scrub first to remove dead skin cells. Then carefully apply the tanning cream over the skin. You might want to wear plastic gloves to prevent orange palms.

Sequence of Application: Body scrub, then sunless tanning lotion.

System Selling:
1. Sunless tan 2. Body scrub 3. Body lotion
1. Sunless tan 2. Sunscreen 3. Body scrub
1. Sunless tan 2. Face moisturizer 3. Body lotion

Selling Hints: Offer sunless tanning applications as a salon body treatment. If the product is not applied properly it can leave streaks from an uneven application. Why not offer a sunless tanning session for your clients?

Patch test the product first. Some products do give off different colors. The original formulations had a noticeable orange cast, but the newer products look very natural. First test a small area that is not visible. Take the product for a test run before applying the golden glow.

After-sun Skin Hydrators

Statement: After you have had your fun in the sun, make sure you condition the skin. The after-sun hydrator helps to replenish the depleted moisture the sun has zapped from the skin.

Application: Generously massage the cream or lotion into the skin.

Sequence of Application: Take a cool shower to remove all traces of sand and oils. While the skin is still slightly damp work the hydrator into the skin. Reapply as the skin instantly drinks up the lotion.

System Selling:
1. After-sun hydrator 2. Sunscreen 3. Body lotion
1. After-sun hydrator 2. Shower gel 3. Body lotion
1. After-sun hydrator 2. Suntan lotion 3. Face mask

Selling Hints: An after-sun hydrator is different from a normal body lotion. The ingredients cool the skin's surface and replenish surface moisture.

Some after-sun hydrators are available in spray or mist formulas. These can be particularly refreshing on the skin especially if the skin is sensitive from sun exposure.

Eye and Lip Protection

Statement: The eye and lip tissue absolutely need extra care. These areas are the thinnest in tissue structure and demand stronger sun protection.

Application: Apply a coat of product over lips and around the eye area.

Sequence of Application: Sunscreen, then eye and lip protection. Reapply every ninety minutes during exposure, more frequently if in the water.

System Selling:
1. Eye and lip protection 2. Sunscreen 3. Face moisturizer
1. Eye and lip protection 2. Sunless tan 3. Face mask

1. Eye and lip protection 2. Suntan lotion 3. Eye cream

Selling Hints: This can be two separate products—one for the eye area and a balm-type product for the lips.

NAIL CARE
Products for Manicures and Pedicures

Get a firm grip on nail and hand care sales. There is a nice balance for nail care sales because many of the items are primers or stock products (base coat, top coat, and tools). For fun and flavor, there are hundreds of colors to choose from. Nail care sales can add profits to the salon. (Fig. 16.7)

Base Coat

Statement: The first step to perfect nails. Base coat is the digit foundation and can prevent chipping and peeling of nail colors.

Application: On a clean nail bed, paint a thin application of selected base coat.

Sequence of Application: Base coat, two coats of color, top coat.

System Selling:
1. Base coat 2. Polish color 3. Top coat
1. Base coat 2. Polish remover 3. Cuticle conditioner
1. Base coat 2. Hand lotion 3. Body lotion

Selling Hints: Base coat is the primer step before adding nail color. Base coat is going to keep the color from flaking and chipping.

Does your client need a base coat with strengthener? With nail protein? With ridge filler? Match the need to your inventory.

Top Coat

Statement: Protect your nails from daily wear and tear. Top coat seals the color and prevents flaking and chipping of nail color.

Application: Using smooth, long brush strokes, paint a layer of top coat over the nail color. Take the tip of the brush and coat under the free edge of the nail too.

Sequence of Application: Base coat, two coats of color, top coat.

System Selling:
1. Top coat 2. Polish color 3. Base coat
1. Top coat 2. Hand lotion 3. Cuticle conditioner
1. Top coat 2. Day color 3. Nighttime color

Selling Hints: Top coat should be reapplied every other day after a fresh manicure for perfect nails.

   Some top coats leave a wet or shiny look after application. Fun product for high gloss shine.

Nail Enamel

Statement: Add a little spice to your life with nail enamel color.

Application: Starting at the back of the nail, make a long fluid brush stroke tight down the center of the nail bed. Add one stripe of color along the center margin.

Sequence of Application: Base coat, two thin applications of color, top coat.

System Selling:
1. Polish 2. Base coat 3. Top coat
1. Day color polish 2. Night color polish 3. Frosted accent color
1. Polish 2. Hand lotion 3. Cuticle cream
1. Polish 2. Lipstick 3. Lip pencil

Selling Hints: If your client is trying to decide between colors, place a piece of tape on the back of her hand. Apply color to tape. Line up three colors for her to choose from. Once the decision has been made gently peel up the tape and you're done. This avoids damaging a manicure to test a new color.

   Put together a color accent package. Include enamel color, matching lipstick, and lip pencil. You might want to toss in the coordinating cheek color as well.

Cuticle Conditioners

Statement: Protect your hands from hangnails and peeling skin by treating your cuticles. Cuticle conditioner is designed to

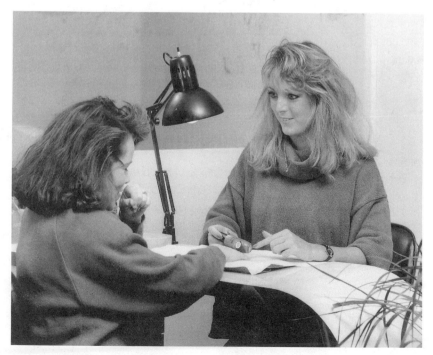

Fig. 16.7 Nail care sales add color and profits to the salon. (Photo by Michael A. Gallitelli on location at Rielms Hair Salon, Latham, NY.)

repair and restore moisture that normal use and abuse of the hands strips away.

Application: When the hands are still damp from cleansing, massage a tiny amount of the conditioner into and around the cuticles.

Sequence of Application: Can be applied as needed throughout the day.

System Selling:
1. Cuticle conditioner 2. Hand lotion 3. Nail polish remover
1. Cuticle conditioner 2. Face moisturizer 3. Body lotion
1. Cuticle conditioner 2. Base coat 3. Polish color

Selling Hints: Cuticle conditioner is easy to forget. With all the other lotions to apply cuticle conditioner is pushed aside. To alleviate this oversight, stash the product on the night stand. Once you are tucked into bed, take a second to apply cuticle conditioner.

Quick Set

Statement: Don't have time to sit tight while the polish is drying? Apply quick set over the nails to speed up the process.

Application:; Once the manicure is finished, wait one to two minutes for the products to set then brush on or spray the nails with the fast-drying agent.

Sequence of Application: Apply one layer of base coat, two layers of nail enamel, one layer of top coat. It's best to wait one to two minutes then spray the nails with quick set.

System Selling:
1. Quick set 2. Polish 3. Hand lotion
1. Quick set 2. Base coat 3. Top coat
1. Quick set 2. Cuticle conditioner 3. Hand lotion

Selling Hints: Prevent ruining a manicure. Quick set saves time as well as nail smears and nicks.

Foot File

Statement: Terrific tool for keeping feet smooth and soft. This super body-buffer sands away rough calluses and buildup.

Application: Working on the trouble spots buff away the thickened tissue. Whisk back and forth over callus.

Sequence of Application: After the foot has been soaked in water for a few minutes, buff away.

System Selling:
1. Foot file 2. Body lotion 3. Cuticle conditioner
1. Foot file 2. Polish remover 3. Polish
1. Foot file 2. Body scrub 3. Body lotion

Selling Hints: This terrific tool helps prevent unsightly buildup on the bottoms of the feet. Use weekly between salon pedicures for maximum results.

Emphasize the importance of filing the feet between pedicures. Instruct the customer on how to use the file while you are administering the foot treatment.

FRAGRANCE

Perfume—the word perfume comes from two Latin words; *per* meaning through and *fumum* meaning smoke. Today, perfume implies a mixture of a solvent or extender with one or possibly hundreds of essential oils, which give the perfume its distinct scent. The ratio is usually eight parts alcohol to two parts essential oils. True perfume is the most expensive in a fragrance collection and is a great base to use in the morning for lasting power.

Eau de toilette—a much thinner dilution of the same materials, containing approximately 5 percent oils.

Cologne or **Aftershave** (for men)—still lighter fragrance containing about 3 percent of the dilution.

Many colognes are available in mist, spray, or dab-on form.

Splash-on—great for after bath when just a hint of fragrance is desired. Most diluted form of fragrance.

Sprays—aerosol forms of fragrance. They are used to lightly mist the body with fragrance.

Statement: Fragrance stimulates the emotions and the imagination. A hint of fragrance should leave a lingering shroud of yourself. Fragrance is the finishing touch. A signature scent completes a person's image statement.

Application: Start by applying the fragrance at the ankles, the back of the knee, the crevice of the elbow, between the breast, the hollow of the throat, and in the hair. As your body warms the fragrance, you will be enveloped in the wonderful aroma.

Sequence of Application: Start by using a scented body shampoo or soak in your signature-scented bath. While the skin is still damp, apply the perfume oil to pressure points. To seal in the fragrance liberally apply matching scented body lotion and finish off with a hint of cologne. This technique is called layering the fragrance.

System Selling:
1. Perfume 2. Cologne 3. Eau de toilette
1. Cologne 2. Bath bubbles 3. Body lotion
1. Body shampoo 2. Body lotion 3. Cologne

Selling Hints: The nose can become quite used to a fragrance. Unfortunately, many of your clients are still using the same fragrance after decades. Your client may lose the ability to judge the quantity to apply if the nose becomes so sensitized to the aroma. Find out how long she has been wearing the scent and suggest different "weights" of the fragrance.

Build a fragrance wardrobe. Match scents for different moods—a fun sport scent, a dramatic power scent, a provocative scent, a work scent. By building a wardrobe of fragrances, the client can enjoy a wide variety of aromas.

Most women tend to dab cologne behind the ears. If you apply the product low on the body and work your way up, you will have the fragrance enveloping the body throughout the day. If you spritz just behind the ears, the only one to enjoy the lofting aroma is the birds.

Excellent sales builder at Christmas, Mother's Day, and Father's Day. If colognes are not a regular item in your inventory line, look to adding a small collection for these three time periods.

TOOLS

Hair Styling Helpers

There is no way around it. Professional tools equal professional results. For your client to look good away from the salon, she needs the proper tools at home to recreate the style you have selected for her. Retailing tools is a natural extension of your service and home care recommendations.

Hair Dryers

If the condition of your client's hair is very dry and damaged, ask her to bring in her blow-dryer from home. You may find that the dryer is the culprit. It may be getting much too hot, especially for fine, delicate hair. See if there are temperature controls and volume adjustments.

A salon-quality dryer may be a bit more of an investment, but if your client wants perfect hair, evaluate the quality of the dryer. Sell the client the investment dryer versus the cheaper one that will need to be replaced every year.

Salon-quality dryers are better and offer unique features such as special styling attachments, cool air flow for maximum curl, and front to back air flow patterns to prevent overheating.

Set up a test bar where the styling tools you have available for sale are plugged in and ready to go. Let the client experiment with the different grades and accessories.

Diffuser

This specialty attachment fits on the end of the blow-dryer. Blowers can aggressively move the base of the hair shaft. The blasts of air from a blower can be too much for some styles. The diffuser evenly disperses the warm air flow from the blower over a large area of the head, without disrupting the curls. If the finished look is for soft, natural-looking curls, the diffuser is a terrific tool.

Curling Irons

If you are dramatically changing the client's style, you may need to recommend a new curling iron to complement the style. Common barrel sizes are mini, half-in., and three-quarters. Check to see if the client has curling iron marks of fish hooks in the hair when she comes in. Does the client need a marcel-style iron to eliminate clamp kinks?

Hot Brush

This is similar to a curling iron except that a brush fits over the barrel of a curling iron.

Air Brush

For a looser style of curl, an air brush may be the ticket. This model of styling tool forces air through the barrel and out the openings. While the hair is wrapped around the brush, it works much in the same way a curling iron adds curl.

Brushes

There are vast differences in the quality and uses of brushes. The basic beauty tool box should include a brush for use when drying the hair, a brush for adding volume and height, and a finish brush for final touches. (Fig. 16.8)

Some shapes include: round, vent, flat or paddle, and curved. Match the brush to the desired look.

When you are shopping for brushes, look for bristles that are firm but not hard. Keep an eye out for knots in the tips of the bristles. Plastic molded bristles sometimes have a small seam where the tip comes together. If the ridge is pronounced, it can pull out or break off the hair.

Combs

Offer options in combs—one for combing out wet hair, one for shaping, and a rat-tail comb for separating and styling. You have choices in everything from plastic to bone combs.

Have the client pull her comb or brush out of her bag. Look over the quality of the tool. It may be a culprit for damaging hair.

Makeup Accessories

If you want to create the perfect flawless face, it is critical to have the proper tools at your fingertips. Look for brushes that have tightly-packed hairs that don't splay out when they caress the skin. Good brushes should fall back into place after use. Check if any hairs shed from the barrel. Run the brush over the inside of the wrist. Good bristles will caress and glide over the skin. Good brushes should feel luxurious. (Fig. 16.9)

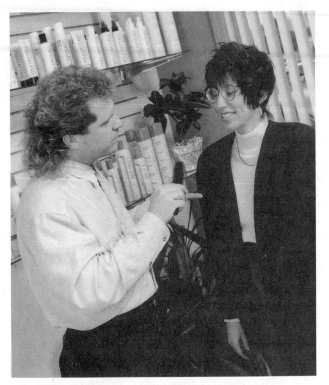

Fig. 16.8   Shopping for brushes. (Photo by Michael A. Gallitelli on location at Rielms Hair Salon, Latham, NY.)

Makeup Brushes

Touch sponge—perfect for blending base makeup and applying loose powder to create a smooth, flawless finish. Packs makeup with staying power.

Powder Brush—for blending cheek color. Whisk through powder blush, tap off excess, and brush back and forth over cheek. For a light finish, dust loose powder over base.

Fan Brush—essential tool for dusting off excess eye color that may flake down on skin. Great for adding accent cheek color. Use to blend and soften eye shadows.

Retractable Lip Brush—paint on lip color. Fills in fine lines of the lip, helping lipstick to stay on twice as long.

Angle Contour Brush—use to create sculpted cheek-bones. Place darker shade of cheek color in hollow under cheekbone.

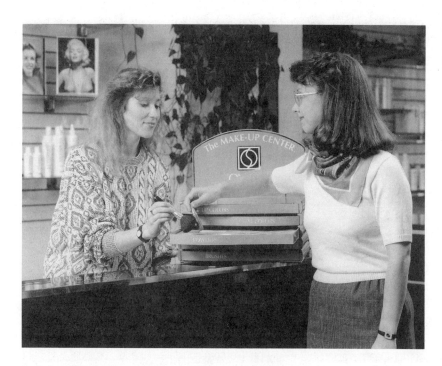

Fig. 16.9 Selling makeup brushes. (Photo by Michael A. Gallitelli on location at Rielms Hair Salon, Latham, NY.)

Rouge Brush—unique brush for lightly dusting on cheek color. Smaller shape helps you kiss the top of cheekbone with highlight color.

Eye Shadow Fluff—for blending powdered eye shadow evenly and delicately on eye area. Perfect tool for placing eye bone color to create shape and definition.

Eye Shadow Angle—grab this tool if you want to line the eye with shadow. Dot color along lash line. Creates soft smudged look. Hot tool for fashion color placement.

Eye Shadow Sponge—super for applying wash of eye shadow color. Another trick is to use sponge for concealing dark shadow under eye. Tap concealer on and blend with sponge.

Fine Eye Liner Brush—delicate brush for drawing on eyeliner, use with cake liner or dampened shadow.

Spoolie—super to separate the lashes. Use to define eyebrows.

Makeup Mirrors

Shedding the proper lighting while applying makeup makes all the difference in the world. Look for a mirror that gives you options for intensity and color variation. It should have options for daylight, office lighting, and home lighting.

Use a makeup light in your retail area to show the difference proper lighting can make. This also gives you a natural lead in for suggesting different looks—office, night, and outdoors. Different looks equal different products equal additional sales.

Hand-held Mirror

It's been said that eyesight is the second thing to go. So to play it safe offer a hand-held mirror for sale. Select one that is two sided with a normal strength on side one and a magnification mirror on the flip side. Great for closeups, checking blending lines for makeup, and catching a rear-view look at the hair. The bonus is that they are super to travel with because of awful hotel lighting and visibility.

PACKAGING YOUR WORDS

Now that you have had some lengthy examples of selling more products, it's time for you to make this part specific for your product mix.

When I made a commitment to retailing, the first project I undertook was to make a product guide for the staff. At the time, I knew the product line but there was a gap in transferring the information.

The solution I designed was to compile a product knowledge guide. And now I'm going to ask you to do the same.

War of the Words

We better start off with what you can and cannot say about products before you compile your product charts. There is a delicate line drawn between a cosmetic and a drug. The difference is in the claims and the results of a given product.

The governing regulatory body is the United States Food and Drug Administration (FDA). The Food, Drug and Cosmetic Act defines cosmetics as: "(1) Articles intended to be rubbed, poured, sprinkled or sprayed on, introduced into, or otherwise applied to the human body or any part thereof for cleansing, beautifying, promoting attractiveness or altering the appearance and (2) Articles intended for use as a component of any such articles, except that such terms shall not include soap."

The Food, Drug and Cosmetic Act defines drugs as, "Products intended for the use in the diagnosis, cure, mitigation, treatment or prevention of disease or products intended to affect the structure or any function of the body." Drugs must be proven safe and effective to a satisfactory level before they are released to the public. Cosmetics are not required to follow suit.

Now this verbal tightrope can be tricky because the products you are selling in your salon are cosmetic items, yet you know for a fact many of the products produce outstanding results. The catch is that you can't claim miracle results or the product crosses the line from cosmetic to drug. The product could be taken away from cosmetologists. The best rule of thumb is to follow your manufacturer's product literature and product knowledge guidelines. Don't ad lib your sales dialogue when it comes to product benefits. I once overheard a sales clerk tell a woman, "This product is so effective, it will not only penetrate the skin, it will penetrate to the bone!" Boy, is that a sales claim or what? Obviously she had no clue what was true of her product and benefits. Please be careful you do not lead your clients down a primrose path for product claims. Guard your words and what you say to your clients.

Claim Substantiations

Follow your manufacturer's guidelines. If the company is touting a certain benefit, it is safe to relay that nugget of information to your client. The major manufacturers spend millions of dollars to prove what their products can and cannot do. The unfortunate side here is that many of the products do produce certain results, but to publicly declare the result is financial suicide. As soon as they say it can do such and such, we can't sell it in salons. I can't stress the importance of guarding your tongue in this department enough.

Product Buzzwords

Earlier in our studies, we talked at length about the differences in the way people communicate—the left brainers and right brainers and the visual, auditory, and kinesthetic people. When you talk to the clients regarding home care products, it's critical that you lace your conversation with buzzwords that massage the client's brain, comfort words they can consciously and subconsciously relate to. Here are some examples for you to include in your sales presentations.:

- Oily—balance, control, fresh, lightweight, lets skin breathe, oil-free, potent, removes shine, shine-free, squeaky clean, won't clog.

- Normal—balance, keeps looking fresh, lightweight, maintains, natural.

- Dry—cleanses gently, conditions, eliminates tight feeling, hydrates, lubricates, protects, supplies moisture, supple, softens.

- General—appears to feel like, alive, beautiful, absorbs, controls, dewy, dissolves oil, elegant, effective, easy, quick, formula, fresh, flowing, feel the difference, glowing, glides, helps to, it works, instant, immediate, luster, light, mild, moist, natural, noticeable, nurtures, nature-based, organic, proof, pure, penetrates, rich, results, refines, safe, scientific, smooth, soothe, softens, see the difference, treat, tends to, texture, vital.

- Seasonal—builds moisture, cooling, calming, glowing, instant repair, lightweight, protection, refreshing, soothing, smooth, sleek, silky, soften, special agents, soothing care, weatherproof.

Make sure you observe the reactions on the client as you occasionally slide the appropriate word into the sales presentation. Notice the physical body reactions.

Product Knowledge Charting

The technical side of the sale requires study in the brands and individual products you are carrying. (Fig. 16.10) One easy way to learn how to sell more products is to compile a product knowledge chart. (See Figures 16.11 and 16.12, p. 217–218, for samples.)

The chart covers every area needed for effective selling as it relates to the product benefits and uniqueness. The product knowledge chart covers:

Statement
This is a brief description for the product. This can be one or two sentences that stress the uniqueness or main reason for using this product.

One-Liners
Frequently when I teach retailing classes, the one objection I hear all the time from beauty professionals is that they need more product knowledge. One way to simplify the multitude of products and ingredient combinations out there is to learn at least one thing that makes Product XYZ different from Product ABC. If you can spill out this one-liner, you will help the client decide between the products.

Application
The application procedures and the directions for using the product are written out. Many products can be used in numerous ways. List the recommended sequence of application per product. If there are alternative uses for the product, note them as well.

FABs
Your clients buy products and services that will benefit them. When it comes to product knowledge, stress the unique benefit the product will offer to your client. Learning to effectively retail products requires that you be familiar with the FAB principle of selling. The FAB stands for feature, advantage, and benefit.

The feature of the product is the physical aspect of the item. This would include the texture, fragrance, feel, packaging, and certain ingredients.

The advantage is what the product does or how it does it. The advantage is the action the specific ingredient has on the hair, skin, or nails.

The benefit is the ultimate result the client wants or needs from your product. The skin will feel softer and smoother; the hair will be shinier and more manageable; the nails will be stronger.

Every product on your shelf can be sold through the FAB technique. This is the perfect place to sell your professional knowledge to the client without becoming overwhelming or wordy.

System Selling
The system selling section gives you three products that are grouped together to help trigger a sale. If the client requests the first item, you then have two additional products to build into the sale.

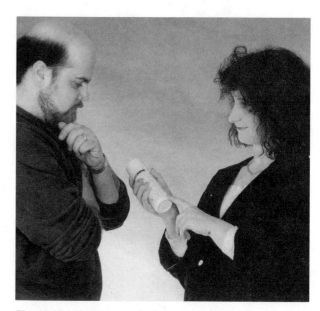

Fig. 16.10 Know the products you are selling. (Photo by Michael A. Gallitelli.)

Selling Hints

Write out suggestions that will make the product sale easier.

MISSION

Use the descriptions provided earlier in this chapter as a sample for your verbal arsenal of information. I am sure you have a certain style you are most comfortable using. Adapt your style to the products listed. The result will be an easier more confident flow of phrases and words to help you get the product off the shelf and into the bag.

Take the form provided and compile the necessary information for every product that you retail in the salon. Doing this exercise may take some time and elbow grease, but the dividend will show in daily sales and commissions.

NOTE: If you are a salon owner, use this as a staff meeting or staff project. Assign X amount of products per person on the staff, deadline it, and in the end you have a completed product knowledge chart book. Schedule a staff meeting where each person presents the assignments to the entire staff. This also gives staff members the opportunity to get comfortable speaking in front of a group.

Product Knowledge Sample Form

PRODUCT $

Recommended type:

Statement:

One-Liner:

Sequence of Application:

Application:

FABS

Feature: Advantage: Benefit:

Product Ingredients:

System Selling:

1.   2.   3.

1.   2.   3.

1.   2.   3.

Selling Hints:

Fig. 16.11   Product knowledge sample form

Information on Product Knowledge Form

PRODUCT   Protective Emulsion $ 14.00

Recommended type: May be used on normal to combination skin. Excellent first moisturizer for couperose.

Statement: Protective Emulsion is a light moisturizing lotion containing proteins, biotin, and dimethicone to maintain skin moisture and provide protection against the elements.

One-Liner: Protective Emulsion is perfect for clients who need moisture and protection without heavy or greasy feel.

Sequence of Application: Protective Emulsion should always follow the cleansing and toning steps. Used with cream wash or cleansing lotion. Toner is freshener or skin tonic.

Application: Using a nickel-size drop, dot Protective Emulsion sparingly over the face and throat. Apply lotion from the cheekbones down and the eyebrows up.

FABS

Feature:	Advantage:	Benefit:
Protect and cushions.	Prevents evaporation that can lead to dry, chapped skin.	Lightweight fluid.
Biotin.	Necessary for cell growth.	Promotes blood circulation to skin.
Natural Proteins.	Cell Growth.	Builds better cells.
Dimethicone.	Invisible veil on surface.	Retards moisture loss.

Product Ingredients:
Water, Mineral Oil, Stearic Acid, Glycerol Stearate SE, Acetylated Lanolin, Alcohol, Dimethicone, Triethanolamine, Hydrolyzed Animal Protein, Paraffin, Cetyl Alcohol, Methylparaben, Propylparaben, Quatemium-15, Biotin, Fragrance, Color FD&C Blue #1, FD&C Yellow #5.

System Selling:
1. Protective emulsion	2. Cleansing lotion	3. Toning lotion
1. Protective emulsion	2. Penetration cream	3. Eye and throat cream
1. Protective emulsion	2. Makeup base	3. Loose powder

Selling Hints:
The dimethicone in the product glides smoothly over skin. Have client try on just one hand, to see and feel the difference.
Great body lotion if the client suffers from dry, flaky patches on the hands, arms, or legs.

Fig. 16.12   Sample information on product knowledge form.

CHAPTER 17

EIGHTY-FIVE COMMON CONSUMER QUESTIONS

This question and answer chapter will give you some standard responses to common consumer questions professionals are frequently asked. Use the answers as guidelines. Adapt the responses so you are comfortable with the dialogue.

It is my desire to supply you with a verbal arsenal of information. If you disagree with some of the responses, that's okay—just modify them to match your beliefs and personal recommendations. These are guidelines, not gospel.

The goal here is to answer the customer's question and close the sale. Do not try to tell customers how much you know about the subject. Tell them what they need to know. Keep it simple and direct.

You will find the question, the response, and a way to bridge back into the sale.

HAIR CARE

1. Does your hair really get used to products? Do you need to switch?

If you were to eat the same food day in and day out, your taste buds would not get excited with the repeated flavor. Your hair can get used to the same products with repeated use as well. Try switching your home care routine at least twice a year for maximum results.

How long has it been since you've switched your home care routine?

2. How do I know what shampoo to buy? They all seem to have extras.

Select your product based on the results you desire and any preexisting conditions. The extras can be the active ingredients. They are higher concentrations of a selected ingredient added to the products to intensify their working power.

What do you want the product to do? Describe the results you are looking for.

3. I want to add shine to my hair. What can I do?

There are new translucent haircolors that add shine and gloss to the hair. The translucent color imparts a healthy sheen, without changing your natural color. These wash out slowly and can be reapplied as desired, plus you won't see any outgrowth.

Are you just wanting to have shiny hair or would you like to alter the color slightly?

4. There are so many styling products. Which ones do I need?

Everyone needs the appropriate cleansing shampoo and conditioner plus one of the following styling aids: a mousse for a light airy look, a lotion for medium control, or a gel for maximum hold. It is best to have two brushes, one for blow-drying and a round one for adding curls to the look. To top it all off, use a finishing spray.

Now, based on your current style, I'd recommend . . .

5. To keep my hair in tip-top shape, how often should I have it cut?

Most hairstyles need to be trimmed every four to six weeks. Consistently schedule your appointment to stay ahead of the uncontrollable droop.

Do you feel your hair grows quickly or slowly?

6. If I use hair spray, my hair gets stringy during the day. Why?

Sometimes using too much spray can weigh the hair down. Avoid spraying the hair into place. Hold the spray can high above the head and with large sweeping circles let the spray gently fall onto the hair.

Let me show you two options for holding your hair in place without it getting stringy.

7. Is there any way to "pump up" fine, thin hair?

The best place to start is with a deep-cleansing shampoo designed to thoroughly rid the hair of all traces of debris that can weigh it down.

Follow the shampoo with an appropriate styling aid for extra body and fullness. When you blow-dry the hair lean over and dry from underneath to add extra fullness at the base of the hair shaft.

For your hairstyle I professionally recommend these two products.

8. My hair takes a beating—weather, beach, and pool. What would you recommend to get it back in shape?

The environment takes a lot out of the hair, and conditioning is a must. Chin length or longer hair needs to be treated with a deep conditioner twice a month. Use a deep conditioning treatment with a protein base and a moisturizer for best results. Intensive hair conditioning treatments can be achieved in the salon or recommended as a home care maintenance program.

This time of year, hair needs a little extra care. The treatment is $15 and I can do it after your shaping. Shall we go ahead and do it while you are here? I'd be glad to mix up a special conditioning treatment if you have an extra fifteen minutes today.

9. I am at the end of my hair and it's split. Help!

Unfortunately split ends have to be snipped away. A simple trim will solve the problem.

How long has it been since your hair was shaped up?

10. How conditioning are conditioning treatments?

Healthy hair is equal to its protein content. Conditioners are available in varying strengths; as detanglers, light, medium, and heavy. Look for conditioners that require at least ten to fifteen minutes of contact time. Deep conditioning is extremely important for beautiful, healthy, shiny hair.

Are you looking for a deep treatment or something you can use after shampooing at home?

11. Can I perm over a perm?

Yes, if the hair has been brought up to condition. Short hair can be permed approximately every three months and long hair every six to nine months.

A root perm is an alternative to perming over a perm. This specialty technique only waves the new growth—a super option for chemically treated hair.

Before I administer any chemical service, I always check the condition of the hair. Determining the quality of the hair determines your final results. Let's analyze your hair.

12. What can I do to defrizz my last perm?

There are many reasons for frizzy hair. Are you using a styling aid even if you air dry your hair? Permed hair needs control and a styling aid like mousse or lotion. The styling aid will hold the hair in place while it is drying. Hair left bare can rub together and rough up the cuticle layer resulting in the frizzes.

Starting two weeks after your perm, allow time to deep condition your hair twice a month. This helps to restore protein and moisture into the chemically treated hair.

First, I'd like to show you this styling aid to use after shampooing.

13. Why didn't my last perm take?

There are a couple of possibilities for a weak perm; it might have been underprocessed, or the hair has gone through a settling process. In a settling process, the curl gradually softens within the first ten days to two weeks. If your curl looked perfect the day of the perm, chances are within a short time your curl will not have the same depth.

How long has it been since you permed your hair? Describe the way you want the curl to look.

14. I've read that you shouldn't perm your hair if you're pregnant.

During the first trimester there is a tremendous amount of hormonal activity. I would hold off on perming until the second term if the client is experiencing morning sickness. After that, the mother-to-be is an acceptable candidate for perming.

Is there any chance that you are pregnant?

15. What can I do to help my perm stay in longer?

I red-flag the brand of shampoo and conditioner you have selected for your home use. Many products can weaken the perm, causing the curl to soften faster than normal.

Let's select the perfect combination of products for your hair.

The second thing is to make sure you are conditioning at home twice a month, starting two weeks after your perm. Healthy hair has to have a proper balance of protein. Conditioning treatments help treat the hair and restore the protein and moisture factors.

Your next visit is in four weeks. I recommend we do a deep conditioning treatment at that time to keep your hair in super shape.

16. Should I cut or perm my hair first? I was told that if you perm first, then cut your hair, the perm will fall out.

I would suggest we trim off the extra length before perming, if you need more than one inch off your hair. Following the perm we'll design and cut the hair to suit your style and finished requirements.

How short do you want to go?

17. If I don't like my new haircolor, what happens then?

We can always modify the color. My experience has been that if we communicate prior to the color application, we both will know what to expect. I don't want any surprises, so if you and I spend time discussing it first, clarifying our objectives, and possibly doing a patch test, the actual color selection process will go beautifully.

Here's a color guide. Based on your natural color, I'd look in this range.

18. Once I start coloring my hair, how long does it last?

I'd suggest you cut and color your hair during the same appointment, which is every four to six weeks. This saves time and trouble and keeps your hair looking its best.

I recommend the product for the results you desire. Highlights are generally touched up every three months.

19. Is haircoloring safe?

Yes! A patch test administered twenty-four hours prior to your appointment is an assurance policy signaling us if you are sensitive to the product before we apply it all over the hair. It is required by the FDA before every application of color.

How soon would you like to color your hair?

20. I want to change my hair color, but I don't know which color would look best. How do you select the color?

The first area I look at is your natural hair shade, then eye color and skin tone. These three areas will be my guideline for the color selection. Successful haircoloring should enhance your natural features and your visual personal statement.

Coloring techniques have improved over the last decade; we can achieve you-only-better looks. A simple rule of thumb is that most people look better with their skin tone two shades darker and their hair two shades lighter.

Have you decided what color family you would like to make your hair?

21. How temporary is temporary hair color?

That depends on the brand of product and its formulation. Some temporary colors are designed to last from shampoo to shampoo. Others stick around for about thirty days. Temporary haircolors are great because you don't have to commit to them. You can change your color as you change your mind or mood.

What did you have in mind?

22. I love to wear hats, but I hate the way my hair looks when I take them off.

Hats are a fun fashion accessory. Treat the ends of the hair with a rich moisturizer after shampooing to control dry fly-away hair. Completely dry your hair before topping it off with your hat. If hair is still damp, the trapped moisture can lead to "hat hair." Try spraying the inside of the hat with a static guard product so your hair will stay in place when you remove the hat. If the hair still has static, spray your hair brush with super hold hair spray, then brush through the hair.

What style of hats do you prefer?

SKIN CARE

23. Is it okay to use eye creams?

The eyelid and surrounding area are the thinnest in tissue structure. The eye area should be treated with extra care and special products.

Apply eye cream sparingly under the eyebrow and in the hollow under the eye. Pat or dot on the eye cream. Never rub the eye cream into the skin.

Many companies make a day and evening treatment for the eyes. The eyes are worth a little extra effort, since the first signs of aging usually surface framing the windows of the soul.

Are you currently using an eye treatment product?

24. My grandmother always used the simplest things for her skin. Why should I be any different?

Your grandmother was lucky. Time has changed things like pollution, stress, environmental damage, ozone thinning, and decrease in the wholesomeness of foods.

Today, product and ingredient technology allow for outstanding advances in product formulations. You have choices your grandmother never even dreamed of having.

There are programs available that are very simple, easy to use, and produce dynamite results. What's your current home care program?

25. Do toners really close the pores?

No! Toners are used to complete the cleansing process. Toners pick up any traces of cleanser, makeup and residue left on the surface of the skin. Many toners have a tightening feeling, but that is the evaporation of alcohol from the skin's surface.

Are you trying to make the pores appear smaller?

26. Will an all-purpose cream do the same thing as one for each facial area?

The problem with an all-purpose cream is that it has cleansing and moisturizing properties. If you cleanse your skin with the all-purpose cream, reapply a little extra as moisturizer, then put your makeup on, I'll wager before long your makeup does a vanishing act. When the cleansing agent comes in contact with other products on the skin, it tends to dissolve what it touches.

What area are you wanting to treat?

27. Do I really need all this skin stuff?

No, but each product does have certain benefits that will help your skin. Start with the basics. Start with a simple program that is comfortable for you. Which collection looks best?

NOTE: Many beauty professionals recommend everything imaginable for the customer to purchase, especially on the first visit. The client is overwhelmed when faced with so many products to use at home. Select the necessary items, and allow the customer to add to her collection a little at a time.

28. What do facial masks do?

Generally they are used for nourishment and treatment. Some masks have sloughing ingredients to whisk away the buildup of dead cells. Others are used to hydrate or add moisture to the skin. Some masks help fight bacteria and calm irritated skin.

For maximum results mask at least three times a week—one time for sloughing and two times for hydrating or balancing, depending on your skin's need.

Describe the results you desire. What do you want the mask to do?

29. I have sensitive skin. Will your products make me break out?

Normally when skin reacts to products, it reacts to the perfume or fragrance in the formulation. Companies today leave out most of the known skin irritants.

Does your skin react to products? What happens to your skin?

NOTE: If the skin is ultrasensitive, don't even risk suggesting your product line. Send your client to a physician for product recommendations.

30. Do bleaching creams really work?

Many of the bleaching creams do lighten the skin, but unfortunately you are on an on-again and off-again schedule with the product. Bleaching creams are not to be used as a daily treatment. You apply them for several days, then discontinue use. The best thing is to apply a sun block daily to prevent the spots from darkening due to sun exposure.

What area are you wanting to lighten? Are you using sun protection daily?

31. Is alcohol drying to the skin?

The term *alcohol* is a little misleading. SD-alcohols and rubbing alcohols can be drying to the skin. However, other alcohol derivatives, such as cetyl alcohol and lanolin alcohol, are safely used in product formulations.

Trust me to recommend your skin products. Do you feel your skin is naturally dry?

32. Is mineral oil bad for the complexion?

Mineral oil has taken a bad rap. Mineral oil itself is not the culprit in skin problems. Years ago mineral oil was processed and laced with other ingredients. There are hundreds of grades of mineral oil, each varying in quality. So if the label lists mineral oil, don't automatically disregard the product.

Are you interested in a cleansing or moisturizing product?

33. How regenerating are rejuvenating creams?

You cannot turn back the clock, but what you do to your skin today affects how the skin will look tomorrow. It has been proven the skin does absorb substances through the surface. The effectiveness of any product is determined by the delivery system and the percentage of active ingredients in the formula. Some claim to affect cellular turnover, causing the skin to act as if it was in its younger days. Other products claim to affect the respiration cycle of the skin.

With any new product, it is necessary to faithfully use the program for at least thirty days in order to fairly judge the products' effectiveness. Cream or lotion will not work in the bottle or jar. It needs to be applied! Your mirror will tell you if it is working.

What are you using at night on the skin?

34. Is soap good for my skin?

Soap is a favorite product for many people. Years ago, advertising implied that skin should be squeaky clean. Healthy skin should feel slightly moist, soft, and flexible, not dry and tight.

Are you a soap-and-water fan?

> NOTE: If you have a stubborn client you can tell her that if she were to repeatedly wash her car with the detergent, certain products would dull the finish of the car. Her skin is definitely more delicate than the exterior finish on her vehicle. You personally would not risk it.

35. Will facials really help my skin?

Yes, but it does depend on what you expect the facial to do. Certain skin treatments will help to eliminate dead skin buildup and pore debris, hydrate and moisturize the skin, relax you and the muscles, stimulate the blood circulation, and help to destress the nerves. Your makeup will go on smoother and more evenly as a result of the facial.

Have you ever experienced a facial?

MAKEUP

36. My pencil liner runs down my cheeks. What am I doing wrong?

How are you removing your eye makeup? Chances are an oily residue from baby oil, greasy makeup remover, or cleanser has been left on the skin.

I strongly suggest a nonoily, eye makeup remover to be used both at night to remove the makeup and in the morning to prepare the eye for your makeup application.

Talk me through your cleansing routine.

37. I am plagued with dark circles under my eyes. What can I do?

Unfortunately, dark circles tend to happen to most of us who are under stress, working late, or just not sleeping well.

Camouflage concealers (pigment-loaded products) can be used under the delicate eye area. Gently tap the concealer in the hollow of the eye, then blend with the ring finger or a clean sponge. After blending, apply a thin layer of base makeup to neutralize the colors, but be careful not to wipe away the concealer. (You can demonstrate this procedure to better illustrate the results.)

See the difference? The technique is quick and easy and all you used was the concealer and sponge. Any questions?

38. What are under-makeup toners?

Under-makeup color toners are used to correct color irregularities in the skin tone. Most color toners come in lavender to brighten the skin; pink to add a rosy, fresh face glow; and green to reduce redness in the skin.

Color toners are to be applied under your normal base makeup. Thinly apply the correct color toner then follow with your normal foundation application.

What color are you trying to correct?

39. Do I really need powder? It seems too dry.

The production of loose powder has been refined over the years and can impart a velvety, smooth finish to your makeup. Powder is designed to absorb ten times its weight in oil and perspiration. Loose powder should be used to help keep your makeup on. The new powder blends will not dry out the skin.

Compact powder is used for touch-ups during the day. It's a convenience item that is easy to toss in a purse or gym bag.

The combination of loose and compact powder will solve your problem. The duo is $17.50. I'll set them aside until you are finished shopping.

40. I want to make my eyes noticeable. What products should I use?

First, we'll start by selecting the proper shades of color for your eyes and skin tone. Make sure the eye shadow pattern is well blended. A fine, smudged line of pencil or eye shadow works great as a liner. Finish off the eye with soft sweeps of mascara.

We have a makeup artist on staff. She offers lessons on applying the right colors and products. She is here Tuesday through Saturday. Which day would be convenient for you?

41. What is the difference between oil- and water-based makeup?

Oil-based products have a concentration of oil in a water-base formulation. Water-based products have a minimal amount of oil dispersed through the water in their formulation.

Do you feel you need an oil-rich product?

42. Why does my lipstick change color?

Before trashing any of your lipsticks, try applying your makeup base over the lips. Outline the lips, then fill in the remaining area with the same lip pencil. Lightly press on loose powder.

Try selecting a lip color that is close to your natural lip tone. Most lipsticks are made with two color components. The first is the true color you see in the tube. The other component provides staying power for the lipstick. Many matte lipsticks have extra holding powder and remain true to their tones.

Let's remove the color you are wearing and try this new technique.

43. How long is it safe to keep eye makeup, especially mascara?

Mascara should be replaced every 90–120 days. Once the tube is opened the preservatives begin to fight the invasion of bacteria and germs.

Eye shadows should be tossed every year to avoid possible eye irritations. Above all, don't share your eye products. Cross-contamination can spread among your products quickly.

How long has it been since you've replaced your eye makeup?

44. I have trouble finding the right shade of base. How can I find one that doesn't leave a ring around the jawline?

Start by selecting the base color in natural light. Daylight is best. Test the color of base along the cheek, jawline, and down onto the neck. You should not see a stripe of color sitting on the skin.

Select a color that is in your natural skin tone family. If you have yellow in your skin, your base will need to have a

yellowish undertone. Women get ring around the jawline when they cross over into another skin tone family, for example if their skin is olive and they select a pink base. Stay within your natural color. Your makeup will look more natural.

Here's a mirror. Let's go over in the natural light and take a look at the base.

45. I'm always in the bathroom reapplying my makeup because it fades by noon. How can I save time?

The best insurance for long-lasting makeup is to invest a couple of extra minutes during the application. Make sure the cleansing product is compatible with your skin type. Cleanse and tone the skin. Skipping the toner can be the fading culprit, because toner completes the cleansing process. Moisturize and apply foundation. Use loose powder (not a compact) generously with a sponge or powder puff and press the powder onto the base to help hold it throughout the day. Loose powder will absorb ten times its weight in oil and perspiration.

Once you have your makeup on, look to see if there are tiny flakes, or if the makeup seems to be setting on the surface of the skin. If so, chances are that the skin needs a good sloughing treatment, either with a home mask or salon skin treatment.

Does your makeup get shiny or does it smear? Or do you notice it setting on the surface?

46. After I've had lipstick on for a while, the color bleeds. What will prevent this?

Outline the lip with a lip pencil that matches the lipstick shade. Trace around the natural lip edge defining the lip line with a sharp pencil. Once that is done, color in the rest of the traced area with the same lip pencil. Take a small amount of loose powder and press onto the lip then follow with the selected lipstick.

Shy away from lip glosses and ultrashear products that like to travel on the lip.

Have you ever worked with a lip pencil?

47. My eye makeup creases throughout the day. I sometimes have to wipe my eyes to blend the colors. What can I do to prevent this?

Cleanse the eye area separately with a nonoily eye makeup remover in the morning. Do not apply your face moisturizer to the eyelid area. Try applying an eye shadow base to the eye prior to shadow application. The base or primer is designed to have the shadows cling to it, thereby holding the colors in place during the day or night. The primer also helps the colors stay true throughout the day.

Here, let's test the shadow base on your hand.

48. Can I wear makeup when I work out three times a week?

Many of us would not want to go to the gym bare faced. Try wearing a sport-weight base and minimal makeup for the workout. Remove all the makeup before enjoying the sauna and steam rooms.

How much makeup do you normally wear to the gym?

49. Is it necessary to let the skin breathe?

Some people feel they need to give the skin a rest from makeup. Maybe they are just tired of putting it on every day. Your skin is the largest organ of elimination, excreting 80 percent of the body's waste materials. It's going to continue doing just that whether you have makeup on or not. If you want to give the skin a rest, make sure you have on a moisturizer and sun protection especially if you are going to be outside.

Do you like going without makeup?

BODY AND FRAGRANCE

50. Why doesn't my cologne stay on?

Try layering your fragrance. Select your brand and invest in the full collection. Start by using the scented bath or shower gel, followed by body lotion and dusting powder, and then spritz your fragrance starting at your ankles and working your way up.

Some skin types are prone to retaining fragrance; others have to invest a little extra effort. Your cologne may tend to be weaker during your monthly cycle due to the hormonal change. If you have been wearing the same brand for months, your nose may have become desensitized to the same smell. Add some variety to your fragrance wardrobe by switching colognes.

Do you change your fragrance or do you always wear the same scent?

51. What is the difference between perfume and cologne?

Perfume implies a mixture of a solvent (usually ethyl alcohol) with one or hundreds of essential oils to impart the flavor or scent. The ratio between perfume and cologne is the dilu-tion of the essential oils, with the cologne being the weakest formula.

Do you prefer perfume or cologne?

52. My elbows and the bottoms of my feet look like crepe paper. How can I smooth out the rough stuff?

The elbows and feet are often neglected areas. Try a sloughing cream at least once a week on the trouble spots. After sloughing, massage in a rich body lotion concentrating on the elbows and feet. This ritual will help keep the rough stuff to a minimum.

Allow me to show you how easy and effective a sloughing mask can be.

53. Are sunscreens higher than SPF 15 any better?

A sun protection factor (SPF) of fifteen means that you can stay out in the sun 15 times longer compared to no protection. At this time, there is little evidence of the inflated SPF numbers working any better than the 15. The best protection is a waterproof sun block of at least SPF 15, reapplied every few hours while you are in the sun or at the pool.

Are you sun sensitive or are you looking for a total block?

54. Are sunless tans really safe?

They are definitely safer than being in the sun. Sunless tanning lotions produce a coloring action in the outermost layers of the skin. Many of the lotions alter the color of the outer surface of dead cells with the coloring agent imparting a tanned appearance.

There are many options for consumers who refuse to expose their bodies to harmful solar rays or for those that simply don't have the time for a sun-baked tan. Use a body sloughing gel first for maximum results. Then follow with sunless tanning product. These products need to be repeated every few days as the outer cells flake off.

Have you every tried a sunless tanning product?

55. I experience dry skin year round. Is there anything that will help dry, flaking skin?

Substitute a gentle body cleanser for soap in the bath or shower. After showering in warm to tepid—never hot—water apply a liberal amount of body lotion directly over the skin, while the skin is still slightly damp. This action helps seal in the natural moisture under the body lotion. Limit your exposure to extremely hot bath or shower temperatures.

Do you prefer to take a bath or shower? There are different products you can use to minimize the dehydration.

56. I love hot showers and saunas. What effect do they have on the skin?

Hot showers and saunas are therapy and stress reducers for many people. The unfortunate side effect of lingering in the water is that exposure and immersion can have a dehydrating effect on the skin and body. Limit your exposure to ten minutes maximum. And make sure to follow the water therapy with body lotion, not body oil.

Have you tried hydrating the skin with a moisture mist while lingering in the sauna?

57. I've been waxing for some time and now I notice ingrown hairs. What should I do?

Waxing can cause the hairs to grow in finer and lighter. When they do, they sometimes have a hard time breaking through the skin surface if there is a lot of dead skin buildup. Try using a body scrub every day in the shower. If ingrown hairs persist, try shaving the day after waxing. The shaving whisks away the outer epidermal cells.

Feel the smoothing action of this body scrub.

58. Will waxing make the hair grow in darker and thicker?

Waxing does not make the hair grow in darker and thicker like shaving. It's a common misconception. Waxing lifts out the entire hair shaft and bulb resulting in the total regrowth of the entire hair. Frequently the hair will start to grow in finer and lighter in color after waxing for four to six consecutive months.

What area of the body are you thinking about waxing?

59. Explain how massage will help my body.

Body massage is an excellent way to reduce the effects of stress in one's life. Massage therapy can work out sore muscles from athletics, kinked muscles that are work related, and allow time for total relaxation.

Massage helps to improve circulation, burn up calories, and soften and condition the skin. The best benefit is private time for yourself. The salon massage is a wonderful hour treatment.

How soon would you like to experience the feeling for yourself?

NAIL CARE

60. My nail polish chips off. What can I do?

Begin your polishing process with a base coat. This pre-

pares the nail bed to help hold the color. Next apply two thin coats of polish and follow with a clear top coat or super sealer. Make sure to wrap the free edge of the nail with the sealer.

I'd like the manicurist to analyze your condition. I'll go get her.

61. My polish takes forever to dry. Why?

Start by making sure that your nails are clean and free of moisture allowing the products to adhere properly. There may have been a residue of oil, lotion, or possibly remover left on the nail bed. When you apply the polish apply very thin coats of color. The polish resists drying when the layers are thick. If you have the time, allow a few minutes between each coat of product.

What brand of polish and remover are you using?

62. I have little white specks on my nails. What causes them?

The little white spots, or leukonychia, can be caused by injury to the base of the nail. As the nail continues to grow, the spots will eventually disappear. Be careful to avoid damage to the base of the nail while buffing, filing, or working on the cuticles.

Professional manicuring treatments can help to reduce the trouble spots. What day in the week is most convenient?

63. I had a frightening fungus flare-up under an artificial nail. What causes this?

Occasionally wearers of artificial nails are plagued with a fungus that has grown under the artificial nail and needs to be treated. Examine your nails closely, and watch for any signs of lifting at the back edge. Water can seep in and become trapped.

One of the best ways to avoid fungus is to schedule your fill-ins close together, at least every two weeks. Many of the problems start if the nails are untreated for three to four weeks.

How often are you scheduling your fill-ins?

64. Is formaldehyde bad in nail products?

Too much of anything isn't good, and formaldehyde is no exception. Some products such as nail hardeners and base coats may have the ingredient in the formula. If you choose to use the product, limit your exposure to three days a week. There are so many exceptional products available that are free of formaldehyde, you may want to avoid the risk.

The nail products available here are formaldehyde free. I'd be glad to help you select some.

65. What causes the ridges to form on my nails?

Nail ridges develop either as a result of physical stress, such as banging your nail, or as a natural outgrowth of the nail itself. The easiest way to reduce the ridges is to apply a product called, aptly enough, ridge filler. This product helps to form a smooth nail surface by filling in the ridges. When you're ready to polish, the color will then glide smoothly over the ridges and fine grooves in the nail surface.

Ridge filler will solve your problem. I'll set the product aside for you.

66. My nails have yellow stains and look terrible. What can I do to get them back to normal?

If the yellowing is caused by a residue from the polish this can be gently buffed away. Some polishes stain the nail bed, so it is best to always use a clear base coat prior to the color application.

I recommend scheduling a short series of weekly manicures. The products and service will help remove the staining. Do you prefer daytime appointments or after work?

67. My hands feel as if they have been in hand-to-hand combat. They are so rough and dry. Help!

Clothes help to protect the body from the elements, but our hands are constantly exposed. I suggest washing the hands with a mild cleansing lotion instead of a harsh soap. Gently pat the hands dry after cleansing rather than rubbing with a towel. While the hands are slightly damp, massage in a nongreasy conditioning lotion. Twice a week apply a sloughing mask, let dry for a few minutes, then gently buff the mask off, rinse with tepid water, and finish with hand lotion.

If you spend a lot of time behind the steering wheel, apply sun block to the backs of your hands to help prevent sun damage piercing through the windshield. Another suggestion is to keep a jar or bottle of cuticle treatment on your night stand. Take a second to massage in the oil around the cuticle as you crawl into bed every night.

What products do you need to treat your hands?

68. What can I do for my feet and toes? It is almost sandal season.

Now is the perfect time to treat your toes to a tantalizing pedicure. Feet are often crammed into socks and shoes several months of the year. A pedicure soak will help soften buildup and prepare the toes for treatment. After buffing, mas-

saging, trimming, and treating, you'll feel like dancing out of the salon.

So if you are dipping your toes in the pool or beach, take time out once a month to treat your feet. How soon would you like to treat your tootsies?

GENERAL QUESTIONS

69. Do I need to keep my products refrigerated?

Some products feel better when applied to the skin if they have been stored in the refrigerator. But if your bath or dressing table is out of direct sunlight and is kept at a constant temperature your products are fine.

Eye makeup remover, toner, and body splashes feel great when they have been chilled then applied to the skin.

70. I am looking for natural, organic products.

Natural, organic products usually have a higher percentage of plant and botanical extracts in the formulations. Even if the product is labeled "natural," there are chemicals in the formula for stabilization and preservation.

Describe the results you desire from your products.

71. Why should I buy professional products that are more expensive than the kind I can buy elsewhere?

When you purchase your products from us here in the salon, you are investing in more than just professional products. Our products have passed the toughest standards for exceptional quality—the manufacturer's standards, the salon standards, and my professional scrutiny before I would recommend them to you or anyone else.

You are also receiving my training, education, and professional recommendation. There are hundreds of products to choose from. I'm here to suggest and recommend the best possible product combination for you and your beauty requirements.

Now for your specific beauty needs.

72. I wear contact lenses. Are there any safety cosmetic suggestions?

Always start by cleansing your hands before they touch the contacts. Apply your cosmetics after you insert your lenses. If you are using powdered products, tap off the excess before taking the applicator to the face. If you are using sprays keep your eyes closed and wait a few seconds for the cloud to settle before opening them. Shy away from lash-extenders or mascara with filaments. They can scratch the eye and the lenses. Replace your eye products frequently to avoid contamination.

How long has it been since you've replaced your eye makeup?

73. I travel frequently and my hair and skin are constantly in a state of flux. What can I do to help normalize the travel trauma?

Your travel kit should include the exact products you use at home. Don't rely on the sample bottles in the hotel room for the same results for your hair and skin. Try to keep as close to your home beauty care routine as possible when you travel.

Several of our manufacturers produce travel sizes in many of their products. Allow me to select the best formulations for you.

74. Can I dilute my professional products?

You can, but I wouldn't recommend it. The formulations are concentrated so you only need a small amount. The companies that manufacture the products invest thousands and thousands of dollars researching the best ingredient formulation and combination. I trust the product just the way it is packaged.

Are you diluting the product because you are at the bottom of the bottle?

75. Are there really any differences in brands of products?

Yes! Just as there are different brands of automobiles, there are differences in the brands of beauty products. Each company has set their own standards of product quality and commitment. In beauty products, you have access to everything from a Yugo to a Rolls Royce.

The ingredients may look similar, but the results will vary. What are the final results you require from your products?

> NOTE: Review your feature, advantage, and benefit information. Learn at least one FAB per product in your lines.

76. Are store-bought products any better than those recipes I can make in my kitchen?

I'm not sure if they are any better, but I do know most of us do not even have time to cook our dinners, let alone daily whip up something for our beauty preparations.

Do you have a specific product in mind?

77. Why are salon chemical services so expensive?

The product cost itself is not so expensive, but the experience on how to administer the service is, and the time commitment involved in the process adds up. There are many do-it-yourself kits for home coloring and perm waving. Thousands of women have tried them only to look in the mirror and discover they have green hair or poodle-looking perms. The risk, upset, and aggravation is not worth saving a few dollars.

Salon stylists are trained in the artistic aspect as well as the chemical application of the procedures. After all aren't you worth it?

78. I want to change my look, but I'm afraid to start.

Many of us have locked into a comfort zone about our appearance. Maybe the best place for you to start is with a gradual shift in your look. If you're thinking about a hair cut, remember it will always grow back. Let's not do anything radical, but gradual.

What changes are you contemplating?

79. Does diet affect my hair and skin?

Eating a candy bar or bag of chips or drinking coffee will not instantly affect your hair and skin. However your general dietary habits and consumption will play a role in your overall health and well-being, which affect your hair and skin. Remember the three square meals a day and drink lots of pure water.

Do you feel your diet is affecting your hair or skin?

80. My eyelashes are so light and fair. Is there anything I can do to make them more noticeable?

Eyelash tinting is a process that darkens the lashes, staining them a deeper color. Tinting is a safe service that will last about four weeks when the color gradually fades. Eyelash tinting is great for people with fair, not-so-noticeable lashes.

How dark would you like to go with your lashes?

81. How do I know which products to choose when there are so many on the shelf?

Staring at the shelves can be overwhelming. As your personal beauty therapist it is my job to recommend the best products for you, based on your needs and desires. Many people have guessed which product might work for them only to get it home and discover it just couldn't do the job. Why waste time and money guessing?

Together we can select a program just for you, through consultation and analysis. What type of look do you want to achieve?

82. Can you make me look like this photo?

We can use the photo as a guide and suggestion. Photos are one dimensional and will look different in real life. If you favor the look represented we can analyze if this is best for your face shape and coloring. I'm delighted that you brought the photo in with you, because I can use it as a guideline.

Tell me exactly what you like about the photo.

83. I've heard that facial tissues can be harsh for removing cleansing products and makeup. Is this true?

Yes. Think about the last time you had a cold. After using the tissues for a couple of days what happened to your nose? My guess is that it became very red, flaky, and sensitive. For general cleansing it is best to use a natural sponge, cloth, or dampened cotton pads. Save the tissue for blotting lipstick and to absorb excess oil during the day.

One item I recommend for cleansing the skin is a natural sponge. Here feel this.

84. How long can I safely keep my beauty products?

Hair, body, and face products can safely have a shelf life of one year. If, however, the product changes color, smell or consistency it is best to discontinue use and discard the product. Products you dip your fingers into have a greater chance of contamination. So pay close attention to the product and watch for any signs of the formula breaking down. Store your products in a cool, dark area and avoid exposure to extreme temperature changes.

Are you noticing any changes in your product?

85. What would you recommend to keep in a beauty bag for the office?

Hair spray, styling gel or mousse, brush, comb, miscellaneous hair accessories, concealer, mascara, lipstick, compact powder, extra panty hose, favorite nail polish, and clear top coat.

Which products from the list do you need for your beauty bag?

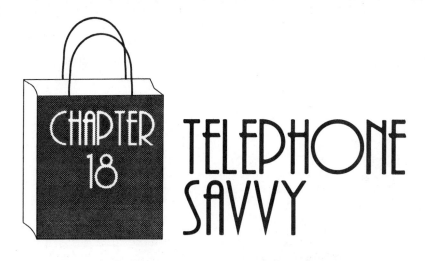

CHAPTER 18
TELEPHONE SAVVY

The manner in which the telephone is handled reflects your entire business. This valuable, useful tool is a direct link to your existing customers and potential clients. Your success at this critical point of contact will determine if the caller will ever walk through the front door. You can't afford sloppy telephone techniques. This chapter will help you build a polished, professional telephone performance.

Handling the incoming calls with skill helps you distance yourself from your competition. Incoming calls will be to:

1. Request information
2. Schedule an appointment
3. Cancel or reschedule
4. Solicit business

TELEPHONE SKILLS

Check Your Attitude

Before you touch the telephone receiver, take a second to adjust your attitude. Make sure you smile as you speak to the caller. Smiling warms up the sound of your voice. This action may sound trite, but the caller is at a disadvantage because he or she cannot see you and therefore can't read your positive body language in person, which would reinforce the weight of your words. You lose 55 percent of your nonverbal personality through the telephone. Your attitude is reflected by the tone of your voice, therefore it must reinforce the positiveness the caller would otherwise be privy to in person. (Fig. 18.1)

Make Call Handling a Priority

Servicing the caller should take priority. Many of your potential customers will have their first experience with your business via the telephone.

One day when I was teaching in a salon I overheard a frazzled staff member say, "If that stupid phone would quit ringing I could get some work done." I was horrified that this comment was even made. I thought to myself if the phone ever stops ringing, her salon is in trouble. In all fairness, there could have been a management problem that needed to be addressed (lack of staff). No incoming calls equals no customers equals no business.

Answer the Call Within Three Rings

Always answer the telephone as soon as possible. Answering by the third ring should become a business goal. When callers are kept waiting images of a closed salon pop into their imaginations.

Apologize if the telephone was not answered promptly. Try using, "I'm sorry to have kept you waiting."

Greeting the Caller

Always answer the telephone with greeting to personalize and warm up the call. Good morning, good afternoon, or good evening are acceptable. Then state the name of the company. This is to reassure the caller that they dialed the right number. "Good morning, (the name of your company)." Then state your

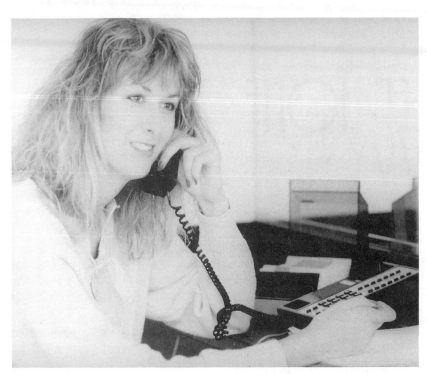

Fig. 18.1   Have a positive telephone attitude.

name. Let the caller have an association or a personality to identify with their call. Your first name is enough, but if you feel you need to establish more credibility your first and last name can be used. "Good morning, Betty's Beauty Salon, this is Martha Howard."

Another reason to state your name is that it saves time. How many times have you heard,

Staff: "Marty's Beauty Boutique."
Caller: "Who is this?"
Staff: "This is Katie."
Caller: "Oh, hi Katie."
Staff: "Who is this?"
Caller: "This is Mrs. Moore."
Staff: "Hi, Mrs. Moore, what can I do for you?"

Now we are finally down to the reason Mrs. Moore called in the first place. Stating your name saves twenty to sixty seconds of valuable telephone and service time.

Never answer the phone with "May I help you?" You better be able to help them; you answered the phone.

"Mary's Salon, Mary speaking" has too many S's. The word "speaking" coupled with a poor telephone or bad connection leads to a snakelike sound through the receiver.

"Good afternoon, thank you for calling Betty's Beauty Box, how may I help you?" is too long. Keep it short and to the point.

State the greeting, your company name, and your name and that's all. "Good morning, Hot Salon, this is Sergio." Then wait; the caller will state his/her business.

Focus on the Caller

Visualize your caller and speak to her as if she was sitting directly across the desk from you. Turn 100 percent of your attention toward the caller. Physically turn your back on surrounding distractions if necessary. Do not talk to others while you are on the phone. Even if you whisper to someone else chances are the caller can still hear you. Focus all your energies toward the caller. The person on the other end is as important as the client standing at the front desk or sitting in your chair. A word of caution: Never slight a client who is physically in front of you to attend to one who is on the telephone. If necessary, take a number and return the call when your business with the client has concluded.

Screening Telephone Calls

Many professionals prefer to know who's calling before they pick up a transferred call. If it is necessary for you to screen calls avoid using, "May I ask who's calling?" This overworked phone phrase makes it appear as if you are the personal bodyguard for the recipient. Soften the bodyguard image by using one of the following:

1. "Who's calling?"
2. "Your name please?"
3. "I'll transfer the call. Your name?"

Putting Callers on Hold

It's inevitable that you will have to put a caller on hold. Your first goal is to transfer the caller to someone who can assist her immediately, but if the caller must be put on hold, first ask if she is able to hold. Never pick up the telephone and automatically put the caller on hold. Once you have agreement, identify how long she will have to wait. "Please hold for ten seconds while I finish the call ahead of yours." When you return to the caller, thank her for waiting.

If the caller's request is going to take some time to fulfill, give her a choice. "It is going to take some time for me to locate that information. Would you prefer to hold or may I call you back?"

Service the Call Now

Try using this technique if the caller requests to talk to a specific person. A client mistakenly feels that she can only talk to a certain person when many times her request is something you could have efficiently handled. If the person requested is not available state, "Richard is with a customer at this time. My name is Sarah and I work closely with Richard. How can I help you?" Then wait for the response.

Find out what action the caller requested and then how you can take care of it. "If you will tell me the nature of your

call, I can direct you to someone who can assist you right now. Thomas is scheduled with clients all day today." Then wait for her response.

If you can accurately state why the person is unavailable, it will help to support your dialogue. "I'm sorry, Cathy is with a client (staff meeting, in production, at a photo shoot, producing a fashion show, whatever)." Never say "They're all tied up." When I hear a person is all tied up, I imagine professionals chained and strung up to their desk or workstation.

Transferring Callers

Once you have identified who the caller would like to speak with, ask if she can wait while you transfer the call. Before you do so, find out the caller's name, the company (if applicable), and what the call is about. Relay the information so when the staff member picks up the phone, he/she can start the conversation with, "Hello Julia, this is James and I understand that..." Internal disorganization and communication gaps show when the caller has to repeat all the information she told the first staff person who answered the phone.

Staff 1:   "Good morning, Carol's Salon, this is Tina."
Caller: "I need to talk with Cary, I'm having a problem with..."
Staff 1:   "Your name is?"
Caller: "Carla Baker."
Staff 1:   "Carla, please hold for one minute while I get Cary on the phone."
Staff (Tina) to Staff 2 (Cary):   "Cary, Carla Baker is on line 1 and is having a problem with..."
Staff 2 to Caller: "Hi Carla, this is Cary and I understand you are having problems with.... Let's see how I can help."

You save valuable time with efficient phone skills, and you save callers mountains of frustration.

Scheduling Appointments

When scheduling appointments try to ask questions that force the caller to make a choice. (Fig. 18.2) All too often in business you hear, "When do you want to come in, we can get you in at 7:00 on Monday, 11:30 on Wednesday, or 6:00 on Friday." Verbally skipping all over the place confuses and overwhelms

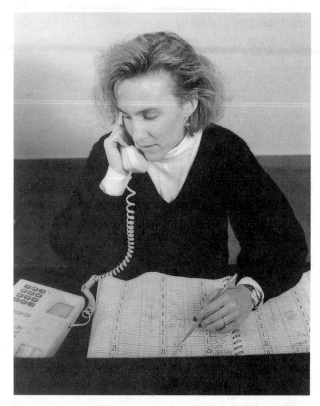

Fig. 18.2   Scheduling appointments. (Photo by Michael A. Gallitelli on location at Rielms Hair Salon, Latham, NY.

the caller. Many callers have a difficult time pinpointing an exact time and day they would like. (The exception to this rule is the analytical, organized client or the pressured professional person who has a specific day or time in mind before she even picks up the phone.)

Remember proper questioning leads the client to the desired result. Take charge and ask questions. State what day, what period of the day and then give them two time options.

- "What day in the week do you prefer?"
- "Do you prefer Tuesday or Fridays?"
- "He's available on Saturday or Monday, which would be more convenient?"

Once the caller has selected a day try,

- "Do you prefer mornings or afternoons?"
- "There is an opening at 9:00 and 11:00, which works best for you?
- "Would you please spell your first and last name for me? I also need a day phone number."

Remember to give the caller choices:

- Question 1: What day?
- Question 2: Morning or Afternoon?
- Question 3: Two time options.

Reconfirm Information

Once the appointment has been secured always repeat the information back to the caller. State the day, date, time, and reference the appointment scheduled for clarification. "Mrs. Schneider, we look forward to meeting you on Tuesday, October first, at 3:30 for your image consultation with Charles."

Message Taking

If you can't service the call and can't transfer it to someone who can help, a phone message is definitely required. "Let me have your name and I'll see that she gets your message." "I'm sorry, Robert is away from the salon today teaching a seminar. Let me take a detailed message for him and I'll personally see that he gets it."

Mastering Message Memos
1. Take detailed, thorough messages.
2. Ask callers to spell their names. Simple names are frequently spelled several different ways. "I can handle Bob but would you please spell your last name for me?" "Please spell your first and last name for me."
3. Print clearly. A phone message can be a valuable piece of information, but it's worthless if you can't read it.
4. Do not abbreviate names, addresses, cities, or even words within the message. If you have an internal code system worked out, that's Okay. Just make sure the same code means the same thing to everybody on staff. For example, does HC mean haircut or haircolor?

5. Always secure two phone numbers, a day and an evening number, where the caller can be reached. Busy professionals are often jammed with appointments during the day and the only opportunity to return phone calls is after normal office hours.

6. Complete the phone message form. Fill in the form as the call comes in. Do not scribble notes everywhere then transfer the information to the phone message pad. Double message taking increases your chance of transferring the wrong information. Don't write messages on the appointment book, matchbook covers, flyers, or tiny pieces of paper. Make sure to use phone message forms that are in duplicate. It never hurts to have a back-up copy.

See Figure 18.3 for a sample message form. Here are the guidelines for filling in the sample message form.

1. Fill in the month, the date, and the day of the week the call came in.
2. List the exact time the call was received.
3. A, B, C, D is the ranking system for coding the importance of the call.
   - A. Urgent, needs your attention immediately.
   - B. Important, priority.
   - C. Need to know, action requested today or tomorrow.
   - D. For your information, not pressing.
4. Fill in the name of the message recipient.
5. Fill in the caller's name and make sure the spelling is correct. Add the phonetic spelling if you feel it's necessary for clear enunciation.
6. List the company the caller represents.
7. Note two phone numbers that are available with extension numbers and the time zone, if necessary. (EST for Eastern Standard Time, CST for Central Standard Time, MST for Mountain Standard Time, and PST for Pacific Standard Time.)
8. Ask for a detailed message. Try to have the caller explain what information is needed—set a meeting, mail a letter, confirm an appointment, schedule a press interview. The information you gather allows the message recipient to prepare the necessary facts before returning the call.
9. Action promised. Detail any and all actions you personally promised the caller. For example, "Mail press kit today." "You will return his phone call today at 5:00."

10. Special notes. Convey the mood of the caller, tidbits from the conversation, or tips the message recipient can use to their advantage for a successful and smooth call back.
11. Does the caller prefer to call again or have his/her call returned? Secure and arrange a convenient time the call back can take place. Obtaining two options will help prevent telephone tag for both parties.
12. Check if you have attached any related correspondence or notes from previous telephone calls.
13. Always sign the phone memo. If there are any questions the recipient doesn't have to play Sherlock Holmes to decode cryptic handwriting.

Handling Different Types of Callers

Slow Talkers
The best way to deal with slow talkers is to give them multiple choice answers. For example: "Did you want to schedule an appointment, have your hair styled, or book a private consultation?" Give them options to select from to help speed up the call.

Fast Talkers
If you can't keep up with fast talkers interject, "Excuse me, I'm having difficulty taking all this information down. Would you please slow down just a bit?"

Foreign Accents
Concentrate extra hard. If you are still grasping for what the caller just said, say "Excuse me, I'm having trouble understanding your question, would you be so kind as to slow down a little? I want to be sure I understand every word." If necessary, have them spell the word or phrase to clarify what they are saying.

Complaints
The client may not always be right, but she thinks she is. Don't panic when you have a complaint call. Be grateful the complaining caller is giving you a second chance to correct or solve a problem. Assume responsibility to the caller, "Gee, I'm sorry that happened, let's see what I can do to solve your problem." Never tell the caller, "Well, you should have done such and

---

PHONE MESSAGE

DATE_____DAY_____

TIME_____:_____am/pm   A   B   C   D

Message for:_____

Caller's name:_____

Phonetic spelling (if necessary)_____

Company:_____

Day phone   (   ) _____–_____ ext. _____

Evening   (   ) _____–_____ ext. _____

Time zone_____

Message:_____

_____

_____

Action promised:_____

_____

Special notes:_____

_____

Caller wants you to return call on:

Date_____at_____:_____am/pm or _____:_____am/pm

Caller will phone you again on:

Date_____at_____:_____am/pm or _____:_____am/pm

Attached:

_____Correspondence

_____Phone notes

Fig. 18.3   Telephone message.

such." Remember, the client has phoned in to have the issue resolved, not to be ignited with negative, prickly comments.

Rude and Angry Callers

Absolutely remain calm and poised. Use your voice to your advantage by projecting a soothing, calming, caring tone. "I'm sorry that happened, tell me what you would like for me to do to resolve the issue. I'd be glad to help." If reasonable, do what they request and follow through.

Obscene Callers

Unfortunately, from time to time, you may be assaulted with an abusive caller. If it is an occasional call, you can ignore the caller and just hang up. If the calls persist you can notify the police department and file a police report and, in conjunction with the police, the telephone company can tap your phone lines. Your lines will be tapped for two weeks during which time you must keep a detailed log of all obscene calls. The telephone company and police department take your information to track the caller and hopefully put an end to the obscene calls.

Phone Faux Pas

Here are five phrases that should be erased from your vocabulary:

1. "I don't know." There may be times when certain facts escape you or you honestly don't know the answer. If so, simply state what you can do to solve or resolve the caller's request. "That's a great question, I'd be glad to find out for you." "Gee, I just drew a blank. Please hold for one minute while I get the colorist on the phone to answer your question."
2. "I can't" or "you can't." I've yet to meet a customer that likes being told they cannot do something. "I can't" translates to "I don't want to." This tiny phrase can erect a barrier between you and the client. Always tell the client what you can do, not what you can't. "Mrs. Brown, the 3:00 time is already filled, I can get you in at 2:00 or at 4:00."
3. "You'll have to." I'm sure you have been on the receiving end of some, short-tempered person who tells you what you must do. No one likes being told they must do some-

thing. Callers can become very defensive especially since you are a faceless person over the telephone. Giving directions or suggestions softens the abrasiveness for the caller, "Margaret, what you'll need to do is this . . ." "Amy, you might try . . ."

4. "No." Avoid using the word no. Rephrase your responses omitting the word no in your answer. If you were to translate English to Japanese you might have a little trouble because there simply isn't a word for no in the Japanese language. Try, "Unfortunately, he already has a full schedule. What other day would you prefer?" "I'm sorry, Debbie only works on Tuesday and Thursday evenings. Which one would be convenient for you?"
5. "I've had a cancellation." Clients should never hear the word cancellation pass over your lips. This reinforces in clients minds that it's Okay to cancel their appointments. Substitute the word reschedule for cancellation. "Earlier I had a customer who needed to reschedule. Would 3:00 be convenient for you?"

TELEPHONE SALES

Scheduling New Clients

Your objective is to match the right client to the right staff member. It is critical to take into account the client's needs, wants, desires, and personality.

- "I have several stylists who are excellent. Do you prefer a male or female stylist?"
- "Do you already know of a stylist that you would like to meet?"
- "Have you been referred to a certain stylist?"

Remember to take into account their personality selling tip-offs.

Interruptions

Avoid receiving or making the phone calls while you are working with a client. The client in your chair is paying for your undivided attention. Don't dilute your service time by talking on the telephone. Your client does not need to overhear what you are saying in your personal or business calls. Only accept and return calls when you are not servicing customers. Remember, if you're on the telephone talking to someone else, you can't sell to the client in your chair.

Rescheduling of Appointments

Unfortunately, clients do call in at the last minute to cancel appointments. Try to reschedule the appointment while they are still on the phone. "I'm sorry you won't be able to make it in today, what other day will work?" (Say this all in one breath and with emphasis on will.) Get them to commit to an appointment time before they have the chance to hang up. Do not ask them if they want to reschedule. Simply ask, "What date will work?" or "What day will be convenient?"

Suggestive Selling

When a client calls in to schedule a service, automatically question what else needs to be done that day.

- "I have you scheduled for your haircoloring on Tuesday, March 17. What additional services will you be needing?"

- "I've got you down for your pedicure on May 3. That week, we are featuring a guest makeup artist from New York. He is scheduling one-hour appointments for new spring makeovers. The session is $45. Would you like to have your makeup updated before or after your color appointment?"

- "I've got you scheduled on August 27 at 4:30 for your hair cut and style. Is it time for your monthly pedicure?"

- "While you are enjoying your manicure, John has time to apply a deep conditioner. You'll only need an extra ten minutes. Shall I schedule your deep treatment as well?"

- "Mrs. Thompson, I know that your schedule is crazy. Why don't we book your facial and manicure to be done at the same time?"

Standing Appointments

Always try to secure a commitment or a regular appointment time with the technician. Save the client time and frustration by helping her select a standing appointment time and day that fits her schedule best. Scheduling in advance allows the client the opportunity to secure her favorite time. "Let's schedule your appointment now, so no one else gets your favorite time." "Now I know, Linda, that Saturday is the only convenient day for you, and Saturdays fill up first, so let's schedule your next three Saturday appointments."

Offer an additional savings to all regularly scheduled appointments paid in advance. "Take an extra 10 percent off your service receipt with any six services scheduled and paid for in advance."

SAMPLE TELEPHONE SCENARIOS

"How much is your perm service?"

Never state the price first. Always start the dialogue by stating what services are included for the fee. Remember that you sell what it does not what it is. Tell the caller the benefits of your product or service before you rattle off the price even if the caller is price shopping. "Our perm service includes private consultation, hair analysis, hair shaping, preperm conditioner, perm application, finished style, and a personal home care guide all for $64. How long has it been since you've had a perm?" You have just educated the caller on the fact that all services are not created equal. They may find another salon offering perms for $45 but be shocked to find that all the extras have add-on charges.

"Do you do facials?"

If you follow this example, I'll guarantee you that your closing rate over the telephone will increase. In my salon, we used to answer that question like this: Of course we do. The facial takes an hour and a half for the first visit. We offer a ten-step treatment that includes consultation, analysis, steam, massage, brush, vac, moisturizing step, galvanic, pore cleaning, and one or two masks depending on your skin." The statement was in fact very true, but I was telling the caller what the facial was, not what it did.

But when I changed our response to the question, our sales went through the roof. "Yes, we do facials. Have you ever had one?" Whatever their response was, mine was "That's great! Are you having any particular problems with your skin?" After they had answered that question, I followed with, "Our treatments are designed to match your skin's needs. The technician will design a treatment based on what your skin is telling

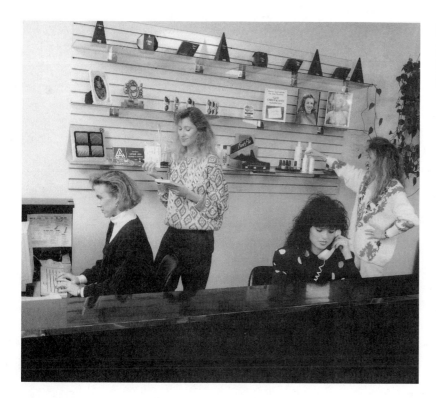

Fig. 18.4 Mission control center. Be prepared at the telephone station. (Photo by Michael A. Gallitelli on location at Rielms Hair Salon, Latham, NY.)

her the day of the facial. She can concentrate on (whatever the stated problem was). The first facial takes ninety minutes. What day in the week is convenient for you?"

"I am looking for Product XYZ. Do you carry it?"

You need to find out if the caller has used this product or if she is just trying to track down the product.

You: "Have you used this product before, or are you wanting to try it?
Caller: "No, I have not tried it, but I have read about the product in a magazine."
You: "What type of hair do you have?"
Caller: "I have very thick, coarse hair."
You: "I'm sorry we don't carry that particular brand of products. However I do have several options of products designed for your type of hair. My name is Joan and I'd love to invite you in to compare the products. The salon offers a complimentary hair analysis. The quick analysis program would tell you exactly what products would be best for your hair. What day would be best for you?"

Another option:

You: "Please tell me what the product is supposed to do."
Caller: Responds
You: "Many products offer those benefits. I have two exceptional products here at the salon, and I've seen super results with both."

"I'm looking for a new place for my beauty services. What is your salon like?"

Find out what the caller is looking for. What services? What products? What did she like most about her current selection and what did she like least? Stress the positive attributes of your business. Ultimately invite the caller in for a tour or consultation. Offer her a chance to meet with the salon director or coordinator.

TELEPHONE STATION—MISSION CONTROL

The mission control center (reception desk) needs to have a place for everything and everything in its place, ready for service and sales. (Fig. 18.4) Supplies needed are:

1. Telephone. There are literally thousands of options from telephone makers. Look for a model that fits your business needs today and still has room for growth.
2. Telephone cord. Invest in an extra long cord, at least twenty feet. You need room to move around without getting strung up by the swirling cord.
3. Telephone cord adapter. This gadget attaches between the telephone and the cord and keeps the cord from twisting. For under $10 you can keep the cord from tangling and knotting.
4. Headsets. Once the sole domain of telephone operators, headsets have emerged as the efficiency device for telephone users. Headsets can:

   - Free up your hands so you can jot notes, schedule appointments, or run the computer.
   - Improve your posture and reduce fatigue.
   - Free you up so that you can move around. The opportunity to be mobile enlivens your voice by letting you roam about and eliminate that rigid phone body posture.

5. Writing material. Always have plenty of paper, working pens, sharpened pencils, and message slips near every single telephone. Nothing sounds so disorganized as, "Hold on while I try to find something to write on." Prevent leaving a bad impression; be prepared and have all your supplies at hand.
6. Sales and advertising literature. Place copies of recent articles, advertising slicks, and reprints from magazines, and have price listings posted by every telephone.
7. A mirror. Place a small mirror by each telephone to remind yourself that you should carry on the dialogue as if the person was staring at you face to face.
8. A small clock. Attach a small clock on or near the telephone. Watch for delays in the amount of time you spend with each caller. Time is money.

I can't stress enough the importance of polishing your telephone skills. Don't take a chance with your sales by overlooking this vital instrument in your salon.

PART THREE
Building Your Business and the Foundation for Success

CHAPTER 19

BUSINESS BUILDERS

Do you believe that you offer an exceptional treatment or service? Do you have outstanding products on the shelf? Do you need more bodies in the front door?

I'm sure you've heard that if you build a bigger, better mousetrap, people will beat a path to your door. Well, I'm here to tell you that if the customers are not aware that you offer the best service and the best products around, they are not going to beat a path to your door to take advantage of them. This chapter will give you ways to build awareness about your business.

Everything is in place—the physical layout is ready to go, the business is organized, and you have all the necessary selling skills. All you need are more customers. It's time to concentrate your efforts on increasing your sales by bringing in more clients. The business-building chapter details five major areas recommended for drumming up customers. In this section I'll share ways to wisely invest your time rather than spending tons of money on advertising.

Areas of opportunity:

- Building your business through publicity
- Building your business through association participation
- Building your business through presentations
- Building your business through publications, especially your own newsletter
- Building your business through personal appearances

BUILDING YOUR BUSINESS THROUGH PUBLICITY

Publicity is the cornerstone for building your business. The goal of publicity is to generate stories and news about your com-
pany to be seen in newspapers, magazines, newsletters, interviews on the radio, and television. The best part about publicity is that it is relatively inexpensive, counting the cost of press-kit production and your own hours of work. My experience has been that excellent press coverage can be more effective than a paid advertisement. The reader understands editorial coverage to be objective and will usually be more impressed by a story in the media than an ad.

For weeks I had been buying advertising space in the local paper and sending direct mail flyers when an article appeared in the business section of the local newspaper. The phone did not stop ringing. I had been investing thousands of dollars for paid ads with moderate results, yet within the first two weeks of the story hitting we scheduled over forty-five new customers. I have never had a paid ad generate more clients than that article. My cost for the article? Only one hour of my time during which I was painlessly interviewed by the writer. I had a copy of the article framed and displayed in our main hallway. As clients would pass, they would comment that the newspaper coverage was the reason they had finally called the salon for an appointment.

There are three characteristics you need to develop for waging a successful press campaign—real news that's worth publishing, contacts, and persistence.

News Ideas with an Angle

Make a comprehensive study of your local print media. What kind of articles do the lifestyle and business editors run in your local newspaper? Study your community. Look for the unique angle that would appeal to your area. Here are some ideas that I have found to be successful. They may or may not work for your community, so study them carefully before offering them to an editor.

- Brand new business, or grand opening.
- Anniversary.
- Unique service.
- Beauty makeovers of women randomly selected by an editor and yourself.
- Beauty classes in the local high school before the prom or graduation.
- Donating your beauty services for a local hospital or nursing home.
- Participation in the Look Good Feel Better program for cancer patients.
- Tie-in with the many churches offering food, clothing, and grooming for homeless people.
- New staff, new management, new owners.
- New products, new treatments, new trends.
- Specialized training.
- Career day.
- Environmental issues.
- Scholarship fund for local students.
- "Official stylist for . . ."
- Sponsor teams, floats, tournaments.
- Judge local, state, national pageants.
- Winning styling competition.
- Special recognition and awards.
- Collection of canned goods or toys during the holidays.
- Delivering flowers and groceries to shut-ins.

I hope you would want to open your heart to a cause or need in your area simply for the greater good, not just the business opportunity. You may elect to do your giving in secret and not use the action as a press opportunity. The choice is yours. It is my goal to simply plant the ideas and seeds of opportunity for you.

Press Contacts

Press relations are a person-to-person activity. Your success rests in your ability to establish a string of contacts, editors and writers who are interested in beauty stories; local, regional, state, and national newspapers, magazines, radio stations, and television stations. Find out the names, titles, addresses, and telephone numbers. Depending on your goal, your contact may be the lifestyle editor, fashion and/or beauty editor, news editor, business editor, president of a group, publisher, show producer, on-air talent, and secretaries (they get the calls through to your contacts).

Now that you have your list of media contacts how do you get their attention? You must first clarify what you do, how well you do it, how your information will benefit their audience, and who you are.

Your next goal is to get their attention, which can be tough. Editors are constantly being sent mailbags full of press information from companies and individuals like yourself who would like to receive a little coverage. They are constantly under time pressure, not to mention pressure from a management that has established editorial policies that may make it difficult for you to get a story through. For instance, if your salon is in Old Town right on the border of New Town, the new town news editor may not be able to use your story because she/he can only print stories from New Town.

Use your creativity to get their attention. You may have success simply by calling and inviting an editor to send a writer in for a service. Or you may need to get really clever to pique their interests and to make sure your information stands out from the crowd.

A real professional in the publicity department is Diane Young of Diane Young Skin Care in New York City. At her third-story salon, Diane had a landscaped terrace where her customers could enjoy their manicures and pedicures out of doors. She created a beauty oasis in the middle of Manhattan. Each springtime Diane sent a "The Terrace is Open" press release tied to a potted geranium that was delivered to beauty editors. Beauty services in a New York garden? That is a news angle even the most sophisticated editor might consider.

Persistence

Work with your contacts. If they reject your ideas, politely ask their reasons and learn from them. Come back with new ideas. Offer to serve as a source of information for their needs, their stories. Become their useful associate.

When you decide to take action with your list of press contacts, the first item you need for building your business is a press kit. If you have the budget for it, consider hiring an art director, particularly one who works with computer-generated type and graphics, to put together a polished look. The art director may create a logo or adapt your present logo for special letterhead paper for your kit. He or she will also be able to advise you on folders, envelopes, labels, photos, type style and size for your releases and camera-ready stories, if they make sense for your market. The kit should include:

1. A fact sheet describing the history of your company and the special services at your salon.
2. Professional photographs and biographies of important people in the business.
3. Press release.
4. Timely feature article, if you have one.
5. Your current newsletter.
6. Calendar of future events.
7. Camera-ready stories and illustrations that could be reprinted as submitted (only if the local paper will run these).
8. Reprints of articles that have already been published.
9. A folder and envelope in the salon's colors for holding all your goodies.

Writing a Press Release

If you're going to submit a press release use the following guidelines:
1. Use the salon's letterhead paper with address and phone numbers in 8 1/2-by-11-inch size.
2. Always use white paper. Easier on the editor's eye and copies come out clearer.
3. On the top left hand side of the page put the name of the contact person (probably yourself). Include your evening phone number. Place the date of the release ont he top right side.

4. Type or set your computer print-out for double spacing to allow the editor to make any necessary corrections.
5. Start a third of the way down on the page allowing room for the editor to insert a headline for your piece.
6. In your first paragraph, or lead, state the who, what, where, when, and why. In case your copy gets cut, all of the important information is in the first paragraph.
7. Use short sentences, third person pronouns, active and direct words. Write objectively. This is not persuasive advertising copy.
8. Be specific and to the point with your information. Try to say your piece in less than four paragraphs.
9. If you have more than one page of copy, tag the bottom of page and end at the very bottom of the last page. Number additional pages at the right hand corner.

BUILDING YOUR BUSINESS THROUGH ASSOCIATION PARTICIPATION

Every community, large and small, has clubs and organizations where you can become involved and participate in the group's activities. Even though some of the organizations listed below are slanted toward personal endeavors, your business can benefit from personal affiliations as well as business organizations. Here are a few categories of clubs and organizations for you to investigate:

- Cause related. I live close to the beach and pier, and there has been a strong effort in the community to save the coastline, especially since the *American Trader* dumped almost 400,000 gallons of oil into the Pacific Ocean. Look into environmental groups.

- Civic Organizations. The function of civic minded clubs is to benefit the local community. Soroptomists, Kiwanis, Rotarians, Junior League.

- Charitable. Organizations are constantly on the lookout for volunteers that can contribute time and talents for their charity. Look to the United Way, American Cancer Society, American Heart Association, March of Dimes.

- Educational. These clubs are formed to assist educational institutions and/or as learning centers. Options: PTA, Alma

Mater, Toastmasters, or any learn-how-to club. Learn a new skill and network for new clients at the same time. You will find educational groups featuring everything from the arts to zoology.

- Professional. Every industry has its own organized association. Check into the chamber of commerce, National Association of Women Business Owners (NAWBO), National Cosmetology Association (NCA), Intercoiffure, Association of Image Consultants International (AICI), Professional Business Women.

- Political. Take a political stand for your favorite local, state, or national political candidate. Energies run high, especially during election year when everyone is pulling and rooting for their favorite candidate. Options: Young Republicans, League of Women Voters, Young Democrats. If this area interests you, the best place to start is by calling your local party office for information. Just remember that this is a double-edged sword. Present customers who agree with you politically will be delighted and you may attract new like-minded customers. But you may lose a few customers who are on the other side.

- Social organizations. Clubs are formed with the sole purpose of providing social interaction. Sororities; fraternities; country clubs; neighborhood block clubs; clubs for tall people, little people, single people, married people.

There are not enough hours in the day for you to become involved in all the organizations. Select one or two clubs that best represent your interests and goals. You need to be very selective when you become involved, if you are wisely investing your time instead of money. Your time could be swallowed up running between meetings and functions if you're not careful. You must ask yourself, where is my time best served? Don't get sidetracked trying to join every club that comes along. Guard your time and select organizations that will help your business grow.

Some clubs and organizations are naturally better places to plant your seeds. Take time out of your schedule and invest in places to work that have fertile soil. You have probably heard the parable of planting seeds, letting them germinate, then after a season the seedling sprouts forth as a reward of your tending and care. When you join a club and become involved

you are planting seeds to germinate new clients for your business. (Fig. 19.1)

Take the opportunity to press the flesh. Give people a firsthand view of your company. Let the people get to know you and become comfortable with you before doing business. Clubs and organizations are the best places to drum up new business, if you use the opportunity to your advantage and work the group. Let me throw in a word of caution. You don't want to be known as a barracuda only looking to make a contact and subsequent sale. You may turn off a lot of the club's members. However, your involvement, properly applied, will stimulate growth for your company.

Once you have found a group or two, you will want to become involved and serve on the local board or governing body. They usually fall into three levels—local, state, and national positions. Every position, every rung of the ladder, brings responsibility and rewards.

When I was in Wichita I became very involved with the National Association of Women Business Owners (NAWBO). My business had been open a year when I did several of the suggestions mentioned in this chapter. Within the second year, I was elected to the local chapter board as secretary. Then I became vice president and by the fourth year in the group I was elected president. Now, my involvement on the local level automatically put me in contact with the national board of directors and its officers. The salon had fifteen newspaper articles that I was listed in or interviewed for as a result of serving on the local board.

I was attending a national NAWBO board meeting in Houston. When I returned to my room there was a message to "call this number immediately." I was shocked when the woman on the other end of the receiver responded, *"USA Today."* She was given my name by the NAWBO administrative office to call me as a source for a story she was preparing on equal access to credit for women in business. Not only were my comments displayed in the trendy newspaper, but the *Wall Street Journal* called for comments as well. Shortly thereafter I received a call asking if I would fly to Washington, D.C., and testify before a Senate subcommittee on the equal access to credit issue.

I am sharing this story with you because it served a great organization, the salon received some great publicity, and it acquired new customers, which is the ultimate goal. Select one or two organizations you can commit to; the rewards will pay off.

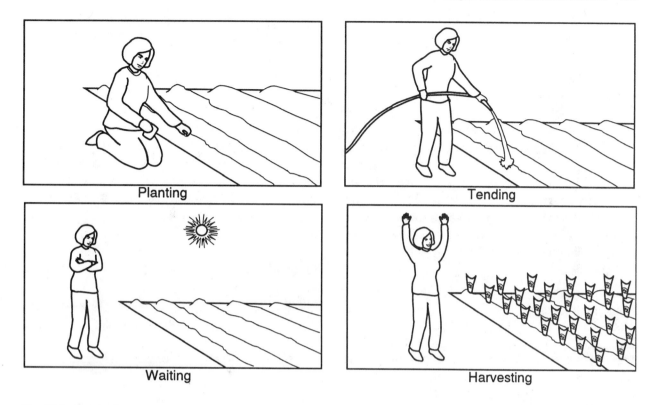

Fig. 19.1   Seeds of success.

Networking

You've selected the organization you want to become involved in. That's great. Here are six tips for making your networking pay off.

Name Badges

When you are networking, the most important thing that someone should remember about you is your name and your company. Always wear your name badge on the right side of your shoulder—the hand you extend to shake—not the left. The reason for applying your badge on the right side is that when you shake hands with someone your eye automatically follows their extended arm. I don't want to have to look to your left shoulder to see your badge while I am shaking your right hand. Doing so breaks eye contact.

   Practice: Find a partner and pretend you are meeting for

the first time. Introduce yourself and shake hands. Notice now natural it is for your eye to look at the other person's right shoulder. Placing the name badge on the right shoulder reinforces your name to the other person.

Take Initiative

Take charge of your responsibility to acquire new clients. The local NAWBO group mentioned earlier conducted a survey of members that chose not to renew their membership. The survey turned up some amazing discoveries: 95 percent of the lapsed members claimed that they just didn't get any business from the group. What struck the surveyors as peculiar was that they could not remember the company names of some of the former members or what most of them were selling. Some of the surveyors could not even remember what the previous members looked like. The lapsed members obviously did not take initiative and work the group because they didn't stick out in our minds. The time is right to speak up and out about your business, talents, and unique selling position after you've become involved.

The Card Trick

When you go somewhere with the intention of networking, always wear a garment with two pockets. Your business cards are placed in your right pocket, along with a pen for making notes. As you collect business cards from others, those are placed in your left pocket. Placing your cards in your right pocket is a natural smooth extension and movement for your arm. Tuck the collected cards in your left pocket to keep them from getting intermingled with your cards you plan to distribute. Separating theirs from yours saves time and keeps you from thumbing through the collected cards to get to one of your business cards.

Food and Beverage

If food and beverages are offered at a function, choose one or the other. It is embarrassing when you are about to meet someone new, and you have a plate of food in one hand and a drink in the other and you're forced to say, "Gee, I'd really like to shake your hand, but . . . ," then you are forced to fumble with your food. Pick one or the other, food or beverage. Never rely on business meetings or networking parties to provide you with your three square meals a day.

Entrances.

When you enter a function for the first time, walk into the room then stop, practically in the doorway. Stop and look around. Many people walk in and head straight to the food table, beverage bar, or, worse yet, the wall. People will notice you if you do the enter and stop for a second technique, then proceed. The next time you are at a function, pay close attention to the front door and watch who uses entrances to their advantage and how people respond to them.

Work a Room

Mix and mingle. Meet new people. Quite often you may gravitate towards those you already know and feel comfortable around. It's a natural instinct to seek out people you already know. Don't pass up the opportunity to meet as many new people as possible, those familiar friends already are familiar with your business.

Challenge: When you network, make it a goal to meet at least three new people you can follow up with after the function either by phone, mail, or in person.

There are professionally organized clubs that bring people together for the sole purpose of networking. One such group is LeTip (a national organization). Check your local area for similar opportunities or take the initiative and start your own referral networking club. These specialized referral swapping clubs are unique because they only allow one business per category. You can feel comfortable and eager to share your information because you won't be divulging your leads and customers to a competitive business.

BUILDING YOUR BUSINESS THROUGH PRESENTATIONS

There are three reasons you invest your time in presentations:

1. To obtain business on the spot.
2. To make an appointment to sell more business.
3. To have a reason for another contact and follow up.

Next to networking, this is the best way to market yourself and business, if it is done properly.

Wondering how to get on the program? Call you local chamber of commerce. Most chambers produce a listing of clubs and organizations for their area that are available for free or a nominal charge ($5–$15). Many of the lists will include the organization's name, address, officers, contact person, and phone number. Target clubs matching your ten best customer list, and contact them for speaking opportunities. One to two programs a month is more than enough for a small business to manage properly.

The length of the program should be kept to a minimum. Schedule consumer programs for thirty minutes at the most. The best results I've had was with a program for a mother-daughter church banquet. Out of the seventy-five attendants, twenty-seven appointments were scheduled as a result of a twenty-minute slide program and short question-and-answer session.

As professionals, we have a tendency to want to tell people everything we know all at one time. Show business people practice a truly simplistic rule; "always leave them wanting more." That is a great rule to follow for presentations too. When you schedule the program insist that the organization be specific in their request for program information. They will usually say that they want to see everything you do. Don't get roped into trying to cover everything under the sun in a short time frame. Make the program short, informative, and fun, such as:

- Eye makeup rather than whole-face makeover

- Fun with scarves rather than wardrobe selecting

- Styling tips rather than hair trends, cutting, perming

- After-five looks rather than complete makeovers

Usually the presentation will be after office hours and the participants have already had a long day ending with a short attention span. There's not time for showing them everything. Besides, this allows you to go back again to the same group with additional programs.

During the program you want the opportunity to generate leads. Make sure if you are investing your time and resources that you have some mechanism for obtaining the names and addresses of those attending. I like to offer a drawing forcing the audience to register for gifts from the company. You win by keeping and working the registration forms and the club wins because you donate one or two outstanding prizes for the group. (See Figure 19.2 for a sample registration card.)

What's the most important time when you make a presentation? The opening? The first five minutes? Introduction? Demonstration? The question-and-answer session? The most important time is the fifteen minutes after you finish. This critical time allows your audience to ask questions and chat with you about scheduling appointments. Make sure you have allowed time to close the sale after every speech or program. If your program is after salon hours, take along your appointment book, and schedule appointments after you finish the program.

NOTE: Don't waste your energy doing presentations if you don't follow up, either by calling the participants and giving them the information they checked off on the form or by mail inviting them to visit your business. If your company doesn't follow up, it's not worth the trouble and time to platform your talents.

BUILDING YOUR BUSINESS BY GETTING PUBLISHED

In the medical community the phrase "publish or perish" can be heard on the lips of administrators nationwide. Most institutions insist their employees continually publish research documents and articles. The main reason is to keep the institution's name before the public and the industry. Well, you don't have to be a doctor to benefit from being published. Some opportunity options are:

Your Own Newsletter

This is my favorite investment for salon promotion. Even for a small salon, a bi-yearly newsletter allows you to share more information with your current and potential clients. Keep in touch with your clients at the beginning of May before Mother's Day and again around Thanksgiving for the winter holiday season. Let your winter letter be your Christmas card.

If your salon has the budget, you may go quarterly, including a fall newsletter at back-to-school time and a spring newsletter just before Easter. Keep the copy informational and educational. Make the newsletter a mini beauty magazine. Working on a computer with the help of your art director, design regular columns. Add photos of your work. Introduce new services and products. Showcase staff members. Include a fashion column. Interview owners of local specialty stores about fashion as it relates to hair, makeup and nail trends. Include a special offer for a new product or service.

The finished product should be mailed to your existing clientele, handed out at seminars and workshops, distributed to potential clients and networking leads, included in your press kits, and also mailed out to all local media.

If you are not a writer, you can hire someone to write it for you. Start out small with a two-page edition, and you can grow with your publication. And remember, desktop publishing on your computer is much cheaper than typesetting.

In my over-enthusiastic approach to spreading the salon message, one of our mailing campaigns meant that six thousand newsletters were distributed. The result was initially outstanding. The phone rang off the wall. And we were booked up for weeks in advance. The down side to that mailing was that potential clients had to wait eight weeks or more to get an

---

REGISTRATION CARD

Program_____Date_____

Name_____

Address_____

City _____State_____Zip_____

Day Phone_____ext_____

Evening Phone_____ext_____

I'd like more information on:

_____Personal Consultation   _____Hair Styling

_____Perms and Color   _____Skin Treatments

_____Makeup Applications   _____Body Therapy

_____Nail Care   _____All of the above

Fig. 19.2   Sample registration card.

---

appointment. It was not smart on my part to mail that many at once.

Pace the success of your publication. Bundle the newsletter in lots of 200–300 to qualify for bulk mailing. Every two to three weeks, mail out a new batch, using the same newsletter. If you really want to make the cash register ring, implement a telephone-calling program to follow the mailing. Have a key person call the recipients to see if they received the newsletter, if they had time to read it, and they knew about special offers for products or services. Close the sale right on the phone.

When you have a successful newsletter with a proven readership and proven response to your product offers, you may be able to reduce the cost of production by selling ad space to businesses that are complementary to your salon—a jewelry store, clothing store, house-cleaning service, day care, auto mechanic shop, car dealership. Target a couple of businesses and try it. You can honestly sell them on the specific target market you are reaching. But, I must warn you that ad sales can be hard work.

To establish the cost of an ad, figure your production cost for one page, half page, and quarter page. If you will have to create the ad for the advertiser, figure in that cost as well. And include the cost of your time in sales and coordination work. Ask each advertiser to sign a contract, outlining all expenses, listing when the newsletter will be mailed, and the quantity of the list.

Contributing Articles

Writing and contributing articles will benefit your business. Target your selections at publications your clients read. It is okay for you to contribute articles for trade publications if that will benefit your business. Remember you must invest your time where it will benefit your business best.

Again, a perfect role model in this department is Diane Young. Over the years, Diane has focused her publicity campaign on consumer publications, and it has paid off. Her business has been open for over seventy-five months and she has been quoted or featured in over seventy-five national consumer publications. The best advice Diane ever shared with me was, "Put your publicity efforts where they will benefit your business not your ego." Many times we get too wrapped up in seeing our name in print, and the end result doesn't benefit the business.

When you have decided to write an article there are two questions you should always ask yourself: How does the reader benefit from my idea, and what do I expect to get for my effort? Be very clear in your objectives. Because time is limited, be cautious where you expend your efforts.

If you are not an experienced writer, you may find it easier to format your article in a question and answer style. Take some of the common questions your clients ask and transfer your responses into an article.

If you are not a writer, and absolutely can't or don't want to write, hire someone else to write the article for you. Many articles you see in the trade publications by prominent industry people are written by ghost writers. It's okay to pay someone to assist your publicity efforts. In fact, you may come out ahead—time, aggravation, and stress versus the dollar investment. (The average investment for ghost writing an article is $200–$500.)

When I found out that a new paper called *Wichita Women* was being established, I contacted the editor and approached her on writing for the paper. The paper agreed and each month I supplied an article featuring the latest service/products/how-tos for their readers. For one year, I invested most of my time and effort into the writing and production of articles as a showcase for my salon. (Fig. 19.3)

Author a Book

Now, I know that can sound like a huge undertaking (and believe me it is) but you could scale it down and write a little six- or seven-page "booklet" to distribute to your clients and potential customers educating them on some facet of your business—at home styling tips, time-saving makeup tips, dress up your wardrobe with jewelry and scarves, skin facts, modifying looks, upcoming trends, body care, makeover magic, beautiful hands and feet, color charting.

Once you have produced your booklet, send it to beauty editors and television and radio stations. How-to educational material can be the start of great free publicity. Tag all your paid advertising with, "Call for our free book on XYZ."

Articles About You

Make contact with beauty editors and producers. Editors and producers are always looking for new, exciting, and unusual sources of information. Make them aware of the fact that you can be a great source of information for them. Once you have established the contact, let them know that you will make it a priority to handle their requests. Quite often they will be calling with a deadline breathing down their neck and need action and your response quickly.

Contributing Photos

A picture is worth a thousand words. As a stylist, writing may not be your forte, but you can submit high-quality photographs of your work. If you are published by a trade publication you can translate that success into excitement within the salon and community. There are hundreds of magazines that publish photographs from stylists all over the world. Stating that your work has been published in other countries such as Spain, Italy, Australia, France, England can and will be very impressive to your customers. (Make sure you frame your work and put it on display in the salon. And also make sure that you and not the photographer owns the rights to the photos.)

BUILDING YOUR BUSINESS THROUGH PERSONAL APPEARANCES

Television

Many local stations produce a talk show. Find out who is the producer and how far in advance they schedule their shows. Then send a letter to the producer with your segment suggestions. Give them three options that will benefit their viewers. Include your press packet, demo video tape if you have one available, and a cover letter. Shoot for at least one show so the producer will be able to view your on-camera appearance.

BEAUTY FOCUS
by Carol Phillips

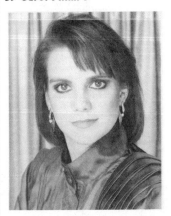

Lost Art of Perfume . . .

Fragrances have been used for thousands of years . . . for worship . . . for medicine . . . to entice . . . to adorn . . . for the pleasure of others or for yourself.

History states that Cleopatra enjoyed perfume so much that the purple sails of her royal barge were saturated with perfume so that the winds would carry her fragrance to announce her arrival.

In the Bible, the beloved of Solomon was described as coming out of the wilderness "perfumed with myrrh and frankincense, with all the powders of the merchant." Song of Solomon 3:6.

Somewhere in the course of time we have truly lost the lovely art of perfume. In our hectic lifestyles "splash and go" does not quite capture the pleasure of fragrance our perfumed civilizations of antiquity enjoyed.

Perfume has always been a secret passion of mine. The more research I do, the more saddened I become because so many of us have deadened our scent awareness. We can readily distinguish between good and bad odors, but in our mass market society the individual preferences and pleasures have been overlooked.

Most of us have selected our fragrance statement by spritzing the arm, waiting a few minutes for the alcohol to evaporate, then deciding whether the girl in the ad is the impression we want to make. By sampling cologne in a "contaminated," meaning multi-fragranced air, it is very difficult to enjoy the excitement perfume should create.

I personally believe that we need to awaken those fragrance receptors. Essences can stimulate thoughts or even open up memories. Once upon a time, perfume was passed down through dynasties, monarchies, and religious hierarchies. As precious as gold, silver and priceless gems, it was known only in the upper echelons of society. Fortunately, times have changed. Now you can create your own signature, experiment . . . enjoy. Here are some fascinating fragrance facts.

1. Egyptians were among the first to truly appreciate the seductive power of fragrance. Women wore vials of perfume as earrings, allowing the fragrance to splash on their shoulders as they walked.
2. The perfumer, referred to as the "Nose," is able to differentiate between 2,000 and 3,000 of the more than 6,000 raw materials and odor harmonies used in creating a fragrance. Custom designing of fragrances is becoming popular in the late 1980s.
3. Jasmine, a prized ingredient, must be harvested just before sunrise, while still covered with the morning mist. If touched by sunshine, it loses 20% of its fragrance potency.
4. Like jasmine, roses must be gathered at sunrise while still moist. It takes over a million roses to yield a single pound of rose essential.
5. Every day you breathe approximately 23,040 times, inhaling and exhaling 438 cubic feet of air. We should take special care to surround ourselves with positive fragrances.
6. A women's sense of smell is more sensitive than a man's and varies during the course of the menstrual cycle. These changes are influenced by estrogen, which increases smell acuity in the first half of the cycle.
7. According to a recent survey conducted by the Fragrance Foundation, scent is a key factor in sexual relationships. The response left no doubt—8.5 females and 7.5 males out of 10 agreed that certain scents can enhance one's sexual activity.
8. Always apply perfume to your pulse points . . . start on the lower extremities . . . ankle, behind the knee, at the waist . . . then apply to the inside crook of the arm, at the base of the throat and of course, the wrists. Wherever you feel a pulse beat, the heat of the body will help to accentuate the fragrance.
9. Never choose a fragrance because you like it on another woman. Fragrance never smells exactly the same on any two people.

Next Month: Long-lasting makeup tips.

Editor's note: Carol Phillips is the owner of Carol Phillips DermaSystems, a complete skin and makeup center in Wichita, Kansas. In 1985 and 1986, Carol was selected as one of the top 100 Entrepreneurs under the age of 30 in the United States. Carol has recently been appointed to the National Cosmetology Association—Esthetic America Educational Committee.

Fig. 19.3 Writing articles for magazines or newspapers gives you the opportunity to showcase your business and reach a large audience.

Arrange to have a video copy of your performance duped from the studio for play in your reception area.

The seasons were changing and the staff had noticed we were getting lots of questions and concerns regarding the clients' skin. "My skin's rough and my makeup is not going on smoothly." It was that time of year when the sluggish, cold days of winter were taking their toll on the skin. If our clients were experiencing problems, I guessed that the viewers of the local talk show were too.

I called the producer and explained about the skin and how a facial could help make the seasonal shift smoother. She agreed to do a segment on the benefits of facials.

The next day she called back. She had an idea. What if we did a facial on the air? The studio would send out a camera crew and do a live remote broadcast from the salon. They would open the show with the model as a before and after, then cut to the salon periodically throughout the broadcast to check on our progress, then show the after-facial model glowing from the treatment. By the time the microphones were disconnected, all three of the phone lines were lit up and kept ringing for twenty minutes with people wanting to schedule appointments.

Some local cable stations also produce shows. One such privately owned network is BLAB-TV. Dr. Mark Lees, from Pensacola, Florida, has his own thirty-minute show that is aired in his target market. I bet you're thinking that your business could never afford such a campaign, but Mark's investment per show is only $350. The price is absolutely phenomenal, but the value gets better. Not only is the show produced for $350, it is also a live call-in show, so there is audience interaction. Plus the station also gives Mark ten free salon commercials per month, plus numerous promotional spots for the show, plus the network is connected with a local radio station, and they frequently have Mark on as a guest. If there is not a BLAB station in your area look for Public Access Television. They are set up similar to the BLAB-TV format.

Radio

I personally love the medium of radio because it allows for quick responses. While you are getting dressed in the mornings, listen to the local station. Listen to the local news and events but also for cues that you could call into the stations.

One morning I was sitting at my dressing table applying my makeup and getting ready for the day when I heard a possible business opportunity. The two DJs were discussing the problems they were having coming up with ideas for Mother's Day gifts. They were tired of giving the same old chenille bath robe. When they went to a song, I called in on the request line to share a few gift ideas. No sooner had I said my name and company when they put me on hold, then from my clock radio I heard, "We have Carol Phillips from Carol Phillips DermaSystems live on the request line with ideas for Mother's Day. Now, here's Carol." We were on the air. The spot lasted about four minutes. The equivalent air time in commercials would have been $432 in my market. The immediate response was out and over the air waves and all for no money. Listen for cues and how you can translate them into a marketing possibility for your business.

Restaurants

Select a restaurant your customers frequent, then set aside time to leave your office and dine out. It pays to be seen. Get out for lunch to help your business grow. Some restaurants offer fashion shows during lunch. This is a great place to find clients who are fashion conscious and would enjoy your looking-good services.

Charity Functions

Use your master ten best list to see where your customers are getting involved. Watch the social section of your newspapers. If the popular club is having a charity function that is where you need to be. Schedule time to get out and socialize, mix and mingle with clients and potential clients at charity functions, auctions, and social events.

Local Sports Activities

Score big points with the community by supporting your local sports team(s). From small-town teams to the Los Angeles Lakers, sports bring people together to rally around the event, the players, and the city.

ABMs

Always be marketing or always be selling. You should always be promoting your business, no matter where you are.

One Friday evening after work, I was pushing my cart through the produce section of the neighborhood grocery store when out from behind the tower of tomatoes, a man yelled, "Hey, are you the makeup lady?" I chuckled to myself because he obviously had seen the talk show I was on earlier that day.

I yelled back, "Yes, I am." He asked if we offered facials for men. By now, we had created a congestion of shopping carts throughout the produce department. As I explained to him the benefits of skin care for men he took out his business card and asked if I would contact his office to schedule an appointment. As we exchanged cards, the on-lookers extended their hands as well, eager to find out how they could have softer and smoother skin too.

After I promised to call his office the following day, I reminded myself that you can always be selling, even between the rutabaga and the radicchio. Take advantage of the Boy Scouts' motto and always be prepared. You never know when you will meet a potential client.

CHAPTER 20

ADVERTISING AND MARKETING

Now that you have the information on setting up the salon to maximize sales and the verbal selling skills, it is time to round up a passel of new clients and to expand your business with current clients. Advertising can do this! Remember, it will only be expensive when it doesn't work. In this chapter, I will share my insights into the tricky business of spending money in the public media to make money.

In the previous chapter, we discussed the importance of marketing your company. We talked over twenty-four options for investing your time rather than big bucks. Publicity, or working with print and broadcast media for the unpaid placement of stories about your salon, is important. It builds goodwill and excitement, but ultimately the message is controlled by media. If you want to control your message, you must pay for it.

WHAT'S YOUR MESSAGE?

What message are you trying to send? How are you going to let the public know? Which public will receive your message? The entire community? A specific segment of that community? As you design your advertising campaign, be very clear on your message and the public that will receive it.

When planning out your message or messages, consider that there are three key areas for you to work with: you and your staff, your services, and your products. The size of the print ad and the amount of broadcast time determines how these areas will be used. For example, it would be best to highlight just one of these areas in a quarter-page newspaper or magazine ad. If you try to squeeze in everything, you will convolute the message and confuse the reader. If you only have thirty seconds of radio time to talk about your salon, focus in on the area that will be important to the listener. Constantly ask yourself, "What is the message I am sending? Is it clear and easy to understand?"

Impressionable State

The first rule to remember is that consumers need to experience your message several times before it will register with them and they can plan to take action. Some top advertisers say that in order to get the audience to act on an offer, the ad or commercial will need to be seen, heard, and experienced twenty-seven times. Every time your salon's message is received, it is called an impression. You will be tired of an ad before it becomes effective.

If you are contemplating the placement of a one-shot ad and you hope and pray for enough response so that the ad will pay for itself save your money. It won't work. You will need to develop a one-year ad plan to grow your company.

Battling the Budget

Budgeting for every area of the salon is important. When it comes to investing your advertising dollars, I want you to work with caution and control. This is one area where advance planning can save you thousands of hard-earned dollars. Granted, an exceptional opportunity may suddenly arise that might be perfect for the salon, and you will want to take advantage of it. A cushion of extra, unassigned dollars will take care of that.

Designated Dollars

Your total marketing budget—advertising, publicity, and special events—should be no more than 3 percent of your gross income. If you are in a very small market, you may choose to go below that figure. If you are in a metropolitan area, you will need to devote more money to marketing. Advertising will take most of your assigned dollars, but as indicated in chapter 19, there are very real expenses in producing press kits. And if you choose to do a newsletter, that project may take almost your entire budget.

Your budget should be fixed. The sign of good promoters is that when times get tough they get tougher. If you go through lean times, don't cut your budget. Scrape by in other areas. If others are slicing their budgets, your company will have the upper hand in exposure.

Budget Breakdown

After you have figured out the amount you will invest in advertising, break down the total dollar amount even further. Budget 60 percent toward activities directed to your present clientele, 30 percent toward attracting potential clients, and the remaining 10 percent as a shotgun approach to the community at large. Using this technique will allow you to target your dollars to attract people who are most likely to purchase your products and services.

MEDIA OUTLETS

In today's market, you have a wide variety of places to invest your advertising dollars. Do you remember studying the history of the midnight ride of Paul Revere in school? The only form of communication in the colony was to ride through the streets announcing that the British were coming. Today, you can't stand on the street corner and yell, "The perms are coming, the perms are coming."

Traditional advertising textbooks consider newspapers, magazines, direct mail, radio, television, outdoor, and transit advertising as the media. And of course, new media like personal computer networks are becoming more and more viable with each passing year. Business cards, brochures, and stationery are usually called collateral, but because they are so important to your business communications, I have placed them first on my list.

Salon Literature

Business Cards

When people think of going into business, business cards seem to be the first item produced. Make sure your cards are straightforward. Tell your message and make it easy for the reader to do business with you. Think of them as minibillboards. You'll need to get your message across in a minimal amount of space. Name, salon name, address, city, state, and zip. Use your area code for telephone numbers, especially if you are in a multilisting area. And include a fax number for your work with vendors and the media. A smart tip is to make your card a fold-over or double-sided. On the flip side, print a map to your location if your salon is difficult to find.

If you give business cards to each employee, bundle them in packs of fifty to a hundred. This will help you monitor employees' marketing. If one box of 500 cards lasts them a couple of years, they are obviously not extending themselves to potential clients for the salon.

Stationery

This includes 8 1/2-by-11 inch letterhead, business-size envelopes, cards for social notes, and thank yous. If you are on a limited budget, make your social card stock the same size as your letterhead envelope.

Your biggest use for letterhead will be to send personal letters to clients and potential clients. Of course, you will send traditional business correspondence on this paper as well.

Here are a couple of personal letter selling tips.

- Stick to one page of copy.

- Announce the arrival of a new staff member, the expansion of services, a change of hours.

- Always include a P.S. at the bottom. Your reader will read the first few sentences, then the P.S., then the signature.

- Picture a favorite client and write directly to her. Keep the language friendly and always clearly state how your information will benefit the reader.

- Use short sentences and short paragraphs to keep the reader's attention.

Social Notes and Thank You's

Card-stock social notes are often the same size as business envelopes. Use these to drop personal notes to clients to thank them for coming in or for referring a new client or to offer new product announcements.

Price Cards

Salons tend to favor price cards or menu cards to post prices. I believe that shoppers want to know how much a product or service will cost. If you list prices, make sure to inform the reader of the differences between services and products. Highlight, foil wrap, low light, frosting, single process, double process—what is the difference? As beauty professionals, we know the answers, but do our clients? Design a price card with service and product descriptions.

Brochures

The salon brochure is an excellent way to tell your salon story in expanded copy. Use consumer-friendly language to describe the salon philosophy, its Unique Selling Position, and why a potential client should select your salon. Also include service categories and photos of services, product philosophy, salon hours, and a map to the salon if necessary.

I was hired by a salon to look at their brochure copy before printing. The basic message was good, the categories were great. The problem was that the copy was written from the salon owner's point of view. In twenty paragraphs, eighteen sentences began with "I." Be careful. It is easy to turn off your readers by inflating your importance. Your message should be how your salon services and products will benefit the customer.

Flyers

One-page flyers are a good way to introduce new products, services, or special promotions. Flyers can be distributed within the salon or can be used as self-mailers. If you are looking for a way to get your message out quickly on a limited budget, check into flyers.

Cross-Merchandise Your Information

Select one or two other businesses that cater to clientele similar to your salon's. Each store exchanges brochures, flyers, and one poster. This will allow you additional exposure to the type of clients you want to attract. Look for fashion, shoe, and jewelry stores as perfect places to merchandise your company.

Create a Lasting Impression

In selecting paper on which to print your letterhead, cards, flyers, and brochures, use an unusual stock. Make it distinctive by texture, color, feel. When the client sees your note in a pretty color among her stack of bills, she will pull your mailing out first. Let color support your salon's message. Make it identifiable with the salon's image and decor.

GETTING MORE BANG FOR YOUR BUCK

Refer back to your ten best customer list. On that list you have an area indicating what newspapers and magazines are read by your most important customer segment and what radio and television shows are watched. There is also a line in the questionnaire that asks how they originally discovered your salon. It makes great sense to put your money and effort into the media selections they cite. When advertising to potential customers, you will want people similar to your best customers.

Newspaper Advertising

You have many options to choose from here: the local daily paper, the regional or community weekly papers, the business news, the neighborhood paper, high school and college papers. School papers are good for promoting prom, graduation, and homecoming services. The rates are exceptionally good. Check to see if there is a women's paper or magazine in your area. What a super place to market your salon!

Two key guidelines for newspaper advertising:

1. Never let the paper create your ad. Many papers will offer to design and produce your ad for free. I shy away from that. You will want your ad to stand out and in my experience, when the paper creates your ad, it turns out looking like every other ad in the paper.
2. Never use a type size smaller than the print the paper uses. The reader will skip over your ad because it will be too hard to read.

Magazine Advertising

You will have many options for magazine ads. Although there are national as well as local and regional magazines on the local stands, the national magazine is not a viable buy for you because of the wasted money spent on readership that will never be able to visit your salon. If you are in a large metropolitan market where a national offers a regional insert rate that, of course, is a different story.

The main advantage of the magazine is its shelf life. Today's newspaper is tomorrow's bird cage liner. If you have a city magazine, this may be a great place to establish your presence in the community. Plus, if the magazine does fashion, health, and beauty stories, your ad takes on even more power.

Radio Advertising

Radio is an intimate form of communication. Rates will vary depending on the program demographics of the listenership. Drive time means prime dollar rates because that is when radio gains its largest audience, but don't let that scare you off. Rates are negotiable. If radio fits into your budget, it can be very effective.

One very successful technique is to select one designated time for your commercial. My favorite was 7:20 or 7:50 A.M. or a time when my clients were driving home and still could stop by the salon. Use ear-stroking words when you create a radio ad, words that stimulate the ear and are pleasing. Use music judiciously, and always use a professional announcer. If the local DJs are doing voice-overs for commercial, only use them if they aren't saturated on the air already. Search for a voice that is easy to understand but distinctive.

Television and Cable

Television is a natural outlet for showcasing your services and products. The drawbacks are often the cost of big-city commercial production and air time. But depending on your city and location, you may be surprised at the rates. Shop around for the time period when potential customers will be viewing. Rates for 2:00 A.M. rates may be $10 for sixty seconds, but what busy, active woman regularly watches television at 2:00 A.M.? The most popular shows, of course, require a bigger bite of your budget. Some local stations can produce your spots, but ask to see a cassette of the station-creative first.

Check cable rates. Cable systems sometimes produce commercials for free when you sign an advertising schedule with them. I like the way cable can target your ten best customer base. Look into talk shows, soap operas, news programs. Viewers of special health and fashion shows already have some interest in looking better. Now, all you need to do is inform them of your business.

Yellow Pages

When potential clients are letting their fingers do the walking, you want your salon to be there under their fingers. I have found Yellow Pages ads either very successful or a total bust. Unfortunately, the only way to tell is to track the results for a year, which you should do with every medium anyway.

Here are some strategies to help your Yellow Pages ad pay off.

- Use size to your advantage. Analyze the size of the beauty ads in your local directory. If most are small, then try one size up from the norm.
- Use bold type and color to catch the eye. A splash of red? It will cost a tad more per month, but color could be the difference between scanning an ad and picking up the phone.
- Make sure your phone number is big and bold.
- Select type that is easy to read. Add some style with the typeface but don't sacrifice artistic design for readability.
- If your location is complicated to find, draw a map.
- Use a distinctive border around your ad space to define it from the others.

When the ad is ready to go to print, read every word and every letter in the word. This is an ad you will have to live with for twelve long months. You don't want a typo or wrong address.

Billboards

Billboards may fill the bill if you are new to the area or as a reminder that you are still in business. For billboards to be successful, keep these tips in sight.

- Before you sign a contract, jump in the car and drive by the locations under consideration. I feel bad for the poor person who bought a billboard off a key freeway in southern California leaving the Los Angeles airport. The problem is that there is a second, smaller billboard directly blocking the view and all you see is the boarder of the bigger billboard. Look into the lighting of the sign.

- Do you need the sign to be visible day and night? If so, you will need light bulbs.

- When you are designing copy for your board, keep the message short and sweet, six to seven words maximum. Remember, readers will be zipping by at fifty-five miles an hour.

Advertising Specialties

One way to get the word out is to distribute items like pens, pencils mirrors, baseball caps, tote bags, calendars, cosmetic bags, combs, brushes, T-shirts, sweatshirts, scratch pads. The items are printed with your business name, address, phone number, and slogan, if space allows. These give-aways should not be your advertising focus, but they can promote goodwill.

One of my favorite give-aways is a calendar for my best clients. The salon vitals are printed in gold on the cover. I was amazed the first year we handed them out. A good percentage of the clients stood at the reception desk and made standing appointments for the year on the spot. Of course, they put the dates right into their new pocket calendars.

Directing Direct Mail

Here are a few tips for making your direct mail campaign more successful.

- You will increase client response if the envelope is hand-addressed.

- Use commemorative stamps or multiple stamps to create attention. Instead of plopping on a basic stamp, try two or three that add up to the postage requirements.

- Once you have written your direct mail piece, review it. Is it the offer, service, product you would want if you were your salon's target customer? Is it exciting?

- Make sure you include your company name, address, and telephone number. I once received a postcard announcing the move of a something or other. I didn't have a clue as to who mailed the piece. There was no return address and no telephone number, just the map to the new location and the move date. What a waste!

Mailing Mania

Mailing lists are available for purchase if you desire to expand your current list. Look in the Yellow Pages under mailing list companies. With today's computers, you can have access to thousands of new people. You can buy addresses for people who have certain credit cards. You can buy selected zip codes, only swimming pool owners, only every other person who lives on the north side of the street. Lists are available for club members, sororities, professional association memberships. You name it, you can get a list for it. The fee for the lists is by the name and varies if you want it on computer disk, mailing labels, or for unlimited use. Check into adding a list for every big mailing you do. Rotate your mailing to see which group produces the best results. At the holidays, check into lists targeted to executives if you are doing a campaign for gift certificates.

CREATING AND PLACING THE AD

If you are the one-person agency for your salon's ads, here are a few tried-and-true tips for selling copy, powerful layouts, media placement, and dealing with advertising salespeople.

Talk to Me

Write to the reader as if you were talking to your best customer face to face. Unlike your publicity releases, you can keep this copy personal with plenty of second person pronouns. "You, You, You." Use everyday words; avoid industry jargon; make the piece easy to understand. If the client has to reach for a dictionary to decipher the copy, you have lost a potential customer.

The Balancing Act

Design your ads to stimulate both the left and right sides of the brain. Look for a balance between emotional words and factual, logical information. Forty-five percent of the population is left brain, 45 is right brain, and 10 percent is balanced.

Words That Sell

A group of psychologists at Yale University once identified key words that will increase the consumer's desire to buy. These words are: you, easy, money, safety, save, love, new, discovery, results, power, and health. I'll add to the list free, complimentary, benefits, now, and yes. Incorporate these words into your ads and salon literature. (See Appendix 2 for a complete list of words that sell.)

The Call to Action

Give the reader a reason to reply now. If you want the most for your money, you want the reader to do something. Tell her exactly what to do. Put a deadline on your offer. Invite her into the salon. "Stop by today to receive a sample of hand and body lotion." "Call the salon today to schedule your complimentary fall makeup consultation."

Critical Review

Select someone outside the industry to review all of your print pieces. When you work with a product or service every day, you know what you want to say, yet important facts can be accidentally left off. A fresh pair of eyes and ears may uncover a key point.

Lost Logo

Take time to reevaluate your type and logo every four years. Type styles can become dated. If you are following trends in fashion, color, art, and music, your salon pieces should tell the public that you are current and up-to-date. Depending on the overall style, you may just need to modify the basic look.

Go Co-Op

If you are stocking a major brand line, see if the manufacturer offers co-op advertising. Many companies will offer you a percentage of advertising dollars or product-credit that you can sell and make your money back. There are guidelines for qualifying. The manufacturer may specify the medium, the size of ad, the art, placement of the company logo, the items to be advertised, or the dates the ad can run. The company may even have targeted a specific area of the country for its co-op program. However if any other retailer in your city carries the line and is receiving co-op, you may well be entitled to it also. Co-op monies can also be used for display and special events.

Perfect Place Setting

Use repetition of ad style and placement for small budgets. One small card store next to the salon was successful with a business-card-size ad that appeared every day in the same location of the paper. The ad was highlighted with a special of the day. Good things can come in small packages.

Referral Requests

As a potential advertiser, you will be presented with possibilities that sound too good to be true. Check them out. Even ad rates that are relatively cheap can cost you money if you have chosen the wrong advertising vehicle. When you are contemplating a new ad buy, ask for a list of businesses that have advertised in the publication or on the station. You can also look in back publications for additional advertisers to contact. Look for businesses that would be trying to attract clients similar to yours and make some phone calls.

A Strategy for Salespeople

Once you have planned your advertising calendar, post the publications and stations you are planning to advertise with at the front desk. This working list can save you tons of time. If an unannounced ad salesperson from a competing publication drops in, your front desk person can request an advertising media kit. She will tell the caller that, after you have read the sales material, you will schedule an appointment if you want to know more.

In some salons, I have seen more advertising salespeople walk through the door than clients. Guard your advertising plan and your valuable service time.

Planning Your Future

You will not only be investing your money in an advertising program but also your time. You may have heard that proper planning prevents poor performance. Schedule an appointment with yourself. Allow plenty of uninterrupted think time. If you take the time up-front to plan your advertising and marketing schedule, you will save yourself future aggravation. (See Figure 20.1 on the following pages for a sample Promotion Calendar form.)

PROMOTION CALENDAR

PROMOTION:_____

PROMOTION GOAL:_____

THEME:_____

_____

TARGET DATE:_____

PRODUCT OR SERVICE FEATURED: _____

_____

BUDGET:_____

INTERNAL MARKETING SELECTED:

_____Point of Purchase   _____Tent cards

_____Posters   _____Banners

_____Feature displays   _____Handouts

_____Signage   _____Flyers

_____Telemarketing

EXTERNAL MARKETING SELECTED

_____Direct Mail

_____Print Ads

          Placement in_____

          Placement in_____

          Placement in_____

_____Billboards

          Location_____

          Location_____

Fig. 20.1   Promotion calendar.

_____TV

    Station_____

    Schedule_____

_____Radio

    Station_____

    Schedule_____

_____Distribution of flyers

_____Group Programs

    Target_____

_____Notices

_____Press Releases

    Publication_____

    Publication_____

    Publication_____

PRINTING REQUIREMENTS:

_____

_____

_____

_____

SUPPLIES NEEDED:

_____

_____

_____

_____

Fig 20.1.

ADDITIONAL INVENTORY REQUIRED FOR PROMOTION:

Product_____

Order Date_____

Delivery Date_____

STAFF ASSIGNMENTS:

Person	Responsibility	Due Date	Follow Up
_____	_____	_____	_____
_____	_____	_____	_____
_____	_____	_____	_____

SUPPORT STAFF:

Person	Responsibility	Due Date	Follow Up
_____	_____	_____	_____
_____	_____	_____	_____
_____	_____	_____	_____

Fig 20.1.

PROMOTIONS

Many business owners want to create special promotions and activities for their business. Unfortunately think time is a rare commodity. Many owners and managers don't have the creative time to come up with tons of ideas and concepts. In this chapter you will find seventy-six different opportunities for increasing your sales. Even established salons need a little shot in the arm, a boost in sales and excitement. Use the ideas as presented or simply use parts of them to create your own plan of action.

Please remember that these promotional ideas are brought to life through all the textbook activities: publicity, advertising, display, special events, and fashion shows. And remember to keep your ideas simple, keep the customers' needs and desires in sight.

FIFTY-SEVEN BUSINESS BUILDERS

1. Makeover Contest

Have clients and potential customers submit photos and letters explaining what they would like to change about their appearance and why they want to have a makeover. Select numerous candidates to undergo the transformation. Make sure you have a photographer on hand to capture the moments. Tie in your makeover contest with a local talk show.

Some possible makeover categories are:

- Mothers-to-be
- New Mothers
- Teens

- College-to-Career
- Working Women
- Sweet Sixteen
- Over-40-and-Fabulous
- Sizzling and Stylish at 60
- Active Athlete
- A Family Affair
- Best Friends
- Mother-Daughter
- Graduation
- Men

The client receives a free gift item (preferably a retail product) with a required minimum purchase. Free travel product with full size works great.

3. Purchase with Purchase

Customers are able to buy a special promotional item at reduced savings. Some companies have used umbrellas, tote bags, trial sizes of products, gym bags, cosmetic bags, clocks, or watches. Make sure that your promotional items are every bit as wanted as those the department store offers.

4. Free-lipstick Cards

The customer may receive a complimentary lipstick with any $15 minimum purchase. The lipstick card is an ideal promotional item to distribute after making a presentation to a group of consumers. Try to keep the minimum purchase to a minimum

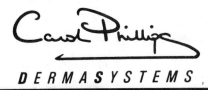

A Special Offer From Carol Phillips

Exchange this card for a complimentary tube of our luscious lipstick with any $15 purchase from the Carol Phillips collection.

DERMASYSTEMS

Fig. 21.1   Free lipstick card.

to create foot traffic for the business. A free lipstick offer entices women to walk into your salon. (Fig. 21.1)

5. Yearly Coupon Card

The object of this promotion card is to establish consistent retail traffic. In order for customers to redeem the coupon for the free gift, they must first make a minimum $25 retail (not service) purchase during the month. The base retail purchase requirement is beneficial for two reasons:

- Once the client starts to enjoy the free gift each month, she becomes accustomed to a little extra present at the end of each visit. Many clients will budget for their minimum requirement and systematically plan to restock their products monthly so they can take advantage of the coupon offer. It is fun for the client to go home with a little treasure.

- The minimum works great as an add-on sales builder. Say the client has selected a few products, but is not up to the $25 level. The salesperson is then in a perfect spot to rec-

ommend, "You are close to receiving the free monthly gift from the salon. What else are you needing today so that we can send Product XYZ home with you?"

Select twelve items you would like to feature for the year. One card is printed annually with twelve windows, one for each month, featuring the selected product, the face value of the item, and the coupon expiration date. You could also break it down and mail the coupon cards quarterly for client contact. Mailing four times a year gives you the flexibility for changing your product selection and features.

In my salon, we would consistently redeem between 125 and 175 coupons a month. Those coupons would generate at least $3,125–$4,375 in additional monthly retail sales. (Fig. 21.2)

6. Free Service with Service

Getting your customers to cross-merchandise to other services is critical. Try offering a complimentary manicure for every new facial customer or a body polish with a full leg waxing service.

Use your imagination to create other cross-overs, but be responsible on your cost of service. Check into your cost per service before you start giving away the farm. Free service with service is ideal for a new staff member that has a special talent and unfortunately lots of available time.

Try a service with service using another but complimenting business. For example, a free wardrobe consultation (using an outside image consultant) with any makeover package.

7. Product of the Month

Select one product to be highlighted each month. Allow for extra display space and have fact sheets on the product available for the client to read. Coordinate your efforts with seasonal activities. For example, feature hand and body lotion when the weather turns cold and it becomes necessary to turn on the heat, resulting in chapped hands.

8. Start a Teen Board

Many department stores have recruited local high school students to serve as advisors and models. Telephone, telegraph, and tell-a-teen is a great way to spread the word about your business to a growing market that spends millions of dollars each year on beauty products. If your salon is located in a mall, speak to the marketing manager about the cosponsorship of a teen board. Offer to do makeovers on the teens and have their photos taken. The mall will use the photos for its promotion and you can use the photos for your promotion and publicity.

9. Out to Lunch

Call and invite three clients out to lunch, brunch, or dinner. Mix new clients with your long-term customers. Select a restaurant that is a popular spot among your customers. Networking among your clientele is a super way to solidify continued business. It pays to be seen.

I was out to lunch with three of my customers when I spotted another table of women staring in our direction. The women would lean in, talk secretly in hushed voices, then turn and refer to our table. Well, I didn't think too much about it until I walked back into the salon. I was amazed to see the three mystery women from the restaurant sitting at the makeup counter being helped by two of our staff members. Makeup

January 96	February 96
Lipstick	*Mascara*
Value – $7.50*	Value – $7.50*
Expires 1/31/96	Expires 2/28/96
March 96	April 96
Nail Polish	*Shampoo*
Value – $7.50*	Value – $8.50*
Expires 3/31/96	Expires 4/30/96
May 96	June 96
Custom Blended Base	*Eye Shadow*
$5.00 Off**	Value – $9.00*
Expires 5/31/96	Expires 6/30/96
July 96	August 96
Lipstick	*Herbal Mist*
Value – $7.50*	Value – $9.00*
Expires 7/31/96	Expires 8/31/96
September 96	October 96
Facial Masque	*Travel Hair Kit*
Value – $13.00*	Value – $9.00*
Expires 9/30/96	Expires 10/31/96
November 96	December 96
Eye or Lip Pencil	*Compact Powder*
Value – $7.50*	Value – $9.50*
Expires 11/30/96	Expires 12/31/96

*$25.00 minimum purchase required

**No minimum purchase required

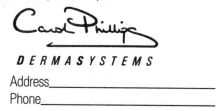

D E R M A S Y S T E M S

Address_____

Phone_____

Fig. 21.2 Yearly coupon card.

was everywhere—all over the counter and all over the three laughing ladies. As I was standing there aghast at the sight, one of the women came over and announced that she had been meaning to come in for months and months and just never got around to it. "Then when I saw you today at the restaurant," she added, "I made up my mind to visit the salon, then my two friends wanted to come. I hope you don't mind." Mind! Of course not! My receipt for the luncheon was $32.95, the three new customers' tab was over $400. I'd say it pays to get out for lunch.

10. Update Your Biography

Take time out to update your biography every six months if you are professionally active. You never know when the press will call and request a copy. Design two styles—one appropriate for tagging articles and photos you have contributed and one detailed biography for your press kit.

11. Schedule a New Press Photo

Call your local photographer and set sometime aside to have a new press photo taken. Have at least twenty-five extra copies made for your press kits. I took a tip from an actor friend and am now having my name, company name, and phone number printed on the bottom of the photo. For the best reprint rates, look in entertainment industry publications. Some companies will reproduce your photos for as little as $69 per hundred.

12. Survival Break

Try a campaign for those clients who need to get away from it all—no work, no kids, no phone, no problem! Half-day packages work best. Offer a haircut, facial, manicure, body massage, makeup application, and remember the cappuccino. A full-day package can be a difficult commitment for working people. Half-days are easier to sneak into their hectic schedules.

13. Body Basics

Schedule your clients for a one-hour body polishing treatment. Offer a special home care gift that includes body scrub, lotion, cleanser, and a loofah. Body basics are ideal for midwinter and after-summer fun in the sun.

14. Hire an Outside Makeup Artist

Bring in an outside makeup artist for three days of makeup lessons and applications. These events help stimulate media interest in the business as well as generate additional makeup sales. Besides, an expert is someone that lives more than fifty miles from you.

15. Men Only

Select one day or evening where your business is open to men only. One lingerie store is reported to keep all women out three nights prior to Valentine's Day so that the men feel more relaxed about shopping in the store. Men can let their guard down if they know others are standing nearby. There seems to be strength in numbers.

16. Save Those Receipts

Maria Minton, Maria Minton Paragon, Charlottesville, Virginia, gave me this idea. Have your clients save their receipts and when they total say $200, the customer is entitled to a gift certificate worth $25. The clients are responsible for accumulating their receipts and keeping tabs on the total. Give them a special printed envelope for stashing their receipts.

17. Makeover Packages

Design three different packages, Minimakeover, Maximakeover, and Head-to-toe makeover. Different price point packages allow more clients to get into the makeover magic.

Minimakeover: Lifestyle consultation, makeup lessons, hair cut and style.

Maximakeover: Lifestyle consultation, skin analysis, facial, makeup lessons, manicure, haircut, perm, and color.

Head-to-toe makeover: Lifestyle consultation, computer makeover, skin analysis, two facials, two makeup lessons, manicure, pedicure, hand reconditioning, haircut, perm and color, products for hair ($30 value).

18. Bridal Registry

Brides-to-be select services and products they would like to receive. Keep a registration list at the front desk. Gift-givers can select from her list or contribute to a full-day beauty package. This is a great idea for personal shower gifts.

19. Bride Packages
Put together a complete beauty program for the bride. Facials, manicures, pedicure, hair styling, photography makeup session, makeup application for the big day—all for one package price. Don't overlook the mother of the bride. Coordinate a mother-daughter bridal special.

20. Beautiful Brides on Location
Many salons are taking their services to the bride the day of the wedding. Rates vary but many are charging an hourly rate with a two-hour minimum. Remember that most weddings are on Saturday, your biggest in-salon moneymaking day, so charge accordingly.

21. Bridal Fairs
Check with local radio and television stations for their schedule of events. Bridal fairs allow you to exhibit your business and possibly become involved in the fashion show production. Don't get trapped in the work room.

22. Gem of an Idea
Give the owner or manager of a local fine jewelry store complimentary manicure gift certificates. The participating jewelry store distributes the gift certificate when a ring of an established size or dollar amount is purchased. The jewelry store creates goodwill because the gift certificate is technically from them, and you obtain a new customer. The client is happy with a new ring, and beautiful hands and nails to show it off.

23. Organize Display Schedule
Change your displays regularly. If your customer revisit cycle is every four weeks, change your displays every three. Outline the themes you want to implement for the year. Plan your work and work your plan.

24. Series Sale
Select one month within the year when you discount your treatment series. Special price incentives and treatment series lock your clients into your business. Salon owner Diane Young claims that she does 80 percent of her yearly business in thirty days. The additional revenues that are generated during the sale are put to work in moneymaking bank accounts. Wouldn't

it be fantastic to have almost your year's revenues ahead of time? You could put the money to work for you.

25. Group Programs
Select twenty-four groups that you would like to target. Two consumer programs a month are excellent ways to recruit new clients. Make sure that you follow up with the attendants either by phone or mail within seventy-two hours after the program.

26. Service with a Friend
Invite your current clients to bring in a new friend to your business. The new client and your regular customer receive 20 percent off the tab.

27. Sneak a Peek
Mail out invitations to your preferred customers and invite them in to preview the season's newest products and trends, before you show the masses. Your preferred clients are allowed to sneak peek twice a year, with the fall and spring collections.

28. Buy One, Get One Free
This one is pretty self-explanatory.

29. Buy One, Get the Second for a Penny
Or a nickel, or a quarter, or a dollar.

30. Mystery Envelopes
One of my favorite stores sponsors a mystery envelope promotion every year. The store's customers are mailed a sealed envelope with a card enclosed for 10–90 percent off. The envelope must be presented unopened to the clerk when the client checks out. The clerk opens the envelope and awards the designated percentage discount on the purchase.

31. Gift Certificates
These should be displayed year around. Frame several certificates and display them through your business. Gift certificates should have a short expiration date (two to three months). The short cycle nudges the recipients into action to redeem the gift before the certificate is stuffed in some dresser drawer. Of course, you can always extend the expiration date if necessary.

32. Career Looks

Circulate flyers among graduating high school and college students. Start your promotion around March. Many students will be looking for a change in appearance and can then request gift certificates from your business as graduation presents. Don't forget to promote the offer in the school's newspaper, which often has affordable ad rates.

33. Giveaways

Radio stations look for gifts that can be given to listeners in exchange for on-air promotions. Donating your product and services is an easy way to get your name out over the airwaves without buying advertising time.

34. Fund Raisers

Your company's services and products make for exciting gifts as door prizes, auction items, and school raffles. Make a list of organizations that you are willing to support for the year and the total dollar amount you are willing to contribute. This master list will help the front desk weed out solicitation phone calls.

35. Frame and Display

Mount all newspaper and magazine articles that have featured you and/or your business. Make copies of the articles that are appropriate for distributing to your clients. Display current articles near the reception desk or cash register. Framed articles proudly displayed on the walls are definitely better business builders than framed artwork.

36. Birthday Cards

Sending clients birthday cards lets them know you are thinking of them. Some people don't like to be reminded, but cards help to trigger the thought, "Well I am getting older, I need to get in to the salon."

37. Back to School (for Faculty)

Mail a special invitation to teachers offering them an incentive to visit your company before school starts. Mail the letters to the school, for most teachers have to report days and weeks ahead of the students. Most back-to-school promotions only offer special savings to the students. Make teachers an offer for their return to the blackboard jungle.

38. Discount Baskets

If you have dead inventory that you want to sell before you have to dust it again, dump it into a bargain basket. For some unknown reason, people like to rummage through things for secret or hidden treasures. If you don't believe me try driving past a few garage sales or flea markets this summer.

39. Have Card, Will Promote

Hand out your business cards everywhere. Leave your card with your tip at a restaurant. Hand one to your bank teller. Put a card in all your local mail. I have even handed them to women that looked like they could be my customers and said, "You women look so good, I would be honored to have you as my customers. Here is my card."

40. A Little Bird Told Me

If your client drops a hint that she would really love to have someone treat her to a certain service, mail a note with the saying, "A little bird told me that . . ." and state the request from your client. Some spouses have even called and ordered the gift over the phone and thanked us for sending the note. They had wanted to do something special but didn't have the foggiest idea what.

41. Wish List

At holiday time hand your clients a wish list form to fill out. They highlight the service, product, size, treatment, color—whatever they would like to receive as a gift. The form has a place for clients to reveal their Santa's name and address. Mail a copy of the wish list to the Santa with a personal note on hassle-free holiday shopping. Clients are delighted that they might actually receive gifts they want.

42. Get Involved in One New Organization

Networking with others in the community can be a great source of information as well as new clients. Select the group carefully and make sure it matches your goals or your ten best list.

43. Reach Out and Touch Someone

Select one day a week that you call several of your clients. Find out how they are doing with the products, new look, or new job or just keep in touch. How many phone calls have you received from someone saying they just called to tell you that they appreciate your business? A short and to-the-point courtesy call can do wonders to anchor clients to your business.

44. Fragrant Bouquet of Success

Weed out a local flower shop and have it send flowers to new, old, sick, and/or promoted clients. A simple bud vase with unusual flowers will do the trick.

Check to see if the florist will discount because of volume or, better yet, donate the expense. The main benefit for the florist is the promotional value of having your clients talking about the gorgeous bouquet that arrived today from XYZ Floral Shop. Think about the office hubbub that is created when fresh, beautiful flowers arrive for you or someone on your staff.

45. Calendar Gifts

During the holidays, give your preferred clients a personal calendar/date book. These can be purchased through an advertising specialty company or local stationery store. Invest in the style that can be imprinted with your company logo and address on the cover. You can even have special monthly stickers made and attached within the calendar redeemable throughout the coming year.

46. Sponsor a Wardrobe/Clothing Seminar

This can be a one day or evening program that focuses on clothing and style. A wardrobe seminar is the perfect opportunity to tie in the beauty business with clothing, accessory, shoe, and jewelry stores. Pool your mailing lists and split the promotional investment with the other merchants.

47. Quarterly Newsletter or Flyer

Make contact with your customers at least every ninety days. Produce a newsletter that informs the client how to do something or features new products and services. The newsletter can be elaborate or simple, but make it informative. (Fig. 21.3)

48. Gift Baskets

Around the holidays, many grocery and floral shops set up a build-your-own-basket promotion. Why not make it available year-round? A few simple supplies and all you need.

49. Spoil Yourself in Grand Style

Take the full-day pamper package and add a few outrageous activities. Schedule your client to be chauffeured to the salon in a stretch limousine. Have hot coffee in the car and her favorite newspaper waiting. At the salon, have a monogrammed, snuggy bathrobe or gown waiting and warm. Take her through your normal beauty rituals. Have roses delivered during the day for the client.

At the conclusion of the salon day, the limousine whisks the pampered person to a private hotel or bed and breakfast inn where the spouse (or significant other) is waiting with chilled champagne and hors d'oeuvres. Establish your price for the day taking into account all the extras. Set a flat fee for everything—the beauty services, hotel, flowers, limousine. You might be pleasantly surprised at the Grand Style takers. This also makes a great publicity release for the "Ultimate Christmas Gift," but be sure to send it to the paper's lifestyle editor by Thanksgiving so that he/she can include it in the annual gift round-up.

50. Movers and Shakers

Read through the local newspaper with a fine-tooth comb. Keep your eye out for people who have been promoted or honored in some way. Clip the article, have it laminated and enclose a congratulations note and a gift certificate for service or product. A warm recognition from your company could just fill your business with movers and shakers from the community.

51. Styling Classes

Schedule a monthly styling class for your customers. The class teaches clients ways to dry, style, and finish their hair at home. Show them how they can change their look. Set up the sessions so clients can learn hair accessorizing with professional guidance. Many clients love the way they look when they leave the salon only to become frustrated and furious when they try to repeat the look the next day. Supplies to have on hand are note paper, pins, styling aids, tools, stations for each of the clients, a flip chart, mannequins, markers, and hair accessories.

52. Trade In and Trade Up

Women are notorious for stashing half-used tubes, bottles, and jars of beauty products. Here's a promotion idea that's

Touch Sponge

Powder Brush

Carol Phillips
DERMASYSTEMS

Beauty News and Views

Fall & Winter

Notes from Carol...

Carol Phillips and staff have been on the move again. On a recent trip to Chicago, Angie Vaughn, Patricia Heald and I attended the Federation of American Aesthetics Congress. We spent several days in the other windy city fulfilling my commitment to you and to our staff, to constantly offer the latest in treatments and products available. One portion of the program during the FAE Congress was an exam for accrediting facialists on an international level. Both Angie and Patricia have spent long hard hours reviewing for the written, oral and practical examination. It was confirmed that Angie passed her certification, making Carol Phillips DermaSystems the only salon in the United States to have more than one current certified aesthetician. I passed the exam in New Orleans in 1982. To date only 13 people have successfully completed the testing. Patricia's results are not yet in but we are confident that there will be three AIACA's to serve you at Carol Phillips DermaSystems. Congratulations to both.

This Fall and Winter are going to be very exciting at Carol Phillips DermaSystems. We have many new services to share with you and many outstanding products. If you have not yet been into the salon, I would like to personally invite you to drop in and see what we are all about. You will be pleasantly surprised.

A heartfelt thank you goes out to all of our customers for your continued support. I look forward to seeing you soon. Remember that I am standing behind every product or service one hundred percent.

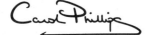

Carol Phillips

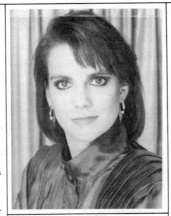

Under Make Up Texturizer

Under make up texturizer is a whole new category of make up that speaks to women at every age. Texturizers are neither make up nor treatments for the skin, but a step in between the two that helps to smooth the skin, diminish tiny imperfections, minimize lines and even wrinkles.

Under make up texturizer is a light clear liquid that should be used over your moisturizer and under your foundation. It cushions in between the two. Everyone of our customers, young or mature, oily or dry, will enjoy the smooth appearance under make up texturizer gives their foundation.

To apply your texturizer, dot several drops over your day-time conditioner. Blend lightly over the complexion, avoiding the eye area, and then dot your custom blended foundation on. Blend as usual.

You will notice a smooth make up appearance and the satiny sheen as your foundation takes on.

INDIGO
The Paisley Colors of the Desert at Sunset

Pima, Comanche, Apache, Navajo, Youque are just a few of the Indian Tribes that live on the American Deserts. They give us their traditional colors which were conceived as they watched the sunset strike out the bright, hot shadings of day. Their brocades and paisleys in intense teals, reds, oranges and purples transcend now to us as we create the FASHION LOOK FOR FALL.

These are the colors and moods seen by our ancestors as they crossed the American Deserts — the Rich Brick, Wedgewood Blues, Frosted Champagnes, Salmons, Apricots, Teals and Purples used in THE FALL FASHION STORY.

In the winter, the sun sets early, its chilly rays illuminating the San Francisco Peaks, powerfully printed in black against the dove grey sky.

All is chilled, and the pearly smudge of sun gives no more warmth than a flashlight.

The autumn sun descends behind the jagged mountains of the desert like a heavy, red ball. The earth seems almost to tremble in a serenade of shadows as soft purple images and streaks of sunlight are left glittering through and across the plains. Soon the sun will be slowly rising again towards the summits in tones of champagne, banana, salmon, and wedgewood blues.

Now, the vanishing sun scowls its signature across the western sky in sizzling raisin tones, wines and cranberries, and before its final disappearance, it takes a last breath with glints and halos of gold, pale green, bone, violet, peach. The sun breathes a last sigh of relief, and a peacock blue tail sears across the sky and is gone.

The earth is left in night — sunset renders an aura of control, mystery and drama. We are so fortunate to be in the land of an unending horizon, allowing us to experience the bold sunrises and soothing sunsets to their fullest.

1

Fig. 21.3   Newsletter.

bound to please your customers. The client brings in any half-used bottles or jars of products and receives 25 percent off every new item. (Fig. 21.4) If she trades in five items, she can select five new items. The real kicker is to put the old products in a clear container with a subtle sign stating "Products our clients used to use." You may even want to purchase a few competitive brands, rough them up, and then stuff them in the basket.

I shared this promotion with Mark Lees of Pensacola, Florida. He opted to offer only a 10 percent discount. Needless to say I received a phone call telling me he was overwhelmed at the response—$10,000 in retail sales for the month. Twelve months later he repeated the trade in and trade up offer and broke the bank with $19,000 in retail sales!

53. Silver System Bonus Card

Clients become "members" of your business. For a flat fee they are entitled to special privileges. The one I set up for the salon offered two sneak-a-peek previews, a free facial the month of their birthday (they pay for one and get the second one in the same birthday month free), 10 percent discount on all skin products, and after completing six monthly facials they were entitled to a free body massage or body facial every six months. Their Silver System card was valid for one year and was $75 dollars. (Fig. 21.5)

54. Bonus Dollars

Diane Narron, Hair Flair, Raleigh, North Carolina, shared this idea she uses for retaining clients. "One offer we make to our good clients is that with every $50 ticket the client receives a $5 coupon that can be used for other services."

55. Frequent Customer Cards

Good salon clients receive a gold card entitling them to receive free services or discounts on products. The promotion awards regular faithful customers with a gift incentive. One idea is to give top customers a gift certificate to an outstanding restaurant. Try to select one a little out of the way (they have to plan and set aside time for the special event).

56. Gift Gifts

Give your customers gift certificates for $5–$10. The gift certificate is made out for a friend or associate of the client. You're really giving the certificate to your customer and she will then give it to a potential customer.

57. Corporate Memberships

Robert Narrone from Salon du Jour, Margate, New Jersey, uses this promotion as a way to build volume sales. "I look for unique businesses in our area with twenty to thirty employees. I'll offer each employee a personal Salon du Jour membership card. The card entitles the employees to 20 percent off products or services—anything in the salon. The membership card is honored for one year. The customers present their personalized card any weekday to receive the membership discount."

UNIQUE AND UNUSUAL PROMOTIONAL THEMES

Following is a collection of unique and unusual promotional ideas and themes. You'll see some old-time favorites but with a new twist. Spice up your business. Create excitement and sales by throwing a theme promotion campaign. Use them as is or modify the ideas to match your business. You will find a theme, the description, and a suggested prop list.

1. Christmas in July

Deck the halls in July. Stage a festive celebration in the middle of summer. Trim the tree. Feature early shopping bonuses. Free gift wrapping (Christmas paper, of course). Serve up the eggnog and a little holiday cheer midyear. Who says you can't have the Christmas spirit year-round?

Prop list: tree, lights, ornaments, tinsel, stocking, Santa and his sleigh, mistletoe, wrapped packages under the tree, holiday potpourri.

2. Lincoln's Birthday

Honest Abe sale. Have clients look to your business for tall savings on this president's birthday. "An Honest to Goodness Sale."

Sample Mailer

Our Copy

For the first time ever, I am inviting you to try my very exciting and special makeup collection with a unique offer.

I challenge you to clean out those boxes and drawers of "can't-wear cosmetics" and bring them to Carol Phillips DermaSystems. For each brand name item you bring in, I will personally give you 25% off any selection you make from the Carol Phillips Cosmetic Collection.

For some, luxury is a bare necessity.

You deserve to have the very best products available and exceptional service at the same time. Why wait?

For 25 days only, you can get 25% off. Starts Jan. 15–Feb. 12.

Here's to a beautiful year—

Your signature here

Fig. 21.4   Trade in and trade up.

_____

is a member of our

SILVERSYSTEM

and receives the following
privileges and services:

- **Private Champagne Showings**
  - Seasonal trends in make-up design
  - Previews of new Carol Phillips cosmetics
- **Birthday Facial Free**
- **10% Savings on Carol Phillips Skin Cleansing Products**
- **SILVERSYSTEM Bonus**
  - After six monthly facials, you receive complimentary Body Facial **or** Body Massage. Two bonuses are possible per each year's membership.

Approved _____

Expirationo Date _____

Jan	Feb	Mar	Apr	May	Jun	Jul	Aug	Sep	Oct	Nov	Dec

Fig. 21.5 Silver system card.

Prop list: replicas of log cabins, stovepipe hat, map of Illinois, Gettysburg Address on parchment paper, Lincoln Memorial.

3. President's Birthday

Sometime in February the nation celebrates the birth of two outstanding leaders in American history: George Washington and Abe Lincoln. Mail special invitations to outstanding leaders in your community. Invite them in to visit your business and receive a complimentary service or gift along with a big slice of cherry pie.

Prop list: cherry blossom flowers, three-cornered hat, stovepipe hat, hatchet, copies of the Declaration of Independence and Gettysburg Address, and of course, the cherry pie.

4. April in Paris

In springtime, the heart turns to flights of fancy and romance. What could be more romantic than April in Paris? Feature a fashion show with French looks. Serve cappuccino and croissants to the clients. Highlight Parisian looks and attitudes.

Prop list: the Eiffel Tower, French music, French designer accessories, silk scarves, perfume, Moulin Rouge posters.

5. Life's a Beach

Sand, sun, and soaring temperatures. Highlight fun-in-the-sun-looks. Team up matching products to help protect the hair, skin, and body. Distribute "Life's a Beach" flyers featuring easy-to-wear looks and protection tips.

Prop list: sand, bucket, little shovel, umbrella, sunglasses, paperbacks, suntan lotion, beach balls.

6. Halloween

Play dress-up. Schedule appointments for clients to have their hair and makeup styled at the salon. Have them bring their costumes and change right there in the facilities. Talk about a total transformation. Ghoulish ghosts and gremlin makeovers.

Halloween is the perfect time to showcase your artistic talents. Hairstyles can run the gamut from fancy to fright night. Showcasing your talents leaves the impression that you also offer special occasion services.

Prop list: ghosts, gremlins, goblins, pumpkins, colored leaves, trick-or-treat bags, candy jars, spiders, webs, and haunting music.

7. Manager's Special

Oops! We goofed. The manager ordered too many XYZ Products. Save money on our overstock. Help! We don't have room to store all this product for three months. We made the mistake, but we're willing to pass along substantial savings to you.

Prop list: memo pad, visor, accountant arm band, dolly with crates of product, wheelbarrow, brown bags.

8. The Boss is Away

The last thing that Mary Sue said before she left for vacation was, "Don't give away the store." While the boss is away, who knows how much fun we'll have? Enjoy extra big savings on

XYZ. While the cat's away, the mice will play. Join us for wine and cheese on Thursday at 7:00 P.M. Signed: The Mice

Prop list: suitcase, vacation stickers, "gone fishin'" signs, fake mousetraps, cheese, wine, crackers, photos of the boss with a scarf covering the photo, suitcases.

9. Secretary's Week

April is the one time out of the year when these office troupers are recognized. Secretaries are the backbone of American businesses. Tell bosses about your nine-to-five beauty day. Plan a full day revitalizing package for secretaries—no phone, no fax, no boss.

Each year the floral industry is the only business that regularly promotes Secretary's Day. It shouldn't come as any surprise that every secretary I spoke to this year received a plant or flowers in honor of Secretary's Day.

Prop list: typewriter, stenographer pad, phone, file folders, phone message pad, noose, and a mannequin tied to the chair.

10. Valentine's Day

Roses are red, violets are blue, I care enough to send you to (your salon). Every client on Valentine's Day receives a long-stemmed red rose from the company. The holder of this gift certificate is entitled to receive (service).

Prop list: hearts, lace, candy, cards, balloons, all red and white, and, of course, roses.

11. Island Days

Come back to Jamaica. If your clients can't escape to the islands in the dead of winter, bring the islands to them. If you are still offering tanning services in the salon, invite the clients in for a tropical tan in January.

Prop list: print shirts and shorts, tropical drinks with the little umbrellas, steel drum music, sand, island hats, bird of paradise flowers.

12. An All-American Special

Baseball, hot dogs, and apple pie. Feature American beauty looks and fashions. Born in the U.S.A. styles and shapes. Set up displays that show you are proud to be an American. Try a tie-in with the local beauty pageant, or sponsor a softball team.

Prop list: picnic baskets; flags; family photos; fireworks posters; anything red, white, and blue; beauty pageant banners.

13. Fourth of July

Support your local community Fourth of July celebrations. Sponsor a float, join in the parade. Take the staff on a picnic.

Prop list: red, white, and blue banners; Uncle Sam posters; flags; straw hats; U.S.A. paraphernalia.

14. World Series

The World Series of 1989 really shook things up when the big quake hit San Francisco. Shake things up around your business with a little baseball excitement. If it is legal in your state, organize a baseball pool with proceeds going to your favorite charity.

Prop list: baseball cards, bats, gloves, hats, jerseys, T-shirts, popcorn, hot dogs, organ music, baseball diamonds, score cards, programs.

15. We're Seeing Red

Feature all products and accessories that are the color red. Target lip, nail, and cheek colors. Tie in your theme by having the staff wear red clothes.

Props: Red brushes, combs, blowers, mirrors, poker chips, scarves, flowers, checker board, Chinese pottery.

16. Anniversary

Eighty percent of all new businesses fail within the first five years. Every year you remain in business is a reason to celebrate. Your festivities could be as simple or as elaborate as you desire. But do celebrate your special day.

Invite your long-time clients in to star in your own company video production. Set up the video camera and have them come in for interviews. Interview them about how they came to find out about your business, how their looks have changed over the years, funny stories they have about you and the staff. This video capsule will be a wonderful treat to play back and watch if you are having "one of those days."

Prop list: cake, celebration, stickers, streamers, bells, memorabilia of days gone by, old photos of the staff and clients, before and after of any business renovation, video camera, blank tapes, lights.

17. Grand Opening

You've decided to participate in the American dream of owning your own business. It's time to celebrate. Schedule your grand opening three to six months after you've opened your doors. Give yourself the opportunity to work out all the kinks and time to put up the finishing touches on the merchandising. Grand opening ideas could be celebrity tie-ins, live radio remote broadcast, a charity benefit, stylathon with proceeds going to your favorite charity, a ribbon cutting ceremony, blessings of the business for staff and clients.

Prop list: a fake key to the city, champagne bottles, streamers, banners, ribbons.

18. Fashion Shows

Fashion shows can include everything from informal modeling to full-scale fashion productions to wardrobe seminars. Fashion shows are hard work and are often time consuming. It's one thing to lend a helping hand, but make it worth your while. Make sure you get more than just a mere mention in the program. Insist on at least ten minutes of stage time to showcase your talents. If possible, commentate the fashion show. Maximize your exposure.

Prop list: your personal well-organized travel kit, also include masking tape, extra extension cord, AC adapters, three-prong plugs, hand mirrors, clips, pins, tissues, towels, high-backed stools to save your back, business cards, any business literature you want to distribute, and model release forms.

19. Discounts

After taking an informal poll of some salon owners across the country, I found that the practice of discounting falls into two distinct camps. Camp one offers discounts only when they want to build up business in another service area. Camp two offers absolutely, positively no discounts. Several of the salon owners felt that on Tuesday it would cost the same amount to give the XYZ service as it would on discount day. They felt that reducing the rate cheapened the perceived value of the service. One owner from New Jersey said, "I would rather treat the client to a complete complimentary service than discount the price."

Before you swing to one camp or the other, first take a look at your customer base. Is your business set up as a specialty store or as a commodity salon?

Note: None of the salon owners I spoke with ever discounted products. One owner said she would "only if the manufacturer and/or distributor made her an unbeatable offer." I'm not saying they're wrong but what if you had a better markup due to manufacturer's incentives, shrewd buying, terms, staff incentives? Could retailing product be discounted to generate additional revenues versus discounting labor intensive services?

CHAPTER 22

PERSONAL SUCCESS

Congratulations! You have made it through. Now all we need to cover is the information that relates to your personal success. The previous information will only prove beneficial if you have the drive and determination to see the tips and techniques through to completion.

In this chapter we will put the finishing touches on your successful progression into selling success. I saved this chapter for last because you are the critical factor in achieving success. All of the information you have learned through this book will grow or die on the vine. It all comes down to your commitment and determination to implement the information.

This chapter is devoted to you. The daily pace you keep is either supporting your success goals or undermining your true potential. In this chapter we will go over key areas for living a successful, productive life.

UNLIMITED POTENTIAL

Attitude and Altitude

The heights you wish to reach are within your grasp. The only thing standing between where you are and where you desire to be is your attitude. However, there is more to building a successful attitude than simply maintaining a positive one. Events that happen in your life first appear in thought form. Guard your thoughts at all times. That nagging, negative voice is determined to sabotage your future success. Head those thoughts off at the pass. Don't give that voice the least bit of room in your thoughts. When you do hear a negative shout or whisper, rephrase the voice into a positive, constructive thought. "Why

bother with Mrs. So and So. You know she will never change her look. Don't waste your breath." Rephrase the doom-and-gloom voice. Give it something to chew on. "Mrs. So and So is coming in today. I am confident she will be receptive to my suggestions for her beauty routine. Today she will readily accept my professional advice and recommendation."

If you doubt that your thoughts are that powerful, have you ever thought of a client you haven't seen in a while and she called you later in the day? How about the time when you told yourself that you needed to get up at a specific time, and you woke up without the aid of the alarm clock? Your mind is incredibly sensitive to suggestions.

One Mind, Two Divisions

Your own mind has two unique divisions; the conscious mind and the subconscious mind. The conscious mind is responsible for your reasoning and cogitative thought. The conscious mind is the choosing center of the brain. This is where you choose the books you read, the house you live in, the clothes you wear, even the person with whom you spend your life. The conscious mind reads the world through the five senses. This part of the brain evaluates your world by tuning into the sight, sound, taste, touch, and smell.

The subconscious mind is the receptive center of the brain. The body's automatic functions are controlled by the subconscious. Thankfully, you don't have to remember to pump blood through your heart. Your body does it for you through the aid of the subconscious mind. The truly mystical occurrence is that the subconscious mind does not evaluate or judge right from wrong. It just absorbs thoughts. The law of nature says that if you plant apple seeds you will grow apples. There is no way in the world that if you plant appleseeds you will grow pumpkins. If the seeds you are planting in the sub-conscious mind are ones that tell yourself you are fat, short, dumb, tired, slow, unhappy, or can't sell, the subconscious accepts them as true and stands waiting and ready for the next message. The subconscious can't look in the mirror and see your sparkling eyes, a muscled physique, or shiny hair. The subconscious just plants the seeds you give it, whether they are true or false.

The rule of mastering your life is that when you change your thoughts you change your destiny. I am sure you have heard the saying, "If you think you can, you can. And if you think you can't, you can't. Either way you are right." That sums up the power of one's thoughts.

Hardy Health

If you plan on staying in the business for any length of time, your overall health will be your measuring stick. This business is too demanding to be fighting poor health. Hear are five areas that are key to living a hardy, healthy life.

Stress Management

In today's hustle and bustle it is virtually impossible to live in a stress-free environment. The trick to a hardy, healthy life is to develop several outlets for dealing with the inevitable stress monsters. Imagine yourself as a sand timer with the top re-moved. As you accumulate stress the sands within the timer eventually fill up the glass cylinder. Before you know it, you have filled the timer up and the sands are spilling all over the place. If you had an outlet for reducing stress you could fill up, dump out, and be ready for more good activity.

Here are some great ways to reduce the levels of stress in your life.

- Meditation
- Deep breathing
- Walking
- Running
- Shopping

- Taking a stroll along the beach or waterfront area
- Having lunch with a friend
- Calling someone you haven't talked to in ages
- Boxing or hitting a punching bag
- Taking a sauna or swim
- Leaving the salon and walking around the block
- Having a cup of tea
- Going to church
- Taking a nap

Find four to five outlets where you can wash away the stress. The reason I am strongly recommending several outlets for you to turn to is that some of your choices may have pa-rameters on the activity.

What are some ways you can reduce the levels of stress in your life? List four to five favorites you can turn to in times of craziness.

Quiet Time

In the salon industry, you are asked to give of yourself for every client. Burnout and boredom arise when you don't have any-thing left to give your clients. One key way to keep your internal battery juiced up is to give yourself a designated quiet time. When I was recovering from burnout, quiet time was one of my favorite activities to rebuild my energy reserve.

What do you do during quiet time? That is entirely up to you. Here are a few ways to treat yourself during the quiet time.

- Read a favorite book that is relaxing to you. I would shy away from thrillers, newspapers, or business books. Look for books that feed the soul and mind during your quiet time.
- Listen to inspirational audio tapes.
- Spend the time in prayer or meditation.
- Take a luxurious bubble bath. Take the phone off the hook and lock the bathroom door.
- Write in your personal journal.

How much time do you need for quiet time? I would love for you to be able to invest at least fifteen minutes in the morn-ing and fifteen minutes at night. You may be saying to yourself that you don't have any time to spare. Keep in mind that your quiet time allows you to function more effectively throughout the day. By being focused and in tune with yourself, your work and those loved ones around you benefit when you sequester yourself for quiet time.

Diet

The amount of energy you require during the day will be provided by the food you give your body. So much has already been written about dieting (and it changes by the minute) that I would never begin to direct your nutritional habits. At this point, however, I would like to encourage you to watch your intake.

I learned to eat quickly as a direct result of going to beauty school. We had thirty minutes from the time we clocked out to go get our lunch, eat it, and be ready to punch back in. Granted, this routine helped to develop my punctuality, but it played havoc with my digestion. The beauty business is a demanding profession. Take for example the pressure of beating the clock and standing on your feet all day. Quite frequently meals are skipped, or we dash out to the nearest fast-food joint and grab food filled with fat and salt. These culprits lead to poor nutrition and subsequently poor health.

I believe we instinctively know what we should and should not be eating. You know your body well enough to listen to its direction. Watch your diet and watch your body respond positively to the improved food sources.

Energizing Exercise

Some people are just naturally athletic and love to exercise. My idea of a good workout is carrying shopping bags out of the mall. To this day, I don't like to exercise, but what I have discovered is that the sense of empowerment and control is truly superior when I force myself to exercise. When I don't work out, I beat myself up for the lack of discipline. When I manage to finish a workout the true sense of accomplishment is as beneficial as the physical results of the exercise.

If you don't like to work out either, try for one week some program to increase your heart rate and stamina. Check with your doctor before beginning any vigorous routine. You can join a gym, take a yoga class, exercise to videos at home, take a hike, go for a swim, ride a bike, jump rope, roller blade, ice skate, take the stairs instead of the elevator. Use a variety of ways to exercise to beat the boredom and droopy buttocks.

Fun Time

All work and no play makes for a very dull person. Make sure you allow time in your day or week for fun and play. One day during a working lunch I was asked what was the most outrageously fun thing I had ever done that was not work related. I didn't have an answer. Some fun things came to mind, but they were all work related. I then realized why my friends had nicknamed me No-Fun-Phillips. Right then and there I made a commitment to add some fun and games into my daily routine.

Life is definitely too short to spend all of our time focused on climbing the ladder of success. The healthy human has a balance of many factors and fun is one of them. I hope you have a good dose of fun activities built into your life. Catch a movie, play a game, go to the amusement park, attend a comedy concert, tell jokes, read the comics, go to the zoo. Laughter is the best medicine, and I prescribe a large daily dose for you.

Time Management

If you could only create time, you would have vast unlimited capabilities for your success. Unfortunately, you are given a limited number of hours in a day and a successful person makes the most out of each and every one of them.

Salespeople get paid for results, not for just putting in time. You have a limited number of working hours, and it is critical that you make the most of them. Please don't get me wrong, I don't want you to cram fifty people into a daily schedule to be more successful. The goal should be to work smarter, not harder. This can be as simple as putting your car keys in the same location so you don't have to call out the national guard every morning when they are lost or organizing your workstation for efficiency and customer service.

Productive time is what counts. Constantly ask yourself, "Am I doing the most productive thing at this moment?" Just think that if you waste 15 minutes a day you have wasted 105 minutes per week, 420 minutes per month, 5,040 minutes per year. That's 84 hours a year wasted! Just think of the productive and fun things you could do in 84 hours.

Get control of your day and schedule. Give yourself plenty of time in the morning for body grooming and head grooming. Making a mad dash to the salon every day is stressful. Set the alarm clock a few minutes early to allow sufficient time to prepare for the day's tasks. Learn to manage your time to its potential.

Personal Appearance

You are a walking billboard to your clients and potential clients. It is your responsibility to set an example for the public. Your fashion statement should reflect the clients you currently have or the type of clients you wish to attract.

People come in all shapes and sizes. Some will be taller and shorter, thinner and fatter. Beauty shines through in all of those packages when the inner glow and confidence shine forth. Set a good example by facing each day knowing you look your best.

Make every day a ten. Have you had a day when you know that you looked great? Didn't everything seem to flow smoother? You had more confidence when you faced your clients. Go through your closet and weed out the garments, shoes, accessories that don't make you feel confident and secure when you put them on. Donate or sell the self-confidence saboteurs from your closet.

I want you to feel and look your best when you are working with clients. When you stand behind the client and look in the mirror I want you to admire the reflection staring back at you. If you need an objective eye hire an image consultant. These professionals can help you with great color selection and figure-flattering silhouettes and will design a shopping plan of attack. Working with the public can be very draining on you emotionally and physically. Knowing that you have that little extra edge can make the day run smoother and with less hassles.

An outstanding woman I have shared many programs with, Ann Mency, shared this dynamite tip with the audience. She told the women in the group to turn the PMS week around. "Instead of pre-menstrual syndrome, use the week as a reminder to Pamper MySelf." Don't wallow in PMS. Do something to pamper yourself. Schedule a facial, have a legitimate hair appointment. Dress to win. Do something special just for you.

As the old phrase goes, "If you don't take care of you, no one else will." Beauty professionals are sometimes the last ones to have a treatment. They are usually getting their hair done at the last minute, and by someone who has already put in a full day and is on the barely-getting-by service. So take time to pamper yourself because your clients are checking you out to see if you are looking good.

DESIGNING A PERSONAL SUCCESS PLAN

There are six key areas in one's life that need to be addressed and balanced for a happy, healthy outlook. The six areas cover the physical, mental, social, financial, spiritual, and career. Take some time and think about what events and activities you would like to accomplish within the next twelve months. You might want to make a dream list of activities. Contemplate your dreams and desires for a two-week period of time. Once the weeks have passed, go back over your dream list and ask yourself if the item listed is something you really would like to commit to over the next year. Make sure these are things that you believe with all your heart are best for you. This should not be a list of should dos, could dos, or other-people-want me to dos. Your list should represent the things you want in your life. For your personal success plan to be useful make sure your dream list is quantitative items. To say you want to be happier this year is great, but how will you know when you achieve your success level? The goals need to have a measurable quality to them. Below you will find a list to help your creativity juices start to flow.

Don't confuse wishes with wants. When you want a thing, you go out and get it. When you merely wish for something, you just wait for it to come.

Jack Klein

Six-Part Balance

Physical

To exercise three times a week. I will design a program that varies my routine every other day. On Mondays I will work out at home with my exercise videos for thirty minutes. On Wednesday I will go to aerobics class. On Friday I will walk around the block before I go to work. By a designated date my weight will be at this level. I will walk the dog every morning for thirty minutes to get in my exercise. I will use the stair master three times a week for twenty minutes.

Mental

I will read twelve new books this year. Out of the twelve, three will be inspirational, three will be business related, three will be on my new hobby or craft, and three will be just for fun. This year I will go to two hair shows and two seminars related to my career. I will sign up and attend a night course of my choice. I will listen to one opera all the way through.

Social

I will host two parties this year for my friends and family and schedule a night out with friends every other week. I will volunteer time or talent to a selected charity. I will get birthday and anniversary cards out on time.

Financial

I want to earn X amount per month. Of that, X percent is in service and X percent is in retail sales. I will deposit 10 percent of my paycheck into a savings account. I will hire an accountant to handle personal financial paperwork. I will present weekly my tithes to my church.

Spiritual

I will devote fifteen minutes in the morning and fifteen minutes at night for prayer or meditation. I will schedule time to go to worship service, write a daily affirmation, read through the Bible in a year, and listen to an inspirational tape every morning while getting dressed.

Career

My goal is to improve rebookings to 85 percent. I will be on time every day and I will not keep clients waiting more than five minutes. I will establish a mentor to guide me on my career path and I will volunteer to mentor someone younger in the beauty field. Within twelve months, I want to be appointed salon artistic director. I will submit six photos of my work to be considered for publication by trade magazines. I will distribute twenty business cards a week to potential clients.

Putting Your Personal Success Plan to Work

The mind remembers pictures better than words. Once you have written out your goals for the year try making a mind map. A mind map is a picture graph of your goals. Start by making a center symbol, then each of the six balance parts has a trunk. Think of the mind map as a tree and each of the six areas as a branch off the main trunk, which is you. On the mind map you can use symbols, pictures, even cutouts to represent your goal. The mind map can be as small or as large as you desire. Use different colored markers or pens for each section of the map. Give each designated area its personal color. (Fig. 22.1)

The trick is to visually reinforce your plan in the conscious and subconscious mind. I like to make a poster-size map for my office and a 8 1/2-by-11-inch size for my notebook to take with me on a daily basis. As you begin each day, take a couple of minutes to study the map. Visualize yourself successfully completing each task or goal. See yourself as having already achieved the desired result.

One outcome of using a mind map is that when the mind has accepted the visual image you are instinctively pulled toward the goal. You might even feel as if you don't have to grab and fight for the goal, but that you have an imaginary hand pushing you along. Map your way to success. If you don't have a map for your life, chances are you may get lost along the way.

WORDS OF WISDOM

There may be days when you just don't feel positive and ready to face the day. Here is a collection of words of wisdom. Allow these words to feed your spirit and help you ready yourself for the tasks ahead.

> Choose a job you love, and you will never have to work a day in your life.
>
> Confucius

> Nothing in life is to be feared. It is only to be understood.
>
> Marie Curie

> I've never sought success in order to get fame and money; it's the talent and the passion that count in success.
>
> Ingrid Bergman

You don't get to decide how you're going to die, or when. You can only decide how you're going to live!

Joan Baez

If one advances confidently in the direction of his dreams and endeavors to Live the Life which he has imaged, he will meet with a success unexpected in common hours.

Henry David Thoreau

People count the faults of those who keep them waiting.

French Proverb

You can't climb the ladder of success with your hands in your pockets.

Anonymous

People who never do any more than they are paid for, never get paid for any more than they do.

Elbert Hubbard

It is impossible to become educated by learning only what we like.

Dr. Frank Crane

All of the significant battles are waged within the self.

Sheldon Kopp

We can only do what we think we can do. We can be only what we think we can be. We can have only what we think we can have. What we do, what we are, what we have, all depend upon what we think.

Robert Collier

The Lord gave us two ends—one to sit on and the other to think with. Success depends on which on we use the most.

Ann Landers

No man fails who does his best.

Orison Swett Murden

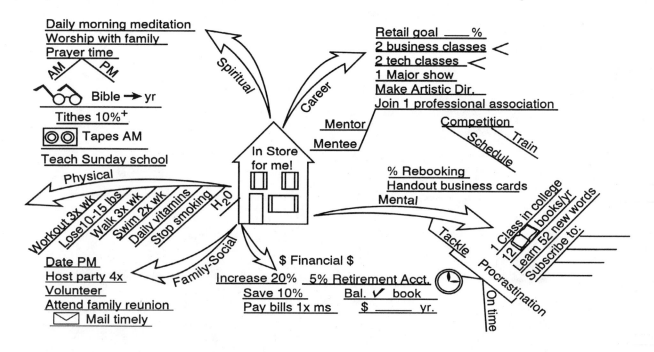

Fig. 22.1a Mind mapping for success (sample).

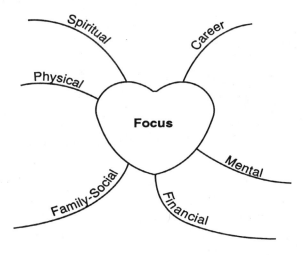

Fig. 22.1b Fill in your keys to success.

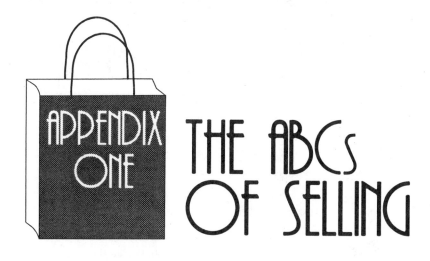

APPENDIX ONE

THE ABCs OF SELLING

The goal of the ABCs of Selling is to give you some quick insights into the attributes and qualities recommended for reaching peak performance. They will be short, simple quips for powerful words that add up to your sales success. If you dare to implement this dictionary of success, the results will be motivational, inspiring, and, of course, life-changing.

A

Ability. Power to perform a skill or talent proficiently. Your ability in sales will skyrocket with a little practice time.

Abundance. More than enough; having your cup overflowing—or chair, or cash register, or client list. Following the suggestions outlined in the book will generate more clients than you can physically service.

Action. As ancient wisdom declares, "The journey of a thousand miles begins with one step." Just do it. Momentum creates momentum.

Appearance. Fifty-five percent of your communication success is based on your nonverbal image and appearance. You do judge a book by its cover. Your attention to detail in the mirror's reflection will have a direct correlation on your level of success.

Attention. Concentrating on the client in your chair. Keep your mind from wandering. Master giving your customers your full, undivided attention.

Attitude. Reflects your position about life, your job, your potential, your mood. As Robert Schuller declares, "Your attitude determines your latitude." Your disposition will either be your glass ceiling or your launching pad to bigger and better things. Only you can determine which one it will be.

Ask. Ask for the order. Ask questions. Speak up and out. If you don't ask you will not find out clients' needs and wants.

B

Belief. Your overall internal conviction. Belief is what you know to be true for you. You must believe in something, or you will fall for anything.

Benefits. How your offer will assist or help solve a problem for the client. They are buying results, not the ingredients in jars. Customers buy the potential of what the product or service will do for them.

Body language. Your conscious and subconscious self is revealed in your natural body movements. Practice positive body language that supports your image and spoken words.

C

Challenge. A task when you must push yourself. Stimulates you to rise above tackling the no-brainers. Testing yourself every day to be just a little better than the day before.

Change. One true constant is your life. People want change. People get excited about it. People are afraid of change. Make the new, the undefined, the unseen your best friend. Because, after all, change is going to happen, whether you are prepared or not, so you might as well have fun with it.

Close. Giving your customer the opportunity to say yes to you or your product or service.

Confidence. Confidence stems from knowing within, a natural result of time and practice. The more you apply this information, the easier it becomes. The addition of lots of little successes will swell your well of confidence.

Consulting. Art of taking into account the client's needs, wants, desires. Learning to ask the right questions. Investigative selling.

Consistency. Calm on a never-ending sea of change. Root to quality control. Comfort zone clients want to cherish when they come to know and expect a level of quality in services, products, and your education.

Conviction. Fierce determination to hold onto your beliefs and philosophy. Gripping fact that you know, that you know, that you know.

Creativity. Release your brain to follow your heart. Every client is different. Use your natural creativity to adjust your presentation and communication to best fit the customer.

Customer. Number one requirement for business. Without these wonderful people, you have no business.

D

Dedication. Concentrate yourself toward your special purpose. Be the best you can be. Set yourself apart.

Desire. A fueled wish for something you want to have happen. Hope. Dreams.

Determination. Unwavering intention. Positive thinking. Exactness of purpose. The will to succeed.

Discipline. Getting the job done. Follow-up and follow-through. Making the commitment and doing the necessary steps to see every task through.

E

Easy. That's right. Selling is easy once you understand the components to completing the sale. If you follow the steps it is easy.

Employee. Person, part of the team working for a company who does whatever it takes to help the business succeed. You'll never hear them say, "It's not my job."

Endurance. Ability to hang in there on bad days. Hanging in there after everyone else has given up the ship.

Enthusiasm. Outward expression of your inner self. Enthusiasm is contagious. It's your energy, your genuine life force.

Excitement. Stirs up activity. Arouses feeling, passions, and a desire to buy. High, not spastic, energy.

Expect. Confident knowing. You must expect to make the sale. If you think you can, you can. If you think you can't, you can't. Either way your expectations chart your course.

Extra. There is no traffic jam when you go the extra mile. Action above and beyond the call of duty. Put forth a little extra—a smile, a kind word, willingness to serve.

F

Faith. Complete trust and confidence in the unseen. Unquestioned belief. Faith is taking the first step without knowing for certain the outcome.

Features. Selling the unique point of view. What sets the goods apart from others.

Focused. Clarity of vision. Flash of insight as the impression registers in the brain. Seeing one thing clearly at a time. Channeled activities.

Follow-through. Critical rung on your ladder of success. Do what you say when you say you will do it. Carry duties/job/function through to completion. No half-finished projects. Mission accomplished.

Fun. By all means have fun, any way, every day. The guidelines and suggestions in this book are written to take the mystery and fear out of selling. Once you know the secrets, it's easy to relax into successful selling.

Future. Take out the shades. Yours is bright, optimistic, unlimited. Your career is a blank book waiting for you to fill in the pages.

G

Give. In this business, you are constantly giving of your-self—your time, your talent, even your money. The universe will give blessings back to you. When you give from the heart be prepared for an avalanche of abundance.

Great. Better than average. Better quality. Above ordinary.

H

Heart. Most people in the beauty business got into it to help people feel better about themselves. That, my friend, is the heart of our business. Every day, you help someone look in the mirror and like him/herself a little better than the day before. What a gift!

Help. Assist the customer to solve a beauty need or problem, and you've made the sale. You're there to help the client, not swindle or talk him/her into something not needed.

Honest. Honesty is the best policy. Your genuine, honest recommendation will show through in the presentation. Customers will intuitively pick up on your honesty meter.

I

I. Least important word in sales.

Imagination. Take a walk around the elephant. Get a new view on things. Use your creativity to find a need and fill it with new applications, new ideas, new products, new services. There are thousands of new ideas floating out there, waiting for you to latch onto them and put them to use.

Integrity. True grit. Honest grit or personal substance. Integrity allows you to look at yourself in the mirror every day and be peaceful and happy with the person you see staring back at you.

Interested. Curious. Inquisitive. Intrigued.

Invest. Invest in yourself, your education, your appearance, your tools. Consider them an investment in your future. Ignorance is expensive.

Involved. Interactive presentation stimulating all of the senses. Hands-on experience.

J

Joy. Unbridled happiness. Pure satisfaction of knowing you helped people feel better about themselves.

K

Knowledge. Keep learning. Keep growing. Your mind is a sponge willing to absorb volumes of education. Know-how. Familiarity with retailing information removes the fear of selling.

L

Learn. Exercise your brain cells daily. Expand your horizons with new facts and techniques. Go and grow!

Listen. Sounds of opportunity. Tune in for potential sales. Actively listen.

Love. You must love what you do. If you are not impassioned about your career, modify it, change jobs, or get out. If you love what you do, getting up in the morning is a true joy.

M

Merchandising. Art of making your business a profitable store. Designing a place where people want to shop. Stocking the shelves with product, not decorating the salon.

Money. Money is great! It is not the root of all evil. If you are uncomfortable with money think of your services and products as being bartered for cash, checks, or plastic. You are given money in exchange for goods and services. Money is a scorecard of your progress.

N

Needs. Client motive. Hot button for making the sale. Genuine request or desire.

Negative. Guard against any negative influence. Negative energy, thoughts, attitude, actions are self-sabotaging.

New. New and improved. Hot trigger word. New clients, new services, new products.

No. Small word. Think of a no as a red flag. The client wants to say yes but simply doesn't have enough information to make a safe decision. No is not a stop signal; it's a tiny word that means you are not done with the presentation.

O

Open. Willingness to experience. Tear down the invisible walls of self-preservation and insecurity brick by brick. Willingness to reach out to others.

Opportunity. Every person you see, meet, and talk to is a potential client, sale, income. Opportunity is always the right time and right place. Don't let an opportunity pass you by.

Outgoing. Verve to make the first move. Introduce yourself first. It's taking the initiative to walk up to a person and extend your help and services.

P

Patience. Most people decree, "Grant it to me," and "I want it now." Quiet peace of knowing all works in harmony for best possible outcome. Strength and internal peace. Not being hurried or frazzled.

Planning. Organizing your time. Inking not just thinking. Scheduling. Filling in the B to Y in the A to Z.

Polished. Smoothing out the rough edges. Personal presentation, being groomed and pulled together.

Positive. Critical that your words, actions, and deeds are confident and assured. Absolutely. Unquestionably. Affirmative. Upbeat. Happy.

Profit. Big bucks left over after your bills are paid.

Potential. Unlimited. Untapped possibilities. The yet to be's.

Presentation. Act of demonstrating or taking the client through a structured explanation.

Products. Silent employees ready and waiting on the shelf, to make you money. Goal is to get them off the shelf and in the bag before you have to dust them once.

Q

Quality. Top of the line. Top dog. Top banana. No rejects.

Questions. Essential component in the selling sequence. Ammunition in fact-finding mission. Questioning leads the customer down the road to saying yes at the end of the journey.

R

Recommend. Based on your years of experience you are able to professionally suggest routines, products, treatments. Your sage experience will be your guide to the prescribed home care and in-salon treatments. Recommending is the same as selling, only it sounds a little softer for the retailing faint of heart.

Retail. Store. Department. Products. Recommended proper home care to continue the salon results.

S

Self-starter. You are responsible for you, and you're not waiting around for someone else to steer you in any direction. Ability to kick start your own success engine.

Sell. Selling is communication and communication is selling. If you can talk, you can sell. Finding out the clients needs, wants, and desires and then providing solutions to problems.

Service. Noun. The commodity you offer such as haircut, facial, manicure, etc.

Servicing. Verb. Putting service into action.

Smile. Exercise your orbicularis oris. A genuine heartfelt smile is the easiest thing to give away. Try flashing a smile that lights up your eyes.

Style. Taking all of the information and putting your personal stamp on it. Giving it your unique twist.

Success. Is not measured by the amount of things you

accumulate. Success is achieved when you do everything you are capable of, not compared to someone else.

System Selling. Double your sales and double your fun with system selling. Selling products two by two.

T

Talk. Put your money where your mouth is. Selling is talking your way to the bank. You are chatting about something; channel the conversation toward products, services and solutions.

Technical. Skill of explaining your professional know-how in a language the client can understand.

Think. Invisible commodity for propelling your success into the stratosphere. Think. Think. Think. Everything you need to know is in your brain. Take time to engage the brain before you open the mouth.

Time. Make the most of every minute. Time is the one commodity you cannot manufacture. Do the most productive thing every given minute.

Thank you. Two extremely important words to say and hear.

Traffic. One objective is to encourage customers to come into the business for the sole purpose of purchasing products on their nonappointment days. Foot traffic adds virtually labor-free sales.

U

Unbelievable. The perfect answer to most questions. How's business? Unbelievable! How's the weather? Unbelievable! Unbelievable works if the real answer is negative or positive.

Understand. Compassion. Empathy. Walking in the other's moccasins. Ask enough questions and actively listening to the responses to get a grip on the client's wishes.

V

Vital. Essential. Pivotal. People rely on you to be a smooth-running cog in the operation's wheel.

Voice. Sound of success. Learn to make your voice work for you.

W

Want. You need food. But you want a deep-dish Chicago-style pepperoni pizza with extra sauce. Desire, wish, or definite fancy.

WIFM. Radio station most clients are tuned into. What's In It For Me. Stress how the product or service will benefit the client, not just your pocketbook.

Win. All activity should be focused around the win principle. The client wins. You win. The salon wins. Everyone wins.

X

X-ray. Study every success and failure. X-ray your attitudes, actions, successes, and failures. You will make some mistakes, but if you investigate what you did wrong you will not repeat the same error.

Y

Yes. A yes today is better than a maybe tomorrow. Positive agreement to your offering.

You. The star in your galaxy. First chair instrument in the success orchestra. Key to unlocking the potential. You make or break your selling potential.

Z

Zest. Exciting quality and flavor that spices up work, relations, family, and life. Go for the gusto. It's the zing and zap of life.

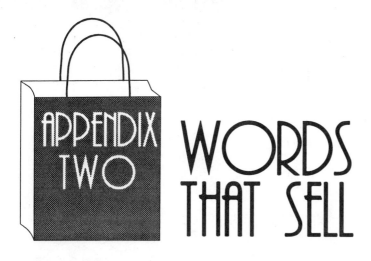

APPENDIX TWO

WORDS THAT SELL

Use the following words to build some sizzle into your product and service descriptions. Use buzzwords that will appeal to the personality of your client.

Appealing

adorable
alluring
bewitching
captivating
delightful
fetching
irresistible
just the right touch
loveable
lovely
luxuriant
memorable
picture perfect
pleasing
satisfying
special
tempting
unforgettable

Big

ample
enormous
generous
grand
great
hefty
huge
jumbo
lavish
massive
numerous
spectacular
substantial
tremendous
unlimited
vast
voluminous
whooping

Comfortable

at ease
casual
cool and comfy
down-home
peaceful
relaxed
restful
serene
smooth as silk
snug
soft as a baby's bottom
soothing
tranquil
unassuming
unhurried
velvety

Complete

a complete package
A to Z
all the right ingredients
everything you need to . . .
everything you wanted
   to know about . . .
extensive
in-depth

Convenient

clarifies
easy access
eliminates the guesswork
fits your schedule
handy
one-stop shopping
right at your fingertips
save frustration
save time
simplifies
transports easily
versatile

Easy

at a glance
clear
easy as one, two, three
fast
in no time at all
instant
it's a breeze
it's a cinch

it's a piece of cake
it's a snap
it's that simple
no fussing
simplified
step by step
uncomplicated

Magnificent

breathtaking
dazzling
drop-dead look
elegant
fabulous
fantastic

marvelous
opulent
striking
stunning
terrific
wonderful

Men's Words

commanding
control
dynamite
electric
high-powered
intense
knockout
manageable
potent

powerful
precision
primitive
rugged
performance
strong
tough
vigor
vitally

Must

critical
crucial
essential
important

invaluable
necessity
urgent
vital

Natural

bouquet
clean
earthy
fresh
light

organic
pristine
springtime
summer's breeze
zesty

New and Improved

a new look
an about-face
better than ever
changed
enhanced
improve on perfection

modified
redesigned
refined
renewed
spruced up

Reliable

established
functional
no-nonsense
practical

proven
secure
trusted

Results

accomplishes
corrects
delivers
does the trick
effective

fixes
gets the job done
produces
works

Self-improvement

a chance to discover
   your hidden beauty
education
expression
growth
hands-on learning

look like a million
move ahead
opens the door
succeed
you'll be glad you did
you'll feel as good as
   you look

harmony
invest in yourself

you'll feel good about
    yourself
you'll learn by doing

Service

advisors
consultation
delivers
helps you
lets you
personal advice

professional advice
solution to your . . .
solves
sound advice
technical support

Status

class
discriminating
elite
prestige
recognized
privy to

selective
the Rolls Royce of
VIP Treatment
you'll be in on
private
you'll join the ranks of

Stylish

bold
chic
classy
current
dapper
daring
debonair
dressed to kill
elegant
flair
funky
glamorous
graceful
in vogue
latest

original
preppie
sleek
slender
slinky
smart
smashing
snazzy
sophisticated
sporty
suave
svelte
tasteful
trendy
unique

INDEX